Nanotheranostics
for Personalized Medicine

Nanotheranostics for Personalized Medicine

Editors

Simona Mura

Patrick Couvreur

University Paris Sud XI, France

World Scientific

NEW JERSEY • LONDON • SINGAPORE • BEIJING • SHANGHAI • HONG KONG • TAIPEI • CHENNAI • TOKYO

Published by

World Scientific Publishing Co. Pte. Ltd.
5 Toh Tuck Link, Singapore 596224
USA office: 27 Warren Street, Suite 401-402, Hackensack, NJ 07601
UK office: 57 Shelton Street, Covent Garden, London WC2H 9HE

Library of Congress Cataloging-in-Publication Data
Nanotheranostics for personalized medicine / edited by Simona Mura, Patrick Couvreur.
p. ; cm.
Includes bibliographical references and index.
ISBN 978-9814713528 (hardback : alk. paper)
I. Mura, Simona, editor. II. Couvreur, Patrick, 1950– , editor.
[DNLM: 1. Drug Delivery Systems. 2. Nanoparticles--therapeutic use. 3. Diagnostic Imaging. 4. Individualized Medicine. 5. Nanomedicine. QV 785]
RS122.2
615.10285--dc23
2015026034

British Library Cataloguing-in-Publication Data
A catalogue record for this book is available from the British Library.

In-house Editors: Amanda Yun/Dipasri Sardar

Typeset by Stallion Press
Email: enquiries@stallionpress.com

Printed in Singapore

CONTENTS

PREFACE

The book — edited by Dr. S. Mura and Pr. P. Couvreur — represents a timely treatise on advances and challenges in the development of nanotheranostics for personalized medicine. The key characteristic of the so-called nanotheranostic approach, aiming to combine both therapeutic and imaging/diagnostic functionalities, results from its strong pluridisciplinarity where chemistry of materials, bioconjugate chemistry, pharmaceutical technology, drug delivery, imaging and pharmacology are talking together. The major ambition of this book is therefore to present an integrated and transdisciplinary description of this emerging concept in the nanomedicine world. Students from bachelors to Ph.D. as well as experimented researchers in academy or industry would have interest in reading this book, even if they are not specialist in the field.

The first chapter shortly introduces the nanotheranostics and their key role for the personalized medicine. The Chapter 2, which describes the high resolution techniques employed for medical imaging is followed by a presentation of the different imaging modality/therapeutic agent couples applied in the oncology field. Design and developments, preclinical results, opportunities and challenges, which arise from the combination of anticancer drug with magnetic resonance imaging, optical imaging, ultrasonography and nuclear medicine are detailed in Chapters 3–7.

Chapter 8 refers to the application of nanotheranostics in gene delivery.

Chapter 9 deals with the nanotheranostics designed and applied for treatment and imaging of cardiovascular diseases.

Chapter 10 provides an overview of recent progresses in the emerging field of stimuli responsive theranostics.

Finally Chapter 11 presents and discusses personalized medicine concepts of practical clinical utility by covering specific tasks in modern pharmacology and pharmaceutics.

On the whole, this book would offer to the reader a clear overview of the progresses in the field of nanotheranostics and their fundamental contribution to the emerging field of personalized medicine. We hope it would open the way to further improvements and to the clinical translation of the nanotheranostic concept in a not too far future.

We would like to thank all the contributors to this book for their enthusiastic participation. S. Mura is grateful to her boyfriend (Alexandre) for his support and constant encouragement. Patrick Couvreur is thankful to his wife (Cecile) and his children Catherine, Marie and Nicolas for their love and affection and moral support. Finally we wish to extend our thanks to the team of the World Scientific Publishing and Imperial College Press who provided the opportunity, the help, and the support for making the idea of this book into reality.

Chatenay Malabry
Simona Mura, Patrick Couvreur

CHAPTER 1

COMBINING IMAGING AND DRUG DELIVERY FOR THE TREATMENT OF SEVERE DISEASES

Simona Mura* and Patrick Couvreur†

Institut Galien Paris-Sud,
UMR 8612, CNRS, Univ. Paris-Sud,
Université Paris-Saclay, Faculté de Pharmacie,
5 rue JB Clément, 92296 Châtenay-Malabry, France
**simona.mura@u-psud.fr*
†patrick.couvreur@u-psud.fr

1. Introduction

Owing to the impressive progresses in material sciences and medicine, a broad range of nanoscale devices (i.e., nanomedicines) has been developed in the last decades for drug administration, transport and delivery with the aim to overcome the limitations of traditional pharmaceutical formulations.[1] Nanomedicines demonstrated the capability to enhance drug properties by (i) offering protection from degradation, (ii) enabling controlled release and biodistribution and (iii) increasing bioavailability. Using lipids, polymers or inorganic material as building block, a large number of systems with different architectures and surface properties has been designed. Surface shielding with a hydrophilic PEG shell prolonged circulation half-life of nanomedicines, thus allowing preferential passive accumulation in tumor tissues due to the "enhanced permeability and retention" (EPR) effect, which is a hallmark of leaky vasculatures and poor lymphatic drainage.[2] In addition, decoration with various ligands conferred specific cell-targeting ability.[3] Attention focused mainly on cancer treatment, achieving important improvements in the therapeutic index of various drugs by increasing the possibility to localize them at the target site and alleviate undesired side effects.[4] Other severe pathologies such as neurodegenerative and inflammatory diseases, lung and cardiovascular maladies, HIV, diabetes can as well benefit from the use of nanomedicines.[5–10] Nevertheless, despite the wide enthusiasm and the promises associated to the presentation of each new nanomedicine, only few of them have been approved for clinical applications and reached the marketplace (liposomal formulation of doxorubicin, (Myocet®, Caelix®) and paclitaxel nanoparticles (Abraxane®), for instance).

Not limited to the delivery of drugs, nanomedicines have been also employed for diagnostic/imaging purposes. Nanoscale systems conjugated with diagnostic agents such as (i) fluorescent molecules (e.g., indocyanine green) for optical imaging, (ii) contrast enhancing agents (e.g., gadolinium, metal nanoparticles, perfluorocarbons) for magnetic resonance imaging (MRI) and ultrasonography or (iii) radionuclides (e.g., 18-fluorodeoxyglucose, In-111 and Tc-99m) for positron emission tomography (PET), computed tomography (CT) and single-photon emission computed tomography (SPECT) have been actively exploited for detecting both primary tumors and metastases. In addition, several inorganic nanoparticles possess intrinsic imaging properties. Undoubtedly, such nanomedicines represent a powerful tool for non-invasive body imaging, but they are devoid of therapeutic action.

In the continuous effort to improve sensitivity and precision in cancer screening/diagnosis as well as the effectiveness of treatment strategies, the combination of imaging and therapy function within a single nanomedicine has received a great deal of attention in the last years.[11–16] The term "nanotheranostics" (or, with a little extent "nano-theragnostics") has been proposed to describe this new class of nano-medicines, which integrates the simultaneous detection and treatment of a disease. Thanks to the advances in the biomedical and nano-technology field, many creative approaches have been proposed to co-deliver imaging and therapeutic agents. The exponential interest in the field of nanotheranostics is attested by a brief review of the articles published on the topic (Web of Science database search during the month of January 2015), which showed more than 1,300 papers published since 2006.

The various available imaging modalities allow monitoring non-invasively in real time (i) the distribution of the nanocarriers, (ii) the release of the loaded drugs and/or (iii) the disease evolution thus gaining insight on the treatment effectiveness. The ultimate goal of the nanotheranostic approach is a monitoring of the disease progression when the treatment is applied in order to overcome the limits of the conventional clinical settings in which imaging is generally performed before/after the treatment.

Efficient combination of imaging and therapeutic agent in the same system is likely to prompt the nanomedicine field toward the personalized medicine.[17,18] Opposed to the idea that "one fits all", personalized medicine aims to tailor the therapy to each specific individual enabling to administer the most appropriate treatments at the right moment at the right patient. In this context, nanotheranostics have the potentiality to revolutionize the way we detect, treat and follow up the progression of a disease allowing for a better outcome. Monitoring in a real time nanotheranostic accumulation at the target site and subsequent drug release, will make possible to screen and thus to distinguish the patients who would potentially benefit from a specific treatment from the ones for which another therapeutic alternative (e.g., conventional chemotherapy, radiotherapy, surgery) must be envisioned.[19] Then, the longitudinal follow up will allow, according to patient's response, to rapidly tune the treatments, which will therefore reflect the characteristic of the disease in that specific individual (e.g., extent of the EPR effect, desmoplastic reaction, resistance, etc...). The feedbacks to the treatment will therefore be obtained in real time and its modification eventually applied without waiting traditional physical endpoints such as the reduction of the tumor volume. In addition, evaluation of body distribution and potential accumulation in healthy tissues would allow to predict the risk of insurgence of undesired side effects and lead to an opportune modulation of the treatment in order to combine the highest efficacy level and the best safety profile. Certainly, nanotheranostics represent a valuable instrument to personalize the treatment protocols, overcoming inter- and/or intra-patient variability, thus enabling a better management of the disease and optimizing the effectiveness of the therapeutic intervention toward cancer and other severe diseases.

Nevertheless, the integration of imaging and therapeutic function in a single agent is not an easy task and many challenges have to be faced before translation of nanotheranostics to clinical settings.[20] Going through the published articles, a plethora of innovative, more or less sophisticated systems is described. Unfortunately, in a large number of studies, nanotheranostics have been evaluated only *in vitro* and a proof of their real value as dual (i.e., imaging/therapeutic) agents is rarely provided *in vivo*. When the *in vivo* assessment has been performed, attention mainly focused on the imaging/diagnostic purposes and the effectiveness of the treatment is only implicitly assumed. Finally, when both functions have been demonstrated in preclinical animal models (mainly rodents) many obstacles still limit their entry into the medical practice.

For instance, a major challenge for the nanotheranostics is the loading capacity of both drug and imaging agents and their requirement in terms of timeline and concentration, which can be extremely different. Another issue relies on the biocompatibility and toxicological profile of the nanotheranostics. It has to be noted that the safety of the building materials does not assure the innocuousness of the resulting multifunctional system, which presents unique pharmacodynamic/pharmacokinetic properties. In addition, many of the currently employed imaging agents show a potential toxicity: the fate after *in vivo* administration and the biocompatibility of quantum dots, gold, iron nanoparticles are still matter of debate. Furthermore, important concerns arise from the physico/chemical complexity of the nanotheranostic and the protocols required for their synthesis/ formulation, which are often hardly transposable to a larger industrial scale. Thus, much research and development efforts still need to be done before nanotheranostics could be effectively introduced into medical practice.

References

1. P. Couvreur, C. Vauthier, *Pharm. Res.,* 1417 (2006).
2. H. Maeda, J. Wu, T. Sawa, Y. Matsumura, K. Hori, *J. Control. Release*, 271 (2000).
3. J. Nicolas, S. Mura, D. Brambilla, N. Mackiewicz, P. Couvreur, *Chem. Soc. Rev.,* 1147 (2013).
4. M. Ferrari, *Nat. Rev. Cancer*, 161 (2005).
5. S. Krol, R. Ellis-Behnke, P. Marchetti, *Maturitas*, 61 (2011).
6. B. Godin *et al.*, *Trends in Pharmacol. Sci.*, 199 (2010).
7. D. Brambilla, B. Le Droumaguet, J. Nicolas, S. H. Hashemi, L. P. Wu, S. M. Moghimi, P. Couvreur, K. Andrieux, *Nanomedicine*, 521 (2011).
8. U. Pison, T. Welte, M. Giersig, D. A. Groneberg, *Eur. J. Pharmacol.*, 341 (2006).
9. B. J. Crielaard, T. Lammers, R. M. Schiffelers, G. Storm, *J. Control Release*, 225 (2012).
10. A. Gaudin, M. Yemisci, H. Eroglu, S. Lepetre-Mouelhi, O. F. Turkoglu, B. T. Dönmez-Demir, S. Caban, M. Fevzi Sargon, S. Garcia-Argote, G. Pieters, O. Loreau, B. Rousseau, O. Tagit, N. Hildebrandt, Y. Le Dantec, J. Mougin, S. Valetti, H. Chacun, V. Nicolas, D. Desmaële, K. Andrieux, Y. Capan, T. Dalkara, P. Couvreur, *Nat. Nanotechnol.*, 1054 (2014).
11. J. R. McCarthy, R. Weissleder, *Adv. Drug Deliv. Rev.*, 1241 (2008).
12. S. M. Janib, A. S. Moses, J. A. MacKay, *Adv. Drug Deliv. Rev.*, 1052 (2010).
13. J. Xie, S. Lee, X. Chen, *Adv. Drug Deliv. Rev.*, 1064 (2010).
14. T. Lammers, S. Aime, W. E. Hennink, G. Storm, F. Kiessling, *Acc. Chem. Res.*, 1029 (2011).

15. B. Theek, L. Y. Rizzo, J. Ehling, F. Kiessling, T. Lammers, *Clin. Transl. Imaging*, 66 (2014).
16. H. Cabral, N. Nishiyama, K. Kataoka, *Acc. Chem. Res.*, 999 (2011).
17. S. Bates, *Drug Discov. Today*, 115 (2010).
18. T. Lammers, L. Y. Rizzo, G. Storm, F. Kiessling, *Clin. Cancer Res.*, 4889 (2012).
19. L. Y. Rizzo, B. Theek, G. Storm, F. Kiessling, T. Lammers, *Curr. Opin. Biotechnol.*, 1159 (2013).
20. T. Lammers, F. Kiessling, W. E. Hennink, G. Storm, *J. Control.* Release, 175 (2012).

CHAPTER 2

INCREASED SENSITIVITY FOR MEDICAL IMAGING USING NON-IONIZING NANOMEDICINE AS CONTRAST AGENTS

Cyrille Richard, Bich-Thuy Doan and Nathalie Mignet*

Paris Sorbonne Cité, Paris Descartes University,
Faculty of Pharmacy, Chimie ParisTech,
Team Vectors for Targeted Therapy and Molecular Imaging,
CNRS UMR 8258, INSERM U1022, 4 avenue de l'Observatoire,
75270 Paris Cedex06, France
** Nathalie.Mignet@parisdescartes.fr*

The search for new contrast agents (CAs) that could help physician to detect a disease or to evaluate the efficacy of a drug is of particular interest in modern medicine. To this end, various probes, with specific imaging properties, are actually actively developed in research teams. Nanomedicine have a role to play in this field thanks to their ability to concentrate a large payload of molecules, and to their surface functionalization which confer them targeting abilities. Some of them have already been approved by drug regulatory agencies and are already used in clinical imaging for magnetic resonance and ultrasound imaging. This chapter will focalize on magnetic resonance, ultrasound and fluorescence imaging. For each technique, we briefly described the method and requirements for the CAs to be developed, and give examples of approved CAs based on nanoparticles some of their applications. The last part of this chapter will present promising nanoprobes with optical imaging properties, which are currently in pre-clinical trials.

1. Introduction

In the recent years, medical imaging has gone through technological breakthrough,[1] in terms of technique, such as faster acquisition, multimodality,[2] molecular imaging,[3] image processing and signal enhancement via contrast agents (CAs).[4]

Radiative imaging such as emission of monophoton (SPECT) or positon (PET) are very sensitive techniques used for serious diseases such as cancer detection or follow-up. Recent reviews on this topic can be find elsewhere.[5,6] In this chapter, we will focus on non-ionizing techniques used in clinic (Magnetic Resonance Imaging (MRI) and Ultrasound Imaging) or about to be used (optical imaging). These techniques are easy to handle and do not need the level of security required for imaging techniques using radioactive probes. Therefore, it is of high interest to use them for early diagnosis, for prediction of therapy response or to monitor in real time the efficacy of a treatment. MRI and Ultrasound Imaging are already used in clinic for example for cancer diagnostic or follow-up, ultrasound is mainly used for pregnancy and heart diseases, and MRI allows the evaluation of injuries to the soft-tissues, of all organs etc.[7–9] The evolution of these techniques towards a higher sensitivity, ultimately enlarge their applications. The evolution of MRI provides the feasibility to follow blood oxygenation, to acquire molecular diffusion, precise quantification thanks to dynamic sequences particularly applied to neuroimaging or oncology.[10,11]

The evolution of the ultrasound techniques such as Doppler[12] and more recently the ultrafast acquisition obtained increases the resolution and as a consequence the number of applications.[13] Both techniques also provide now the possibility to obtain physico-chemical parameters of the tissue using the elastography as a means to define with more precision the elasticity of a tissue in particular for fibrosis detection.[14–16] With the goal to increase the sensitivity of these techniques, molecular CAs have also been proposed. Several molecular agents reached the market for MRI, such as Dotarem, Multihance, Magnevist.[17,18] Recently, CAs based on nanoparticles, also called nanomedicine, have emerged as an efficient means to increase the signal to noise ratio and the pharmacokinetic of molecular CAs.[19] Indeed, the possibility to entrap and concentrate molecular CAs within a core should eventually lead to an increased signal. Alternatively, inorganic nanoparticles presenting intrinsic properties to increase the signal have also opened new avenues for contrast enhanced imaging.[20] Finally, nanomedicine also provide means to obtain specific CAs thanks to their surface functionalization.[4] The three different sections underneath describe the interest, development and marketed nanotechnologies proposed as CAs for MRI, ultrasound and optical imaging.

2. Nanomedicine as CAs to Increase the Sensitivity of MRI

MRI provides anatomic and functional information about tissues based on water proton signal and contrast. Enhanced contrast between normal and diseased tissues could strongly benefit from the use and development of CAs.[21] There are two main class of MRI CAs. Paramagnetic agents, such as oxide (IO) nanoparticles affect primarily T_2 relaxation time and lead to hypo-signals. Paramagnetic T_1 agents, such as gadolinium (Gd^{3+}) accelerate T_1 relaxation and lead to brighter MRI signals.

Clinical Gd CAs have low molecular weights (500–1000 $gmol^{-1}$). These agents allowed MRI with enhanced contrast. After intravenous injection in humans of Gd^{3+} complex, its early distribution phase is completed within a few minutes ($t_{1/2} \approx 10$ min). It is an advantage for diagnosis purpose that CAs stay in the blood stream for a long time, so that high-resolution images can be obtained and targeting can be optimized before final liver capture or kidney clearance. Novel CAs are needed with longer residence life times in the body. Another limitation of the actual small molecular CAs is their rapid tumbling rate, which decreases the relaxivity values, contributing to a reduced signal level. Stoichiometric interactions between a targeted CA with cell receptor lead to a nanomolar range concentration of the Gd^{3+} complex *in situ* which is under the sensitivity detection of the MR CA.

2.1. *Principle of MRI contrast agents*

How MRI contrast could be obtained from these two main MR CAs? MRI contrast is based on the reduction of the T_1 or T_2 water relaxation times induced by dipolar or other magnetic interactions between generally protons spins with the magnetic centers of Gd^{3+} ions or IO nanoparticles for example. Detailed relaxation theory can be found in the literature.[21] As a consequence, after spin magnetic excitation by radiofrequency pulses, MR water signal can be recorded. The signal intensity results the intensity results from the spin return to the thermodynamic equilibrium following the classical Bloch physical formalism[22] (Figure 1). Then, specific MRI sequences and timing parameters of the sequence:time repetition (TR) and Time of Echo (TE), could be finely tuned in order to modify the MR signal in function of the T_1 or T_2 values of the water recorded spins. The way the spins intensity evolve in function of the MRI sequence (TE or TR) timing parameters can be modeled as shown in Figure 1. For example, a Gd^{3+} complex CA will strongly decrease T_1 value and the choice of a short TR weighted image will supply a hypersignal from these spins. Superparamagnetic CAs such as IO nanoparticles will decrease T_2 and T_2* values, and a T_2 weighted image obtain with the choice of a long TE will provide a hypo-signal.

The first class of MRI CAs we are presenting here is the Gd^{3+} complex-based scaffolds.

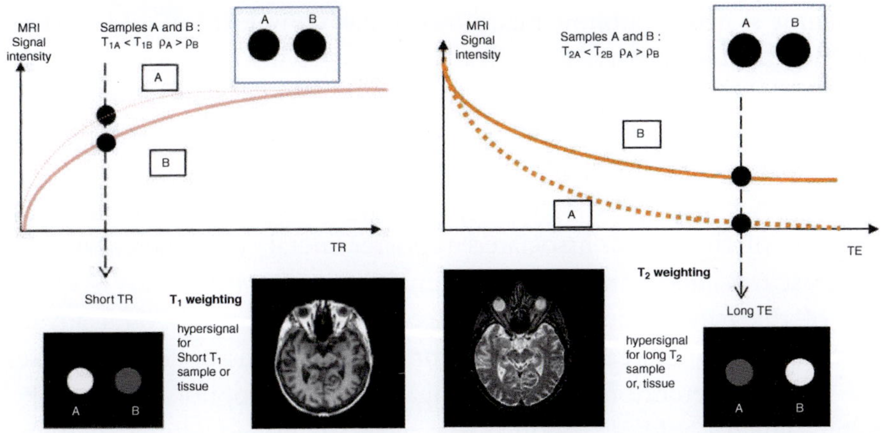

(a) (b)

Fig. 1: (a) MRI T_1 weighting: MRI signal evolution curve in function of TR sequence parameter and T_1 values. (b) MRI T_2 weighting: MRI signal evolution curve in function of sequence TE parameter and T_1 values.[23]

In the past decade, there has been great demand for a new class of CAs that satisfies the following characteristics: (1) high contrast ability, (2) intracellular uptake or cellular interaction for imaging cellular distribution and functions, (3) nanoparticulate or macromolecular form for enhanced sensitivity,[24] (4) easy surface modification with targeting agents for applications in molecular and cellular imaging, and (5) favorable pharmacokinetics and dynamics, efficient distribution to biological targets, and safe clearance from patients with minimal side effects.

Much effort has also been devoted to the improvement of the efficacy of CAs with new intermediary weight Gd complex CAs with optimization of parameters influencing solvent relaxivity such as rotational correlation time, hydration number, Gd–H distance, water exchange rate.[25–28] Indeed, one crucial point is the rate of water exchange which determines the number of protons involved in the relaxation process governing the overall proton relaxivity. Gd CAs in current clinical use (r_1 ~4 $mM^{-1}\cdot s^{-1}$) do not possess sufficiently large relaxivities for molecular imaging since r_1 values greater than 50 $mM^{-1}\cdot s^{-1}$ are generally required.[29] Moreover, slowing down the rotational motion by applying slowly tumbling macromolecular complexes would lead to an increased relaxivity. Chemical exchange with saturation transfer MRI CAs (CEST, lipoCEST)[30,31] have also been recently developed and have proven to be intelligent enzyme or pH sensitive activated contrastophor *in vitro* and *in vivo* in preclinics.

Another way to improve the efficacy of CA is to increase the amount of the carrier-associated reporter metal, thus increasing the contrast ratio and enhancing the signal intensity with the same quantity of the nanoparticle carrier. This strategy presents several advantages. It locally increases the amount of Gd-contrastophors, increases the vascular retention by modifying the contrastophor pharmacokinetic, which could also reduce the cytotoxicity and ultimately allow functional imaging. Macromolecular complexes have been prepared by conjugation of Gd^{3+} chelates to biomedical polymers such as polypeptides, polysaccharides, dendrimers and proteins.[32] Commercial clinical contrastophors are divided in two, weak and strong protein binding scaffolds. For instance, agents such as Multihance, Gadovist or Vasovist (*cf.* Figure 2) are able to bind to albumin to supply high relaxivity CA.[33] One of the biggest drawbacks of these macromolecular agents is their unstability because Gd^{3+} ions might be able to leak out of their chelates due to their longer residence in the body as compared to a small molecular weight CA. Nanocarriers should also been preferentially degradable. It is therefore necessary to design and construct nanosized architectures with high relaxivities, but also higher stability.

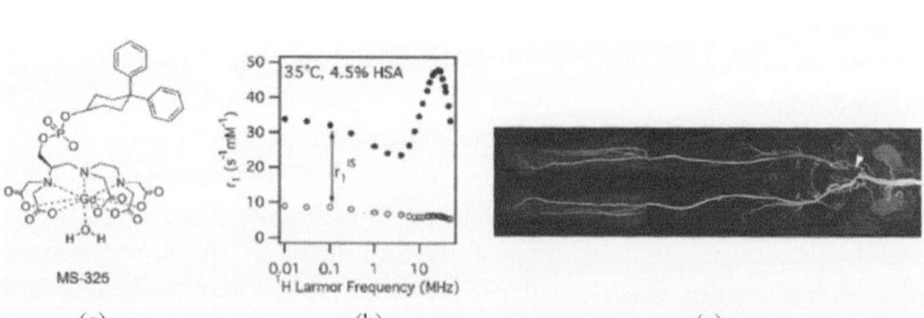

(a) (b) (c)

Fig. 2: Gd complex CA in clinics, example of Vasovist for enhanced sensitivity. Figure adapted with permission from P. Caravan,[34] copyright 2009 American Chemical Society.

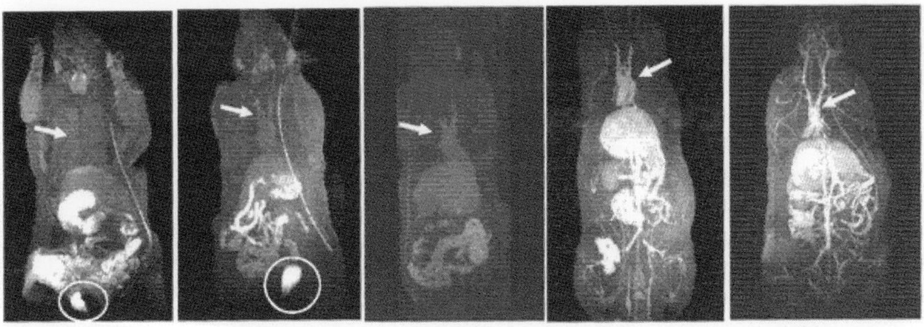

Fig. 3: Comparison of whole body MR image on rodent with different Gd complexes sizes from small molecular with Omiscan and Vasovist to nanoparticular scaffolds with Gd Nanoparticles obtained using a 3T MR instrument.[47]

In this context, various contrastophors have been proposed such as biopolymer conjugates,[35] porous nanoparticles,[36] inorganic nanoparticles,[37–39] dendrimers,[40,41] micelles,[42] liposomes,[43,44] onion like vesicles.[44] Globally, nanoparticles reported in the literature led to relaxivity improvement as compared to currently approved molecular agents[43,47] (Figure 3). Moreover, targeted liposomes bearing Gd^{3+} complex have also shown to increase the MR contrast as the desired site.[45,46]

The second class of CA are composed of IO derivatives (USPIO, MIONs). Magnetic nanoparticles made from IO, present the advantage to be non-toxic and biodegradable, and have received the authorization for inflammation and liver metastase imaging. The development of targeted CAs on nanoparticles such as superparamagnetic particles to increase the sensitivity of molecular MR imaging techniques is essential for biological investigations with significant potential for clinical translation. Potential applications of ultra-small iron oxide nanoparticles (USPIO) are more and more documented, such as heart transplantation,[48] atherosclerotic lesions,[49] or brain lesion imaging.[50]

In clinics, Gd chelates CAs are mostly in use to provide perfusion information and contrast enhanced images allowing new insights to the physiopathology of diseases.[54] We differentiate non-protein-binding

(Gadovist, Magnevist, Prohance...), weakly (Primovist) and strong protein binding (Vasovist) CAs which provide increasing efficacy due to enhanced relaxivity. The relaxivity at 20 MHz is respectively 5.8 to 45 $mM^{-1}\cdot s^{-1}$.

Superparamagnetic nanoparticles such as Endorem, Cliavist, Resovist (Ferucarbotran Bayer Schering) have been extensively used for liver metastases imaging in clinics but are no longer available. They provide high r2 relaxivity of about 150 $mM^{-1}\cdot s^{-1}$ at 20 MHz or 100 MHz.

2.2. *Some MRI CAs applications*

Superparamagnetic and paramagnetic micro- or nanoparticles that are functionalized with targeting ligands have been extensively developed[51,52] for diagnosis.

Molecular MRI studies with target-specific CAs have shown the capability for *in vivo* detection of molecular markers after experimental stroke. Earlier detection of brain metastases is critical for improved treatment. Sibson *et al.* have developed a targeted MRI CA based on microparticles of IO that enables imaging of endothelial vascular cell adhesion molecule-1 (VCAM-1).[53] The objective was to determine whether VCAM-1 was up-regulated on vessels associated with brain metastases for early detection of these tumors. Early up-regulation of cerebrovascular VCAM-1 expression was evident on tumor-associated vessels in murine models of brain metastasis. Metastases were detectable *in vivo* using VCAM-1-targeted MRI 5 days after induction (<1,000 cells, Figure 4). At clinical imaging resolutions of 1 mm^3 voxel (two or three order of magnitude higher than for rodents), the amount of cells will be two or three order of magnitude higher (10^7–10^8 cells), we could expect then to detect the labelled cells enabling a clinical translation of the metastase detection using this VCAM-1 MPIO molecular MRI method. Another example of molecular MRI concerns USPIOs functionalized with fucoidan ligands which were designed to target P-Selectin in activated platelets, enabling to visualize by MRI arterial thrombi on rats models.[55] (Figure 4).

Gd^{3+} complex have also been covalently coupled to lipids to form Gd-liposomes able to supply a high payload of Gadolinium (50,000

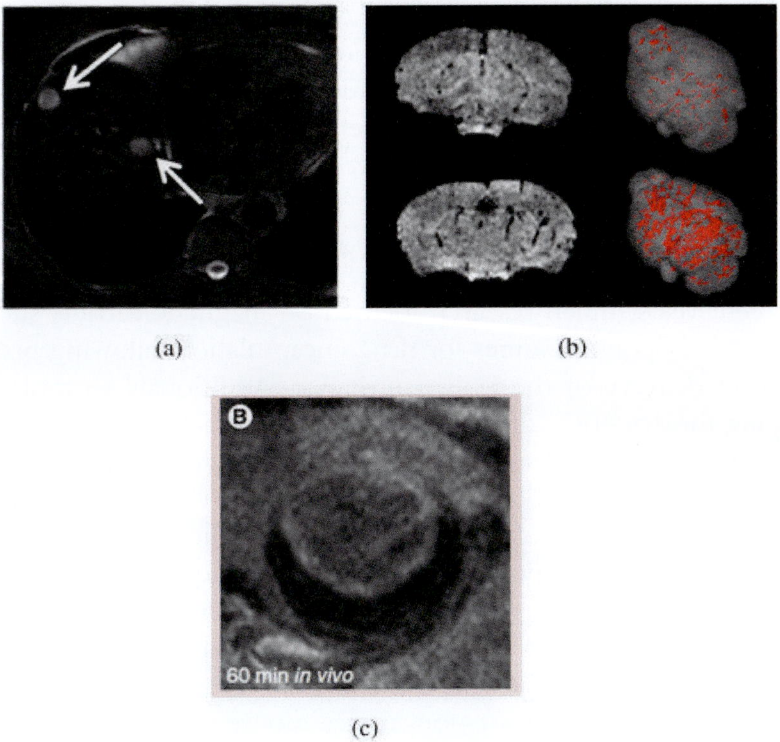

Fig. 4: (a) Hepatic metastases detection using IO CA in clinics.[54] (b) MPIO VCAM functionalized for brain metastases detection *in vivo* on rats (Sibson *et al.*)[53] (c) Atherosclerosis detection using USPIO functionalized by fucoidan.[55]

Gd^{3+}/particles) and functionalized with anti-fibrin monoclonal antibody for detecting vulnerable plaques.[56]

Liposomes with high payload of Gd^{3+} complex associated with RGD ligands have demonstrated to be efficient for $\alpha_v\beta_3$ integrins mapping *in vivo*.[43] Gd^{3+} complex CAs with enhanced r_1 relaxivities due to protein interactions have been developed to detect myeloperoxidase expressed consecutively to inflammation in rodents.[57]

Via ratiometric approach, the MRI response of CEST CAs may be rendered independent of the concentration of the CA and smart, responsive specifically to the presence of an enzyme.[31] For example, a self-immolative spacer has been grafted to a CEST Yb CA,[31] in the presence of the β-galactosidase, it is cleaved which frees an NH exchange site; the difference in exchange rates of this amine protons leads to a change in the PARACEST effect, evidencing in the MRI images the presence of the enzyme. *In vivo* preclinical applications for pH or sodium studies demonstrated a CEST effect related to pH using intrinsic CEST proteins[58] or a clinically approved CA[59] in tumoral tissues.

2.3. *Approaches using MRI CA*

In recent years, much research focused on magnetic carriers such as liposomes or polymersomes for drug encapsulation, allowing protection and delivery of the active substance. Additionaly to molecular imaging for diagnosis, drug coencapsulated with the CA will provide theranostic platform ideal for personalized medicine strategy. Enhanced sensitivity imaging probes should make it easy to control the adequate targeting and pharmacokinetics of the drug to the pathological site.

For example, IO liposomes loaded with manque un espace doxorubicin targeting with anti-mesothelin monoclonal antibody were able to decrease tumor growth.[60] Multifunctional nanoemulsions[61] have been prepared to provide a theranostic multimodal and efficient antitumoral therapy on a colon cancer mouse model. It carries IO nanoparticles, NIR Cy7 dye at the surface and a glucocorticoid hydrophobic Prednisolone Acetate Valerate (PAV) for therapeutic purpose. PAV loaded emulsions induced a significant inhibition in tumor Figure 5.

Magnetic liposomes offer opportunities as theranostic systems. The prerequisite for efficient imaging, tissue targeting or hyperthermia is high magnetic load of these vesicles. Ultra magnetic liposomes (UMLs), may encapsulate IO nanoparticles in an exceptional volume fraction of up to 30%.[62] This remarkable magnetic charge provides UMLs with high magnetic mobilities, MRI relaxivities, magnetic guidance and heating capacities for magnetic hyperthermia, and among all, drug release via High Intensity Focused Ultrasound (HIFU). UMLs suitable for systemic delivery have been developed and characterized by an outstanding loading potential for magnetic nanoparticles and monitoring features by magnetic guidance demonstrated *in vivo* on tumor bearing mice using MRI.[62,64]

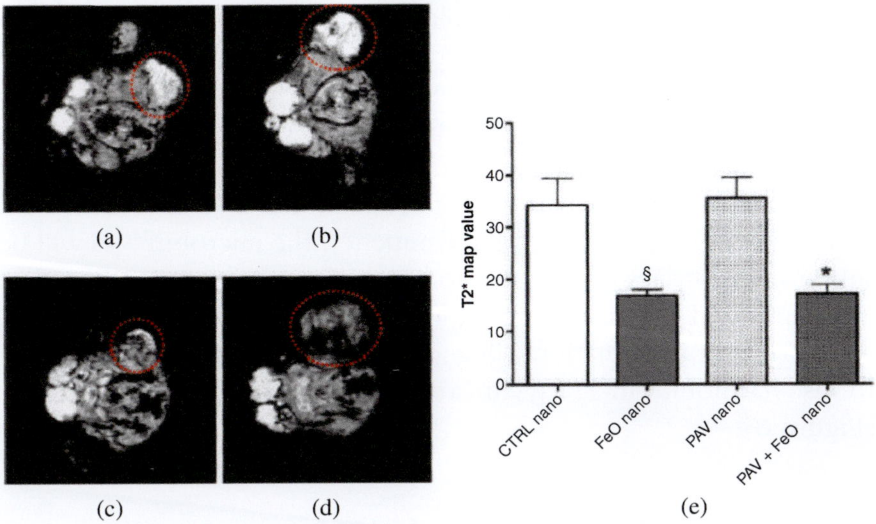

Fig. 5: *In vivo* MRI of tumor bearing mice with theranostic PAV nanoemulsion (PAV, IO CA). Hypointense tumors indicate the IO accumulation.[61]

Enhanced sensitivity MRI CA at different magnetic field strengths have been extensively developed with intermediate sizes but in particular thanks to a high payload of contrastophor of Gd^{3+} complex or more efficiently IO particles. As MRI imaging technique is widely used in clinics, targeting and drug delivery features confer a clear advantage for therapeutical purpose with potential clinic translation.

3. Nanomedicine as CA to Increase the Sensitivity of Ultrasound Imaging

3.1. *Concept of CEUS*

Contrast-enhanced ultrasound (CEUS) associates to the conventional medical sonography to provide dynamic vascularization acquisition post-intravenous injection of CAs. As the blood and tissues present similar echogenicities, discerning the interface between blood and tissue is not obvious with traditional ultrasound. Increasing the difference of echogeneicity in the blood flow and the tissue enhances the contrast and eases the diagnosis.

The CAs used are microbubbles small enough (around 3 μm) to cross the pulmonary capillary barrier and strictly reflect the intravascular flow. An increased contrast is obtained thanks to the reflection of ultrasound waves, which modifies the wave behavior and induces differences with the soft tissue. The signature of the ultrasound backscatter obtained from the microbubbles is easily identified. Under a certain range of applied frequency, the microbubbles will be submitted to cycles of compression and dilatation, which will reflect the ultrasound waves. If the compression is lower than the dilatation, these cycles of deformation will generate harmonics, which is referred to as harmonic imaging in a nonlinear stationary regime[64,65] (Figure 6).

3.2. *Composition of microcrobubbles*

Microbubbles are constituted of a gas core stabilized by a shell (Figure 7). Among the gas proposed, one can find air, nitrogen or a mixture of both. However, these first filled microbubbles lasted less

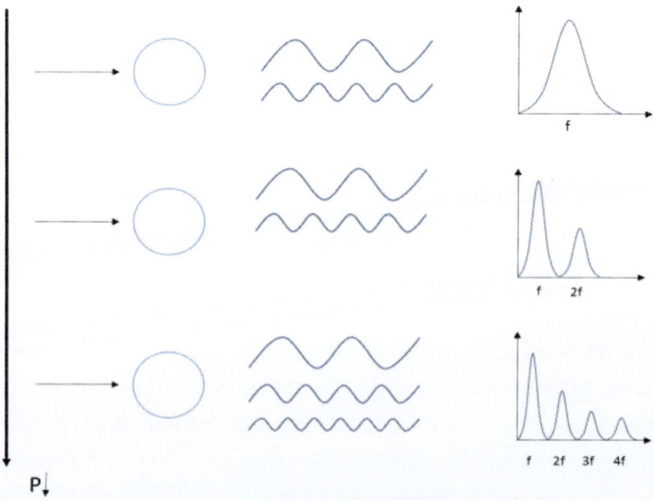

Fig. 6: Nonlinear oscillation of microbubbles relatively to the amplitude of the pressure applied.

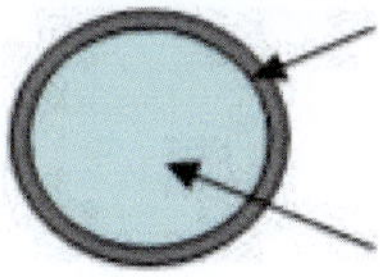

Fig. 7: Schematic representation of a core shell microbubble.

than 1 min in the circulation. This is why, insoluble gases in aqueous media, such as sulfur hexafluoride, or perfluocarbons such as perfluoropropane, perfluorobutane, perfluoropentane or perfluorohexane have been proposed. Extension of the microbubbles half-life has been obtained with these cores. For instance, the BR38 microbubbles made with C_4F_{10} were reported to have a 10 min circulation half-time in mice.[66] To be able to oscillate under the applied energy, the shell of the microbubbles should be deformable. Several shells have been proposed, such as lipidic amphiphiles, protein (albumin) or polymers.[67–69]

3.3. *Microbubble characterization*

3.3.1. *Response to ultrasounds*

Several parameters are crucial to obtain contrast enhanced ultrasound, such as the properties of the backscatter signal in particular when the ultrasound pressure amplitude leads to nonlinear oscillations of the microbubbles.[70] As a consequence of this nonlinear behavior, the scattered signal will be composed by multiple number of the transmitted frequency called harmonics. This harmonic content is the intensity. Therefore, a quantitative analysis of the harmonic intensities as well as the harmonic resonance frequencies are required.[71] Determination of the resonant frequencies of CA microbubbles is an important factor for ultrasound contrast imaging and therapeutic techniques. Indeed, matching the resonant frequency of a CA to the transmitted frequency provides optimized conditions for generating acoustic radiations. The optimal resonance frequency and pressure to be applied is fully dependent on the microbubble composition and microbubble size.[72] The subharmonic imaging technique relies on the bubbles' subharmonic response which can be optimized by utilizing a transmitted frequency of twice the CA's resonant frequency.[73] The resonant frequency should be determined but as of today, there are no perfect system, each group using its own made system. The resonance frequency of commercial CA is fortunately in the range of diagnostic cardiac ultrasound (1–3 MHz). In vascular imaging (7–12 MHz) corresponding to the main applications for CAs, ultrasound and microbubble resonance frequency are not optimally matched, which makes microbubble detection challenging.[74] Moreover, the nonlinear theory would require additional information on the CAs themselves which are not always easy to obtain in practice.[75]

It appears though a general consensus on the fact that the resonant frequency of the lipid-shell microbubbles is decreasing when the size of the microbubbles increase, and that this frequency decreases when the acoustic pressure increases. Now, the dynamic of the nonlinear oscillation is dependent on the nature of the shell.[72] Jimenez compared the ratio of the second to the first harmonic as a function of amplitude of the pressure applied and the microbubble radius relatively to the linear values of microbubbles made of non-encapsulated gas. The results showed rather different behavior from albumin, vs polymer or lipid shell MB (Figure 8). The influence of the driving pressure amplitude was found to be very small for albumin and polymer shells, while the linear vs nonlinear discrepancies was significant for lipid shell MB.[76] Caroll *et al.* also showed that an albumin or polymer shell could stabilize the response to prevent the transition into a chaotic regime throughout the typical clinical range of pressure and frequency, while lipid shell, such as sonazoid MB, just delayed this transition.[77]

3.3.2. *Physico-chemical characterization of microbubbles*

All these data and theory are based on the fact that microbubbles are perfectly characterized. Although, from the physico-chemical point of view, this is not so obvious. Sennoga *et al.* reported a comparison of three methods just to determine the size and the number of the MB formed in a commercially available composition.[78] Electro-impedance

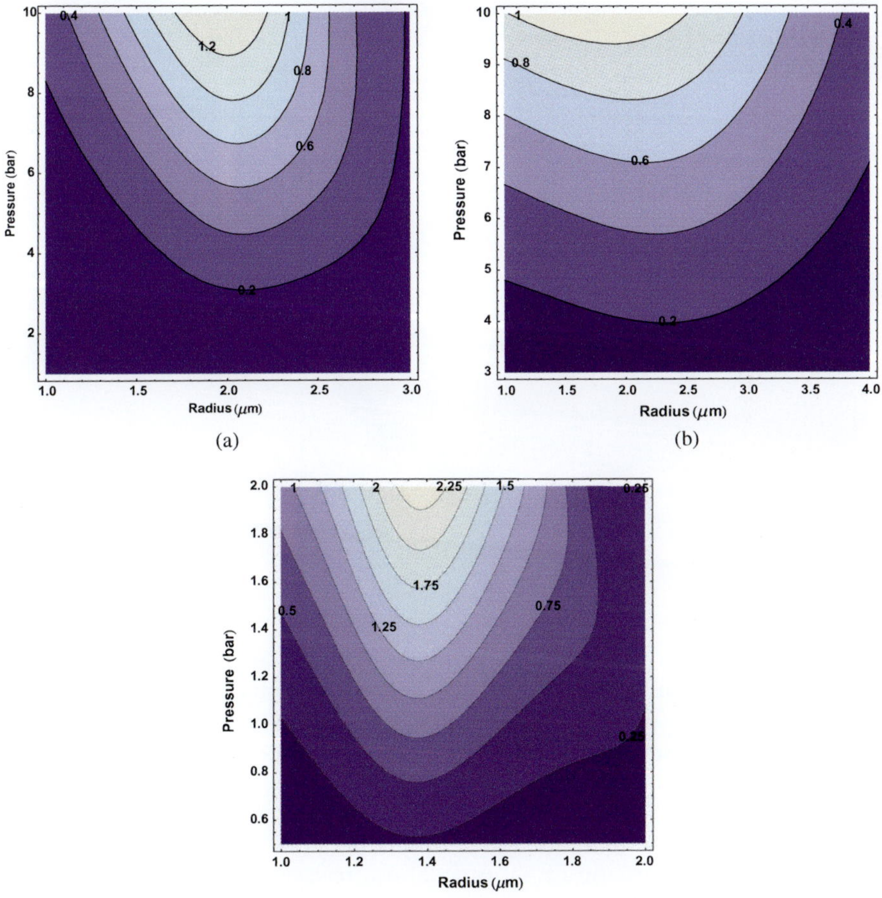

Fig. 8: Contour plot of the ratio of second to first harmonic scattering cross-sections as function of the initial inner bubble radius $R1$ and the pressure amplitude pA for (a) albumin-shelled bubbles in water (b) polymer-shelled bubbles in blood; (c) lipid-shelled bubbles in water at a driven frequency f=3 MHz[72], Copyright from Elsevier Jan 06, 2015.

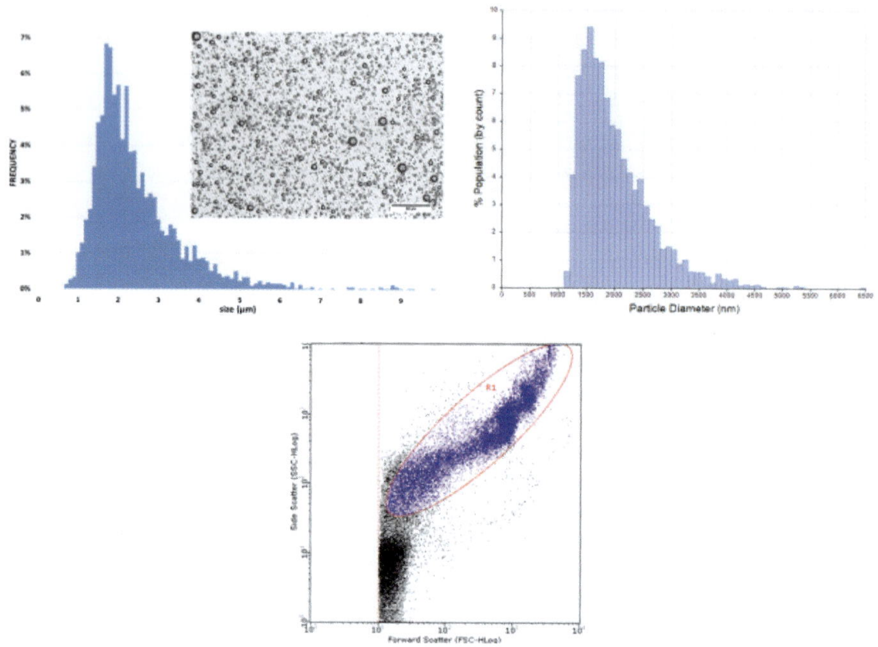

Fig. 9: Comparison of physical methods to characterize the size of microbubbles. From left to right: comparison of positively charged microbubbles by optical microscopy, Tunable Resistive Pulse Sensing and Flow Cytometry. The three methods reflect a typical distribution of MB.

volumetric zone sensing (ES), optical microscopy and laser diffraction were compared. The conclusion of the study was that no single method is fully suited to both sizing and counting of microbubbles. We also recently performed a thorough study comparing dynamic light scattering, optical imaging, flow cytometry and tunable resistive pulse sensing as means to characterize the size and number of positively charged microbubbles (Figure 9). These numbers can be approached but protocols should be optimized in order to take into account the rapid evolution of the sample (Manta, in preparation). Gas filled MB are indeed floating, leading to foam. As a consequence, the size distribution is increasing as a function of time. Stabilization of the MB while maintaining their ability to oscillate is therefore the challenge to take up into MB formulation to increase the number of MB amenable to the market.

3.4. *Commercially available microbubbles*

Initially composed of air surrounded by galactose and palmitic acid Levovist (Schering AG, Berlin, Germany), the ultrasound CAs evolved towards prolonged half-life and higher contrast efficiency thanks to the use of heavier gas as described above. We can find Sonovue (Bracco International, Amsterdam, Netherlands), Optison and Sonazoid (GE Healthcare, Amersham, Buckinghamshire, England), Imagent (Alliance Pharma, Ca) and Definity (Bristol-Myers Squibb, Billerica, MA) which are respectively composed of sulfur hexafluoride, octafluoropropane, a mixture of perflexane and nitrogen, and octafluoropropane. The shell retained for the commercially available microbubbles are mostly lipid shells apart from Optison which has an albumin shell.[79] For a more detailed description of the commercially available microbubbles, please refer to Correas *et al.*[80]

3.5. *Medical applications*

Conventional grayscale ultrasound is used to obtain anatomical information. To obtain informations about the blood flow, Doppler US can be performed, however, Doppler US is limited to relatively large vessels due to a low signal-to-noise ratio. It cannot evaluate the blood flow of microvessels and tissue perfusion. US CAs overcome this limitation thanks to their physical properties, increasing the signal to noise ratio. Observing the enhancement in all the vascular phases, it is possible to differentiate between morphological variants of the parenchyma, this is true for the heart, but also for the liver and the kidney. Sonovue was thus approved for microvascular structures (heart and focal lesions in the liver). Sonazoid can be used both for vascular-phase and liver enhancement coming from Kupffer cell uptake. Similarly, renal lesions can be evidenced by contrast enhancement which will be a different enhancement as compared to the normal parenchyma.[81] Tumor thrombosis can also be evidenced if there is an enhancement in the arterial phase.[82] Hepatocarcinoma can also be detected at earlier stage using contrast enhancement as an early tumor enhancement corresponds to tumor hypervascularity. Therefore, liver applications such as hyperplasia, colon rectal cancer and hypervascularized hepatocellular metastases can be detected, thanks to enhanced ultrasound contrast.[83,84] Furthermore, a real-time CEUS method has recently been developed to assess the skeletal muscle microcirculation which could be used to study patients with peripheral arterial occlusive disease.[85]

Along with works on microbubbles development, acquisition methods and software have evolved to lead to a routine application of dynamic CEUS. The objective is a routine medical quantification of tissue perfusion and objective parameters of various disease state.[86] For instance, prediction of tumor response to chemotherapy has been reported. Analysis of tumor vascular architecture after vascular CEUS was improved taking advantage of individual pixel intensity. This allowed identifying large, medium and small tumor vessels using sonovue microbubbles. Such a protocol on cycles of docetaxel chemotherapy showed vessel enlargement first, than an antiangiogenic effect.[87] Another reported interest is the use of enhanced-contrast ultrasound to accurately diagnose incomplete radiofrequency treatment. This was proposed for liver and renal carcinoma. The specificity of residual tumor vasculature was shown using CEUS, in particular for highly vascularized foci.[88,89]

The limit of the technique is that using harmonics and frequencies at low mechanical index reduces the spatial resolution and the overall image quality. A better knowhow is still required to avoid few difficulties such as the choice of the needle diameter (>20G), the correct positioning of the probe, the length of insonation leading to MB destruction.[88]

3.6. *Targeting with microbubbles*

Targeting ligand binding to receptors expressed in vascular diseases and preferably available from the lumen can be conjugated to microbubbles, to enable the selective accumulation of the microbubble complexes to the diseased tissues. Targeted CEUS can potentially have many applications in both medical diagnostics and medical therapeutics. This statement was written by de Jong and co-workers in 2000.[74] Today, the first clinical trials using targeting microbubbles have been performed. Comparison of non-targeted vs VEGFR2-targeted lipid filled microbubbles showed that the non-targeted microbubbles are quickly washed out, while the targeting microbubbles specifically adhere to their receptors.[90] The use of targeted microbubbles could expand the diagnostic capabilities of current vascular ultrasound imaging by detecting specific molecular processes that play a role in the pathophysiology of vascular disease.[85] Obviously, inflamed tissues, tumors, thrombus appear attractive targets for functionalized microbubbles. MB targeting the receptor $\alpha v\beta 3$ with echistatin was shown to be retained more preferentially within human primary glioblastoma (U-87 MG) xenografted tumor microcirculation, and showed higher tumor margin localization as compared to non-targeted microbubbles.[91] Other adhesion molecules have already been targeted such as VCAM, E, L and P-selectin.[92,93]

3.7. *Theranostic approaches using microbubbles*

Finally, ultrasonography could also be used to localize the microbubbles in order to apply an adapted external stimulus. This is what could be achieved using HIFU, but also for drug delivery. This is seen as a means to target drug or gene delivery. Few examples have already appeared with creative engineered microbubbles to transport as much as possible gene.[94–97] Association of USPIO to microbubbles have also been propose to attract the MB at the site of interest where the sonoporation could then be applied.[98]

Advances in these new concepts which were not even considered 10 years ago, allow a rational hope for the future of these innovant technologies.

4. Nanomedicine as CAs to Increase the Sensitivity of Optical Imaging

4.1. *Concept of in vivo optical imaging*

Compared to the two other imaging modalities presented in this chapter, optical imaging is in its early stage of clinical applications.

Optical imaging becomes a promising technique in pre-clinical studies and for certain clinical applications. Optical imaging is a physical technique based on the detection of photons either emitted by an excited fluorophore (which can be a molecule, a protein, a macromolecule, a nanoparticle), in that case we talk about fluorescence imaging, or by the emission of photons produced by a chemical reaction between an enzyme and its substrate (such as luciferase and luciferin), in that case it is called bioluminescence. When a fluorophore is excited by UV, visible light, gamma or X-rays, electrons move from the ground (S_0) state to a higher energy singlet state (S_1, S_2). Since different electrons have different energies (rotational and vibrational), the transition to a singlet state demands change to an equivalent vibrational or rotational energy at a higher electrical state. During this process, the electron loses a part of its energy, generally through thermal decay (non-radiative energy decay) and, as a result, a lower energy photon is emitted. Among the main advantages of optical imaging we can cite its high sensitivity and the possibility to perform real-time imaging, its low cost, easy to use transportable systems available now, and the lack of ionizing radiations. Fundamental barriers to optical imaging are high light scattering, auto-fluorescence and high absorption by hemoglobin in the mid-visible band. Thus, depending upon the wavelength of light employed, different penetration depths can be achieved. For instance, UV-visible spectral range photons are strongly absorbed by tissue chromophores, deoxy (Hb) and oxyhemoglobin (HbO_2), limiting its penetration. On the other hand, near-infrared light (650 to 900 nm) achieves the highest tissue penetration due to minimal absorbance by tissues in this spectral region[99] (Figure 10).

Thanks to their particular properties, nanomaterials are largely explored in nanomedicine, and nanoparticles-based optical probes are actually intensively studied since they show great improvement compared to their molecular counterpart, notably in terms of light stability, and circulation half-life. Moreover, their surface modifications allow enhance cellular and tissue uptake of nanoparticles.[100] This book chapter section will highlight the characteristics and uses of some NIR-nanoprobes (Quantum dots (QDs), dye-doped silica, gold nanoclusters (NCs), up-conversion nanoparticles (*UCNP*) and

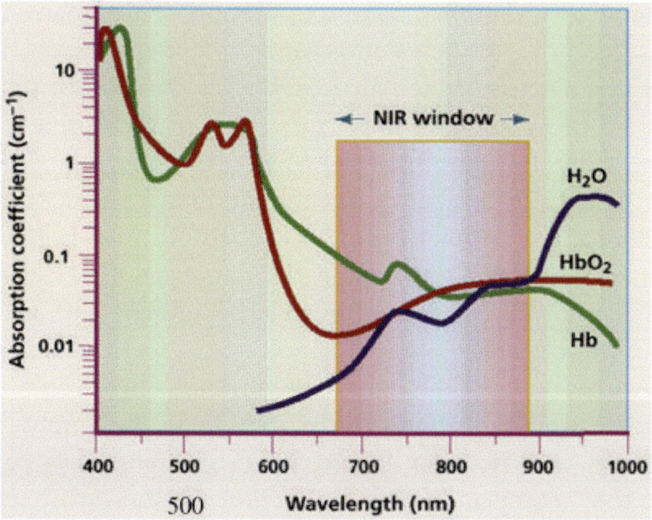

Fig. 10: The NIR window, ideally suited for *in vivo* imaging. Reprinted with permission from Weissleder *et al.*[99] Copyright 2001, Nature Publishing Group.

persistent luminescence nanoparticles (PLNPs)) with potential for bioimaging applications.

4.2. *Optical imaging nanoprobes*

This section highlights the main characteristics of some NIR-nanoprobes.

4.2.1. *QDs*

QDs are luminescent semiconductor nanocrystals with diameters of about 2–20 nm composed of IIIA–VA, IIB–VIA, and IB–VIIA group elements.[101] QDs provide a new class of biomarkers that could overcome the limitations of organic dyes, notably in terms of photostability, that luminesce due to quantum confinement effects. In semiconductors, the overlap of atomic orbitals leads to the formation of valence and conduction bands separated by an energy gap. Upon excitation of a semiconductor, an electron is promoted from the filled valence band to the empty conduction band. This creates a positive vacancy, called hole, in the valence band. The spatial separation (Bohr radius) of this electron-hole pair (exciton) is typically of the order of 1–10 nm for most semiconductors and quantum confinement arises when one of the dimensions of the object becomes the order of exciton Bohr radius. Fluorescence in semiconductor nanocrystals is due to the radiative recombination of an excited electron-hole pair. Both excitation and emission depend on the nanocrystal size. As a consequence, their optical properties are size-dependent and governed by these quantum effects.[102]

Meanwhile, before QDs can be used in non-invasive *in vivo* imaging in patients, the current composition with toxic elements (Cd, Hg, Pb, Se, Te, As, etc.) needs to be altered.[103] Several groups have shown that these toxic components strongly influence the cytotoxic effect of QDs, due to their eventual release into the cellular environment.[104] In most of the cases, naked QDs are susceptible to photo-oxidation, thus, need to be capped by a shell. The shell should be transparent and structurally similar to the core material to efficiently confine the excitation to the core. For instance, encapsulation of CdSe core by ZnS shell reduces the photochemical bleaching and dramatically increases its quantum yield.[105] Initially, chemically synthesized QDs could not be employed for bioimaging applications because they did not disperse well in water, since ZnS or TOPO (trioctylphosphine oxide)-coated QDs are hydrophobic in nature. For biological applications, QDs have to be coated with amphiphilic copolymers, block copolymers, or other water-soluble ligands to enhance their biocompatibility,[106] derivatized with mercaptoacetic acid, encapsulated into phospholipid micelles,[107] or coated with modified poly(acrylic acid).[108]

4.2.2. *Dye-doped nanoparticles*

Rapid photobleaching is one of the main problem of organic fluorescent dyes. Numerous photochemical reactions occur in the cellular environment that lead to photodegradation of the dye.[109] The encapsulation of the dye into a matrix (such as silica or calcium phosphate) is one strategy to maximize *in vitro* and *in vivo* stability. This minimizes oxygen access, increases chemical stability and allows surface modification of the shell to enhance cell uptake. The dye encapsulated within the matrix is the source of the fluorescence.[110] This allows imaging process to be performed over extended periods of time. The most common organic NIR dyes are Cy5.5, Cy7, ICG, methylene blue.[111] The fluorescence emission spectrum of these dyes is between 650 nm and 900 nm, a region where the fluorescence has better tissue penetration and lower tissue absorption[112] (Figure 10).

The surface of these nanoparticles can be easily modified by covalently grafting biomolecules such as proteins, peptides, antibodies, oligonucleotides, etc., using conventional silane-based chemistry[113] allowing the use of dye-containing NPs as fluorescent probes for *in vivo* imaging.

4.2.3. *Gold nanoclusters*

Gold (NCs are novel fluorescent materials that are made up of tens to hundreds of Au atoms. They have intermediate composition between bulk and molecular regimes, where electronic band structure of the bulk gets modified to discrete electronic states as a result of quantum confinement.[114] However, it is relatively difficult to synthesize and stabilize clusters. Two main strategies have been reported so far for the synthesis of NIR Au NCs. The first strategy is to use specific capping agents-thiolate ligands, which can bind on the Au surface, leading to the formation of Au NCs protected by thiolate ligands.[115] The other approach is based on the use of macromolecules, such as proteins.[116] Gold NCs, as a class of metal-containing materials with unique optical properties,[117] are highly attractive for detection and cell imaging due to their low toxicity, bright fluorescence, lack of intermittency and low photobleaching as well as their ultra-small size.[118]

4.2.4. *UCNP*

UCNPs are rare-earth doped materials, mainly containing ytterbium (Yb), erbium (Er) or thulium (Tm) elements, wherein Yb^{3+} acts as light absorber (sensitizer) and the Er^{3+} or Tm^{3+} acts as emitter (activator).[119]

Distinguished from traditional fluorescent probes and NP-based fluorescence probes as mentioned above, UCNPs can be excited by low-energy radiation, resulting in higher energy emission. This anti-Stokes mechanism provides a highly efficient strategy to eliminate the background signal, especially advantageous for *in vivo* imaging. In addition, UCNPs are excited in the NIR allowing deeper tissue penetration. In general, the UCNPs present many advantages, including narrow-bandwidth emission, a long lifetime, tunable emission, high photostability and high resistance to photo-bleaching.[120] Furthermore, the limited background auto-fluorescence and light scattering which allows light penetration in deep tissue, will also make UCNPs attractive optical CAs for *in vitro* and *in vivo* bio-imaging applications.

4.2.5. *PLNPs*

Persistent luminescence is the property of some materials that emit light for minutes, sometimes hours and days, after the end of the excitation. Such materials are mainly used in traffic signs, emergency signage, watches and clocks, luminous paints, as well as textile printing.[121] Our group recently pioneered the use of this optical property for *in vivo* bioimaging applications in living animals.[122] To achieve this goal, the persistent luminescence material should possess at least two criteria: an emission located in the tissue transparency window, and a nanometer size. Indeed, contrary to most of the conventional optical probes such as fluorescent molecules, QDs, dye-doped nanoparticles which require continuous excitation to fluoresce, PLNPs possess the ability to store the excitation energy and to emit light for a long period of time. This property is of particular interest for *in vivo* bio-imaging applications since it will allow complete avoidance of the autofluorescence signal coming from endogeneous chromophors which are also excited when exciting classical fluorescent probes. In 2003, Wang *et al.* reported the synthesis of $MgSiO_3$ doped with Eu^{2+}, Dy^{3+} and Mn^{2+} showing persistent luminescence properties at 660 nm.[123] This composition initiated the development of near-infrared PLNP from our group. The first PLNP developed[124] was

$Ca_{0.2}Mg_{0.9}Zn_{0.9}Si_2O_6$, doped with Eu^{2+}, Dy^{3+} and Mn^{2+} followed by two others:[125] $CaMgSi_2O_6$ doped with Eu^{2+}, Pr^{3+} and Mn^{2+} as an improved optical imaging probes in terms of intensity of luminescence and $ZnGa_2O_4$ doped with Cr^{3+}, which could be, contrary to the two first silicate-based PLNP, followed over extended period of time (> days).[126] Examples of *in vivo* bioimaging applications using PLNP are reported in the next section.

4.3. *In vivo optical imaging examples*

This section highlights some *in vivo* applications of the optical nanoprobes described before.

4.3.1. *QDs*

The use of QDs as luminescence probes has significantly increased since the first examples from Alivisatos[127] and Nie's groups.[128] QDs can be surface modified with targeting moieties to specifically recognize and bind tumor cells. A variety of targeting groups have been developed for the modification and functionalization of NPs, such as small molecules,[129] peptides,[130] affibodies[131] and antibodies.[132] Gao *et al.* first described the multifunctional QDs for cancer targeting and imaging *in vivo*. Their QDs contain an amphiphilic triblock copolymer for *in vivo* protection, targeting-ligands for tumor antigen recognition and multiple PEG molecules for improved biocompatibility and circulation. Subsequently, several research groups performed similar experiments and have confirmed that multifunctional QD probes allow sensitive and specific imaging of cancer cells *in vitro*, such as using RGD-modified QDs.[133]

4.3.2. *Self-illuminating QD*

Fluorescent QDs require excitation from external illumination sources to fluoresce. This requirement may limit their application for imaging living subjects, due to the tissue auto-fluorescence. To overcome this challenge, QD conjugate that can luminesce without the need for external excitation have been prepared.[134] These self-illuminating QD conjugates were prepared by coupling carboxylate-presenting QDs to a mutant of the bioluminescent protein Renilla luciferase. The energy released by luciferase–luciferin reaction can be transferred to QDs via resonance energy transfer, leading to light emission by the QD. These self-illuminating QD conjugates can emit long-wavelength (from red to near-infrared) bioluminescent light in living cells and in living animals, even in deep tissues.

4.3.3. *Dye-doped nanoparticles*

Until now, the most commonly used dye-containing NPs for *in vivo* fluorescence imaging are silica NPs[135] or calcium phosphate nanoparticles (CPNPs).[136] Silica NPs are biocompatible and non-toxic and have high potential applications in bionanotechnology. The hydroxyl groups on their surfaces can be chemically modified with amines, carboxyls, or thiols using conventional silane-based chemistry. These chemically modified silica shells can be easily conjugated with other chemical groups to increase the functionality, stability, dispensability, and biocompatibility. Incorporation of visible dyes into the silica NPs has been widely used for bioimaging.[137] Calcium phosphate is a biomineral mainly presents in the teeth and bones. It has been widely used to synthesize CPNPs for effective delivery of targeted genes or drugs.[138] CPNPs are produced with synthetic methods to achieve colloïdal stability and proper particle dispersion, with well-defined particle sizes and morphology. Further surface modification with polyethylene glycol (PEG) render these CPNPs more efficient for *in vivo* bioimaging.[139]

4.3.4. *Gold nanoclusters*

To date, some researchers have proposed Au NCs as a new class of ultra-small, biocompatible fluorophores for applications *in vivo*.[140] Wu *et al.* presented the first example using ultra-small BSA-stabilized Au NCs for *in vivo* imaging. It was found that the NIR fluorescence and high photostability of Au NCs could be significantly distinguished from the background. Lin *et al.* synthesized water-dispersible fluorescent Au NCs capped with dihydrolipoic acid (AuNC-DHLA) and modified with PEG, bovine serum albumin (BSA), and streptavidin for bioimaging.[141] It has also been reported that the PAMAM-encapsulated Au nanocluster has discrete absorption and fluorescence properties that are size tunable from the UV (Au_5) to the NIR (Au_{31}).[142] After tail vein injections, the fluorescence of Au NCs was immediately visualized over the whole mouse body and remained visible in the circulation even at 5 h post injection. Furthermore, this probe could accumulate at tumor sites with significant fluorescence signal because of the EPR effects.[140] These studies demonstrate that NIR Au NCs are promising nanomaterials for *in vivo* fluorescence imaging.

5. UCNP

Recently, lanthanide-doped UCNPs have been used as potentially promising probes for molecular imaging, due to their unique photoluminescent properties and good biocompatibility. Studies of non-specific target imaging based on UCNPs demonstrated that 50 nm of $NaYF_4$:Yb/Er UCNPs could be employed for *in vivo* imaging in rats.[143] After excitation with a 980 nm NIR laser, the nanoparticles could be detected up to 10 mm under the skin, deeper than the depth reached through the use of QDs. These results provided promising examples for *in vivo* optical imaging at a deeper tissue level for performing minimal invasive imaging in real-time. Compared with QD-based fluorescence imaging, UCNPs showed significantly higher *in vivo* detection sensitivity.[144] Li's group successfully prepared ~8 nm hexagonal Gd-doped $NaLuF_4$-based nanocrystals with bright up-conversion luminescence emission, which could be effective as a luminescent probe for monitoring whole-body of a mouse with an excellent detection limit of 50 cells.[145] The same group also developed RGD-modified UCNPs as luminescent labels for targeted imaging of U87MG (human glioblastoma, high integrin $\alpha v\beta 3$ expression) *in vivo.*[146] Recently, Prasad *et al.* also provided a new approach for *in vivo* imaging by using $NaYF_4$:Yb/Tm-based UCNPs as high contrast photoluminescence imaging probes, with promising light penetration depth up to ~20 mm in mouse.[147]

5.1. *PLNP*

The first demonstration that the light level produced by PLNP was sufficient to yield a localizable signal, without auto-fluorescence background, was reported in 2007 using $Ca_{0.2}Mg_{0.9}Zn_{0.9}Si_2O_6$ doped with Eu^{2+}, Dy^{3+} and Mn^{2+}. The excitation of 100 nm-sized PLNP suspensions before its injection was accomplished by direct exposure to a 6-W UV lamp for 5 min and the injected mice was immediately placed on its back and observed with a highly sensitive photon counting system (Optima, Biospace Lab, Figure 11). Surface modification was realized to modify both the PLNP's tropism.[148–150] A limit of this first generation of PLNP ($Ca_{0.2}Mg_{0.9}Zn_{0.9}Si_2O_6$, doped with Eu^{2+}, Dy^{3+} and Mn^{2+}) was its relative short emission lifetime after UV excitation (about 1 h). The observation time after excitation was extended to 5 h, thanks to a better understanding of the persistent luminescence phenomenon associated with these nanomaterials and the synthesis of an improved silicate-based PLNP.[125] However the excitation of such nanoprobes using UV light, precluded long-term imaging (>few hours). This limit was overcome by the same group with the discovery of the persistent luminescence property of $ZnGa_2O_4$ doped with Cr^{3+}. Contrary to the silicates-based PLNP, the zinc gallate nanoparticles doped with Cr^{3+}could be activated after animal administration using a visible light emitting diode (LED). This property allows to activate

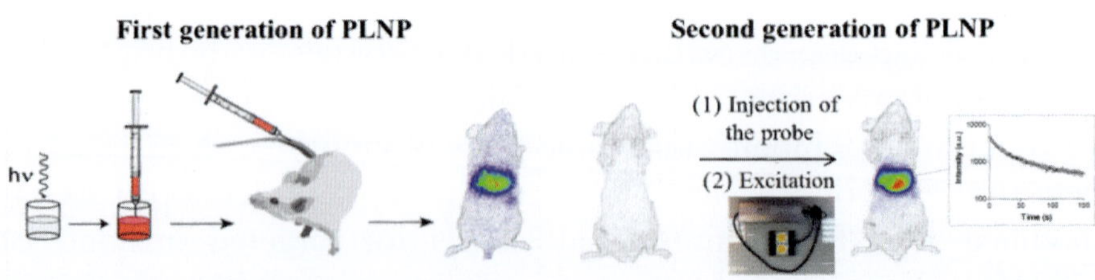

Fig. 11: Principle of imaging with the two generations of persistent luminescence nanoparticles.

probe at any time after its administration, allowing to performing very long term imaging (> days)[126] (Figure 11). Surface modifications of these nanoprobes was realized to enable *in vivo* tumor imaging and to follow the fate of label cells with high target to background ratios.

As presented above, nanoparticle-based optical imaging probes have been widely investigated these last years. In parallel, advances in technologies (lasers, cameras) have enabled the development of high performance instrumentation for near-infrared *in vivo* imaging. Taken together, researches on innovative nanoprobes and advances in the instrumentation should foster the translation of nanoparticle-based optical imaging probes to clinics.

6. Conclusion

The innovation in nanoparticular CAs has led to marketed products for medical imaging. As the innovation has been led in parallel to the evolution of imaging techniques, the field of application has been enlarged for MRI and ultrasound imaging CAs. As the fluorescence technique is getting to the surgical room, no doubt that fluorescent or luminescent nanoparticles will find their way to the imaging market. In all cases, the final objective in health is to detect earlier, with acute precision for faster and more reliable diagnostic for the patient care. The advantages of these non-radionuclide-based techniques are their cost effectiveness and easy handling for ultrasound and fluorescence imaging, its spatial resolution for MRI. Obviously, all need to still go through improvements, but the combination MRI with ultrasound or fluorescence imaging and CAs allows to get the full requirements of spatial resolution, quantitation and sensitivity. Multimodality is not a vain word for nanoparticles which have the possibility to not only combine CAs within one nanoparticle, but also to target a specific molecule. Multimodality can also come from the techniques themselves such as MRI/HiFu hybrids or photoacoustics combining ultrasound and optical imaging. These new developments will require new engineered imaging agents to overcome current limitations or enlarge the applications of these emerging techniques. The advances in imaging quantitation, taking into account the specific properties of the CAs will also further enhance the sensitivity of contrast enhanced imaging.

References

1. J. V. Frangioni, *J. Clin. Oncol.*, 4012 (2008).
2. T. E. Yankeelov, T. E. Peterson, R. G. Abramson, D. Izquierdo-Garcia, L. R. Arlinghaus, X. Li, N. C. Atuegwu, C. Catana, H. C. Manning, Z. A. Fayad and J. C. Gore, *Magn. Reson. Imaging*, 1342 (2012).
3. M. A. Pysz, S. S. Gambhir, J. K. Willmann, *Clin. Radiol.*, 500 (2010).
4. R. Toy, L. Bauer, C. Hoimes, K. B. Ghaghada, E. Karathanasis, *Adv. Drug. Deliv. Rev.*, 79 (2014).
5. C. J. Koch, S. M. Evans, *Adv. Exp. Med. Biol.*, 285 (2003).
6. V. Kumar, D. K. Boddeti, *Recent Results Cancer Res.*, 189 (2013).
7. K. D. Patel, K. W. Abeysekera, M. Marlais, M. J. McPhail, H. C. Thomas, J. A. Fitzpatrick, A. K. Lim, S. D. Taylor-Robinson, E. L. Thomas, *Expert Rev Gastroenterol. Hepatol.*, 91 (2011).
8. M. A. Rutherford, *Curr. Opin. Obstet. Gynecol.*, 180 (2009).
9. W. Sepulveda, R. Ximenes, A. E. Wong, F. Sepulveda, P. Martinez-Ten, *Best Pract Res Clin. Obstet. Gynaecol.*, 593 (2012).
10. G. K. Aguirre, J. A. Detre, *Neuroimage*, 1279 (2012) 1279–1285.
11. M. Ohana, T. Moser, A. Moussaoui, S. Kremer, R. Y. Carlier, P. Liverneaux, J. L. Dietemann, *Diagn. Interv. Imaging*, 17 (2014).
12. N. S. Anavekar, J. K. Oh, *J. Cardiol.*, 347 (2009).
13. C. Demene, M. Pernot, V. Biran, M. Alison, M. Fink, O. Baud, M. Tanter, *J. Cereb. Blood Flow Metab.*, 1009 (2014).
14. E. Bavu, J. L. Gennisson, M. Couade, J. Bercoff, V. Mallet, M. Fink, A. Badel, A. Vallet-Pichard, B. Nalpas, M. Tanter, S. Pol, *Ultrasound Med. Biol.*, 1361 (2011).
15. L. Juge, B. T. Doan, J. Seguin, M. Albuquerque, B. Larrat, N. Mignet, G. G. Chabot, D. Scherman, V. Paradis, V. Vilgrain, B. E. Van Beers, R. Sinkus, *Radiology*, 436 (2012).
16. R. Sinkus, K. Siegmann, T. Xydeas, M. Tanter, C. Claussen, M. Fink, *Magn. Reson. Med.*, 1135 (2007).
17. T. Frenzel, P. Lengsfeld, H. Schirmer, J. Hutter, H. J. Weinmann, *Invest. Radiol.*, 817 (2008).

18. M. F. Tweedle, *Eur. Radiol.*, 225 (1997).
19. M. Mahmoudi, V. Serpooshan, L. Laurent, *Nanoscale*, 3007 (2011).
20. D. Sosnovik, R. Weissleder, *Curr. Opin. Biotechnol.*, 4 (2007).
21. A. S. Merbach, L. Helm, E. Toth, in *The Chemistry of Contrast Agents in Medical Magnetic Resonance Imaging*, John Wiley & Sons, Hoboken, USA 2013.
22. E. M. Haacke, In *MRI, Physical Principles and Sequence Design*, Wiley-LISS, Hoboken, USA, 1999.
23. B. Doan, S. Meme, J. Beloeil, in *The Chemistry of Contrast Agents in Medical Magnetic Resonance Imaging*, Wiley; 2nd edition, 2013.
24. G. M. Nicolle, E. Toth, H. Schmitt-Willich, B. Raduchel, A. E. Merbach, *Chemistry*, 1040 (2002).
25. J. Bridot, A. Faure, S. Laurent, C. Rivière, C. Billotey, B. Hiba, M. Janier, V. Josserand, J. Coll, L. Elst, R. Muller, S. Roux, P. Perriat, O. Tillement, *J. Am. Chem. Soc.*, 5076 (2007).
26. H. Roberts, M. Saeed, T. Roberts, A. Mühler, D. Shames, J. Mann, M. Stiskal, F. Demsar, R. Brasch, *J. Magn. Reson. Imaging*, 331 (1997).
27. R. Sethi, J. Ananta, C. Karmonik, M. Zhong, S. Fung, X. Liu, K. Li, F. M, L. Wilson, P. Decuzzi, *Contrast Media Mol Imaging*, 501 (2012).
28. E. E. Toth, S. Vauthey, D. Pubanz, A. E. Merbach, *Inorg. Chem.*, 3375 (1996).
29. G. M. Nicolle, E. Toth, K. P. Eisenwiener, H. R. Macke, A. E. Merbach, *J. Biol. Inorg. Chem.*, 757 (2002).
30. D. Castelli, E. Terreno, D. Longo, S. Aime, *NMR Biomed.*, 839 (2013).
31. T. Chauvin, P. Durand, M. Bernier, H. Meudal, B. T. Doan, F. Noury, B. Badet, J. C. Beloeil, E. Toth, *Angew. Chem. Int. Ed. Engl.*, 4370 (2008).
32. H. Hifumi, S. Yamaoka, A. Tanimoto, D. Citterio, K. Suzuki, *J. Am. Chem. Soc.*, 15090 (2006) 15090–15091.
33. S. Laurent, L. Elst, R. Muller, *Contrast Media Mol. Imaging*, 128 (2006).
34. P. Caravan, *Acc. Chem. Res.*, 851 (2009).
35. K. Nwe, D. Milenic, L. Bryant, C. Regino, M. Brechbiel, *J Inorg Biochem.*, 722 (2011).
36. A. J. Villaraza, A. Bumb, M. W. Brechbiel, *Chem Rev.*, 2921 (2010).

37. G. H. Gao, J. W. Lee, M. K. Nguyen, G. H. Im, J. Yang, H. Heo, P. Jeon, T. G. Park, J. H. Lee, D. S. Lee, *J. Control. Release*, 11 (2011).
38. E. Nakamura, K. Makino, T. Okano, T. Yamamoto, M. Yokoyama, *J. Control Release*, 325 (2006).
39. C. Richard, B. T. Doan, J. C. Beloeil, M. Bessodes, E. Toth, D. Scherman, *Nano. Lett.*, 232 (2008).
40. H. Kobayashi, S. K. Jo, S. Kawamoto, H. Yasuda, X. Hu, M. V. Knopp, M. W. Brechbiel, P. L. Choyke, R. A. Star, *J. Magn. Reson. Imaging*, 512 (2004).
41. M. Polasek, P. Hermann, J. A. Peters, C. F. Geraldes, I. Lukes, *Bioconjug. Chem.*, 2142 (2009).
42. G. J. Strijkers, W. J. Mulder, R. B. van Heeswijk, P. M. Frederik, P. Bomans, P. C. Magusin, K. Nicolay, *Magma*, 186 (2005).
43. W. J. Mulder, G. J. Strijkers, G. A. van Tilborg, A. W. Griffioen, K. Nicolay, *NMR Biomed*, 142 (2006) 142–164.
44. B. Doan, S. Crauste-Manciet, C. Bourgaux, H. Dhotel, L. Jugé, D. Brossard, D. Scherman, M. Bessodes, C.-A. Cuenod, N. Mignet, *New J Chem.*, 5190 (2014).
45. A. Morawski, G. Lanza, S. Wickline, *Curr. Opin. Biotechnol.*, 16 (2005).
46. D. Sipkins, D. Cheresh, M. Kazemi, L. Nevin, M. Bednarski, K. Li, *Nat Med.*, 4 (1998).
47. T. Bui, J. Stevenson, J. Hoekman, S. Zhang, K. Maravilla, R. J. Ho, *PLoS One*, 5 (2010).
48. Y. L. Wu, Q. Ye, D. F. Eytan, L. Liu, B. L. Rosario, T. K. Hitchens, F. C. Yeh, N. Rooijen van, C. Ho, *Circ Cardiovasc Imaging*, 965 (2013).
49. K. Tsuchiya, N. Nitta, A. Sonoda, H. Otani, M. Takahashi, K. Murata, M. Shiomi, Y. Tabata, S. Nohara, *Eur J Radiol*, 1919 (2013) 1919–1925.
50. B. T. Farrell, B. E. Hamilton, E. Dosa, E. Rimely, M. Nasseri, S. Gahramanov, C. A. Lacy, E. P. Frenkel, N. D. Doolittle, P. M. Jacobs, E. A. Neuwelt, *Neurol.*, 256 (2013).
51. D. Hogemann, L. Josephson, R. Weissleder, J. P. Basilion, *Bioconjug. Chem.*, 941 (2000).
52. J. R. McCarthy, R. Weissleder, *Adv. Drug Deliv. Rev.*, 1241 (2008).

53. S. Serres, M. S. Soto, A. Hamilton, M. A. McAtee, W. Shawn, M. D. D. Robson, O. Ansorge, A. B. Khrapitchev, C. L. Balathasan, T. Weissensteiner, D. C. Anthony, R. P. Choudhury, R. J. Muschel, N. R. Sibson, *Proc. Natl. Acad. Sci. U S A*, 6674 (2010).
54. C. Heilmaier, A. M. Lutz, N. Bolog, D. Weishaupt, B. Seifert, W. J. K., *Radiol.*, 724 (2009) 724–733.
55. M. Suzuki, L. Bachelet-Violette, F. Rouzet, A. Beilvert, G. Autret, M. Maire, C. Menager, L. Louedec, C. Choqueux, P. Saboural, O. Haddad, C. Chauvierre, F. Chaubet, J. B. Michel, J. M. Serfaty, D. Letourneur, *Nanomedicine* (Lond), 1 (2014).
56. S. Flacke, S. Fischer, M. J. Scott, R. J. A. Fuhrhop, J. S. M. McLean, P. Winter, G. A. Sicard, P. J. Gaffney, S. A. Wickline, G. M. Lanza, *Circulation*, 1280 (2001).
57. J. W. Chen, M. Querol Sans, A. Bogdanov, Jr., R. Weissleder, *Radiol.*, 473 (2006).
58. G. Liu, C. Bettegowda, Y. Qiao, V. Staedtke, K. Chan, R. Bai, Y. Li, G. Riggins, K. Kinzler, J. Bulte, M. McMahon, A. Gilad, B. Vogelstein, S. Zhou, P. Van Zijl, *Magn. Reson. Med.*, 1690 (2013).
59. L. Chen, C. Howison, J. Jeffery, I. Robey, P. Kuo, M. Pagel, *Magn. Reson. Med.*, 1408 (2014).
60. L. Deng, X. Ke, Z. He, D. Yang, H. Z. Gong, Y. X. Jing, J. Yao, J. Chen, *Int. J. Nanomed.*, 5053 (2012).
61. A. Gianella, P. A. Jarzyna, V. Mani, S. Ramachandran, C. K. B. Claudia Calcagno, J. T. Wouter, J. R. Dijk, V. L. Thijssen, A. W. Griffioen, G. Storm, Z. A. Fayad, W. J. M. Mulder, *ACS Nano*, 5 (2011).
62. G. Béalle, R. Di Corato, J. Kolosnjaj-Tabi, V. Dupuis, O. Clément, F. Gazeau, C. Wilhelm, C. Ménager, *Langmuir*, 28 (2012).
63. I. Brigger, J. Morizet, G. Aubert, H. Chacun, M. J. Terrier-Lacombe, P. Couvreur, G. Vassal, *J. Pharmacol. Exp. Ther.*, 928 (2002).
64. A. A. Doinikov, P. A. Dayton, *J Acoust Soc Am*, 3331 (2007).
65. M. Emmer, A. van Wamel, D. E. Goertz, N. de Jong, *Ultrasound Med. Biol.*, 941 (2007).
66. M. Schneider, B. Anantharam, M. Arditi, D. Bokor, A. Broillet, P. Bussat, X. Fouillet, P. Frinking, I. Tardy, J. Terrettaz, R. Senior, F. Tranquart, *Invest. Radiol.*, 486 (2011).
67. K. W. Ferrara, M. A. Borden, H. Zhang, *Acc. Chem. Res.*, 881 (2009).

68. E. Pisani, N. Tsapis, J. Paris, V. Nicolas, L. Cattel, E. Fattal, *Langmuir*, 4397 (2006).
69. L. Shan Molecular Imaging and Contrast Agent Database (MICAD) 2004.
70. S. Sirsi, M. Borden, *Bubble Sci. Eng. Technol.*, 3 (2009).
71. E. Stride, in *Front Neurol Neurosci*, Karger, Basel, 2015.
72. J. Jiménez-Fernández, *Ultrasonics*, 52 (2012).
73. S. Zhao, M. Borden, S. Bloch, D. Kruse, K. Ferrara, P. Dayton, *Mol. Imaging*, 135 (2004).
74. N. de Jong, P. Frinking, A. Bouakaz, F. Ten Cate, *Ultrasonics*, 87 (2000).
75. J. U. Voigt, *Methods*, 92 (2009).
76. E. Stride, N. Saffari, *Proc. Inst. Mech. Eng. H.*, 429 (2003).
77. J. Carroll, M. Calvisi, L. Lauderbaugh, *J. Acoust. Soc. Am.*, 2641 (2013).
78. C. A. Sennoga, J. S. Yeh, J. Alter, E. Stride, P. Nihoyannopoulos, J. M. Seddon, D. O. Haskard, J. V. Hajnal, M. X. Tang, R. J. Eckersley, *Ultrasound Med. Biol.*, 834 (2012).
79. S.-H. Seol, J. R. Lindner, *J. Cardiovasc. Ultrasound*, 101 (2014).
80. J. M. Correas, L. Bridal, A. Lesavre, A. Mejean, M. Claudon, O. Helenon, *Eur. Radiol.*, 1316 (2001).
81. A. Granata, L. Luca Zanoli, M. Monica Insalaco, M. Valentino, P. Pavlica, P. P. Di Nicolo, M. Scuderi, F. Fiorini, P. Fatuzzo, M. Bertolotto, *Clin. Exp. Nephrol.*, Oct. 29 (2014).
82. Y. E. Chung, K. W. Kim, *Ultrasonography*, 3 (2015).
83. M. Ronot, V. Vilgrain, *Best Practice & Research Clinical Gastroenterology*, 795 (2014).
84. F. Tranquart, J. M. Correas, V. L. Marcus, P. Manzoni, V. Vilgrain, C. Aube, A. Elmaleh, L. Chami, M. Claudon, M. Cuilleron, B. Diris, F. Garibaldi, O. Lucidarme, D. Marion, C. Beziat, A. Rode, J. P. Tasu, H. Trillaud, A. Bleuzen, A. Le Gouge, B. Giraudeau, E. Rusch, *J. Radiol.*, 109 (2009).
85. D. Staub, S. Partovi, S. Imfeld, H. Uthof, T. Baldi, M. Aschwanden, K. Jaeger, *Vasa*, 17 (2013).
86. F. Tranquart, L. Mercier, P. Frinking, E. Gaud, M. Arditi, *Ultraschall Med.*, S31 (2012).

87. K. Maheo, S. Chevalier, S. Vibet, P. Bougnoux, S. Richard, S. Serriere, A. Bleuzen, F. Tranquart, C. Goupille, *Breast Cancer Res Treat*, 1013 (2012) 1013–1125.
88. M. J. Dill-Macky, P. Burns, S. Wilson, *AJR Am J Roentgenol*, S287 (2006).
89. C. Hoeffel, M. Pousset, M. O. Timsit, C. Elie, A. Mejean, S. Merran, F. Tranquart, A. Khairoune, D. Joly, S. Richard, O. Helenon, J. M. Correas, *Eur Radiol*, 1812 (2010).
90. J. Bzyl, W. A. Rix, C. Grouls, I. Tardy, S. Pochon, M. Siepmann, T. Penzkofer, M. Schneider, F. Kiessling, M. Palmowski, *Eur Radiol*, 1988 (2011).
91. D. B. Ellegala, H. Leong-Poi, J. E. Carpenter, A. L. Klibanov, S. Kaul, M. E. Shaffrey, J. Sklenar, J. R. Lindner, *Circulation*, 336 (2003).
92. T. Bettinger, P. Bussat, I. Tardy, S. Pochon, J. M. Hyvelin, P. Emmel, S. Henrioud, N. Biolluz, J. K. Willmann, M. Schneider, F. Tranquart, *Invest. Radiol.*, 516 (2014).
93. J. R. Lindner, J. Song, J. Christiansen, A. L. Klibanov, F. Xu, K. Ley, *Circulation*, 2107 (2001).
94. A. Delalande, M. Postema, N. Mignet, P. Midoux, C. Pichon, *Ther. Deliv.*, 1199 (2012).
95. K. Ferrara, R. Pollard, M. Borden, *Annu. Rev. Biomed. Eng.*, 415 (2007).
96. R. R. Sun, M. L. Noble, S. S. Sun, S. Song, C. H. Miao, *J Control Release*, 111 (2014).
97. R. Suzuki, T. Takizawa, Y. Negishi, N. Utoguchi, K. Sawamura, K. Tanaka, E. Namai, Y. Oda, Y. Matsumura, K. Maruyama, *J. Control Release*, 137 (2008).
98. S. T. Kang, C. K. Yeh, *Chang Gung Med J*, 125 (2011).
99. R. Weissleder, *Nat. Biotechnol.*, 316 (2001).
100. T. L. Doane, C. Burda, *Chem. Soc. Rev.*, 2885 (2012).
101. A. P. Alivisatos, *Science*, 933 (1996).
102. A. M. Smith, *Acc. Chem. Res.*, 190 (2010).
103. J. Y. Chang, S. R. Wang, C. H. Yang, *Nanotechnol.*, 345602 (2007).
104. A. M. Derfus, W. C. W. Chan, S. N. Bhatia, *Nano Lett.* 11(2004).
105. M. A. Hines, P. Guyot-Sionnest, *J. Phys. Chem.*, 468 (1996).
106. J. Gao, K. Chen, R. Xie, S. Lee, Z. Cheng, X. Peng, X. Chen, *Small*, 256 (2010).

107. B. Dubertret, P. Skourides, D. J. Norris, V. Noireaux, A. H. Brivanlou, A. Libchaber, *Science*, 1759 (2002).
108. X. Wu, H. Liu, J. Liu, K. N. Haley, J. A. Treadway, J. P. Larson, N. Ge, F. Peale, M. P. Bruchez, *Nat. Biotechnol.*, 41 (2003).
109. J. K. Jaiswal, H. Mattoussi, J. M. Mauro, S. M. Simon, *Nat. Biotechnol.*, 47 (2003).
110. S. Santra, B. Liesenfeld, C. Bertolino, D. Dutta, Z. Cao, W. Tan, B. Moudgil, R. A. Mericle, *J Lumin*, 75 (2006).
111. S. Luo, E. Zhang, Y. Su, T. Cheng, C. Shi, *Biomaterials*, 7127 (2011).
112. K. Licha, C. Hessenius, A. Becker, P. Henklein, M. Bauer, S. Wisniewski, B. Wiedenmann, W. Semmler, *Bioconjug. Chem.*, 44 (2001).
113. S. Santra, D. Dutta, G. A. Walter, B. M. Moudgil, *Technol. Cancer Res. Treat.*, 593 (2005).
114. E. S. Shibu, M. A. H. Muhammed, T. Tsukuda, *J. Phys. Chem. C.*, 121680 (2008).
115. X. Yuan, Y. Yu, Q. F. Yao, Z. Q., J. Xie, *J. Phys. Chem. Lett.*, 2310 (2012).
116. J. P. Xie, Y. G. Zheng, J. Y. Ying, *J Am Chem Soc.*, 888 (2009).
117. T. P. Bigioni, R. L. Whetten, O. Dag, *J Phys Chem B.* 6983 (2000).
118. R. A. Sperling, P. R. Gil, F. Zhang, Z. M., P. W. F., *Chem Soc Rev.*, 1896 (2008).
119. W. Feng, L. D. Sun, Y. W. Zhang, F. Wei, S. Ling-Dong, Z. Ya-Wen, Y. Chun-Hua, *Coord. Chem Rev.,*1038 (2010).
120. Y. Liu, D. Tu, H. Zhu, X. Chen, *Chem. Soc. Rev.*, 6924 (2013).
121. T. Kano, Luminescene Centres of Rare-Earth Ions. Shionoya, S., Yen, W. M., Eds. CRC Press, Boca Raton, FL, USA, 1999.
122. Q. le Masne de Chermont, C. Chaneac, J. Seguin, F. Pelle, S. Maitrejean, J. P. Jolivet, D. Gourier, M. Bessodes, D. Scherman, *Proc. Natl. Acad. Sci. USA*, 9266 (2007).
123. X. J. Wang, D. Jia, W. M. Yen, *J. Lumin.*, 34 (2003).
124. Q. le Masne de Chermont, C. Richard, J. Seguin, C. Chanéac, M. Bessodes, D. Scherman, *Proc. of SPIE*, 7189 (2009).
125. T. Maldiney, A. Lecointre, B. Viana, A. Bessiere, M. Bessodes, D. Gourier, C. Richard, D. Scherman, *J. Am. Chem. Soc.*, 11810 (2011).

126. T. Maldiney, A. Bessiere, J. Seguin, E. Teston, S. K. Sharma, B. Viana, A. J. Bos, P. Dorenbos, M. Bessodes, D. Gourier, D. Scherman, C. Richard, *Nat. Mater.*, 418 (2014).
127. M. Bruchez Jr., M. Moronne, P. Gin, S. Weiss, A. P. Alivisatos, *Science*, 2013 (1998).
128. W. C. Chan, S. Nie, *Science*, 2016 (1998).
129. M. Geszke, M. Murias, L. Balan, G. Medjahdi, J. Korczynski, M. Moritz, J. Lulek, R. Schneider, *Acta Biomater.*, 1327 (2011).
130. J. Gao, K. Chen, R. Luong, D. M. Bouley, H. Mao, T. Qiao, S. S. Gambhir, Z. Cheng, *Nano Lett.*, 11 (2004).
131. J. H. Gao, K. Chen, Z. Miao, G. Ren, X. Y. Chen, S. S. Gambhir, Z. Cheng, *Biomaterials,* 2141 (2011).
132. X. Gao, Y. Cui, R. M. Levenson, W. Leland, K. Chung, S. Nie, *Nat Biotech.*, 969 (2004).
133. B. Atmaja, B. H. Lui, Y. Hu, S. Beck, C. W. Frank, C. J. R, *Adv Funct Mater.*, 4091 (2010).
134. M. K. So, C. Xu, A. M. Loening, S. S. Gambhir, J. Rao, *Nat. Biotechnol.*, 339 (2006).
135. R. Kumar, I. Roy, T. Y. Ohulchanskky, L. A. Vathy, E. J. Bergey, M. Sajjad, P. N. Prasad, *ACS Nano*, 699 (2010).
136. A. Tabakovi, M. Kester, J. H. Adair, *WIREs Nanomed. Nanobiotechnol.*, 96 (2010).
137. W. H. Tan, K. M. Wang, X. X. He, X. Zhao, T. Drake, L. Wang, R. Bagwe, *Medicinal Research Reviews*, 621 (2004).
138. M. Kester, Y. Heakal, T. Fox, A. Sharma, G. Robertson, T. Morgan, E. Altinoğlu, A. Tabaković, M. Parette, S. Rouse, V. Ruiz-Velasco, J. Adair, *Nano Lett.*, 4116 (2008).
139. S. V. Dorozhkin, M. Epple, *Angew. Chem. Int. Ed.*, 3130 (2002).
140. X. Wu, X. X. He, K. M. Wang, C. Xie, B. Zhou, Z. Qing, *Nanoscale*, 2244 (2010).
141. C. J. Lin, T. Y. Yang, C. Lee, H. Sherry, R. Huang, A. Sperling, M. Zanella, J. K. Li, J.-L. Shen, H. H. Wang, H. I. Yeh, W. J. Parak, W. H. Chang, *ACS Nano*, 395 (2009).
142. J. Zheng, C. W. Zhang, R. M. Dickson, *Phys. Rev. Lett.*, 077402 (2004).
143. D. K. Chatterjee, A. J. Rufaihah, Y. Zhang, *Biomaterials*, 937 (2008).

144. L. Cheng, K. Yang, S. Zhang, S. Mingwang, L. Shuittong, L. Zhuang, *Nano Res.*, 722 (2010).
145. Q. Liu, Y. Sun, T. S. Yang, W. Feng, C. Li, F. Li, *J. Am. Chem. Soc.*, 17122 (2011).
146. L. Q. Xiong, Z. G. Chen, Q. W. Tian, T. Cao, C. Xu, F. Li, *Anal Chem.*, 8687 (2009).
147. M. Nyk, R. Kumar, T. Y. Ohulchanskyy, E. J. Bergey, P. N. Prasad, *Nano Lett.*, 3834 (2008).
148. T. Maldiney, G. Byk, N. Wattier, J. Seguin, R. Khandadash, M. Bessodes, C. Richard, D. Scherman, *Int. J. Pharm.*, 102 (2012).
149. T. Maldiney, M. U. Kaikkonen, J. Seguin, Q. le Masne de Chermont, M. Bessodes, K. J. Airenne, S. Yla-Herttuala, D. Scherman, C. Richard, *Bioconjug. Chem.*, 472 (2012).
150. T. Maldiney, C. Richard, J. Seguin, N. Wattier, M. Bessodes, D. Scherman, *ACS Nano*, 854 (2011).

CHAPTER 3

MRI T2 WEIGHTED THERANOSTIC NANODEVICES AND CHEMOTHERAPY

Sophie Laurent[*,†], Luce Vander Elst[*,†], Dimitri Stanicki[*] and Robert N. Muller[*,†]

[*]*Department of General, Organic and Biomedical Chemistry, NMR and Molecular Imaging Laboratory, University of Mons, 19 Avenue Maistriau, 7000 Mons, Belgium*

[†]*Center for Microscopy and Molecular Imaging (CMMI), 8 Rue Adrienne Boland, 6041 Gosselies, Belgium*

This chapter presents and compares the different principal methods to prepare superparamagnetic iron oxide nanoparticles (SPION). An important step for biomedical applications is the stabilization with biocompatible non-toxic coating. Numerous ways are proposed in literature using small charged molecules or polymers. The applications described here are focused on the drug delivery associated to magnetic resonance imaging (MRI) to follow the therapeutic aspect and to control the efficiency of the treatment.

Theranostic devices are defined as systems which combine the modalities of diagnosis and therapy. These materials allow to diagnose by imaging or to follow a real-time medical treatment and to deliver therapeutic drugs in the same time.[1,2]

Among numerous nano-systems, magnetic nanoparticles such as SPION have gained significant attention.[2,3] These SPION present a lot of advantages as (i) their intrinsic magnetic properties for magnetic resonance imaging (MRI),[4] (ii) their lack of toxicity[5] and (iii) their surface coated with biocompatible coatings allowing specific targeting for molecular imaging.[6,7] These properties open large possibilities for biomedical applications: *in vivo* medical imaging, tissue repair, hyperthermia, drug delivery, biosensor, ...[8–11] This chapter is focused on the study of SPION as nanocarriers for drug delivery.

One of the most important problems to overcome is the physiological barriers to allow access to cellular target. After intra-venous injection, blood can induce SPION agglomeration or interactions between SPION and plasma proteins, extravascular matrices. Thus, there is a real problem for reaching the target tissues. Another problem is the blood–brain barrier (BBB). Only nanoparticles with sufficiently small size and appropriate physicochemical properties can pass through the BBB. Biodistribution, pharmacokinetics and *in vivo* cellular uptake are directly linked to the physicochemical properties of the SPION (hydrodynamic size, charge surface, shape, coating nature or morphology). For example, hydrodynamic size influences the SPION concentration in the blood vessel[12,13] and affects their clearance from circulation.[14–16] Small nanoparticles (diameter <20 nm) are excreted renally,[14,17] medium sized ones (30–150 nm) are accumulated in the bone marrow, heart, kidney and stomach,[17] while large nanoparticles (150–300 nm) are found in the liver and spleen.[18] A review has suggested that BBB crossing is influenced by several physiochemical properties and not only by the size of the nanoparticles.[19] It has been shown that anisotropically shaped nanoparticles can avoid bio-elimination better than spherical ones.[20]

Charge and hydrophobicity affect biodistribution by interactions of nanoparticles with plasma proteins, immune system, extracellular matrices or non-targeted cells.[21] Hydrophobic nanoparticles have short circulation times due to adsorption of plasma proteins (opsonization) which can lead to recognition by the reticulo-endothelial system (RES), followed by removal from circulation. Positively charged nanoparticles can also bind with non-targeted cells leading to non-specific internalization. Hydrophobic groups on the surface can induce nanoparticle agglomeration after injection, leading to rapid removal by the RES. To limit these interactions, surface engineering has led to the development of stealth nano-objects. Surface modifications with molecules like the hydrophilic polyethylene glycol (PEG) have been shown to reduce the potential for opsonization through steric repulsion, prolonging NP circulation times.[21]

1. Preparation of Magnetic Nanosystems

SPION can be obtained by top-down (mechanical attrition) or bottom-up (chemical synthesis) approaches. Among these two procedures, chemical routes allow to produce nanoparticles with better control of composition and size.[22] Solution chemical methods include standard iron chloride co-precipitation, thermal decomposition, hydro-thermal synthesis, co-precipitation in constrained environments, sonochemical methods and polyol synthesis. Some reviews on these methods have been reported.[2,4,23] Each method has its own advantages and disadvantages. The most common preparation method involves the mixing of ferric and ferrous derivatives, generally chlorides[24] or sulfates[25] in aqueous solution. The precipitation occurs after the addition of a base (NaOH or NH_4OH) to a solution of ferrous and ferric salts under inert atmosphere at ambient temperature or at high temperature. The main advantage is the ability to produce iron oxide nanoparticles in large quantities. However, the control of the size distribution and of the shape is not efficient. The adjustment of some parameters[23,26–28] such as pH, ratio between Fe (II) and Fe (III) concentrations, ionic strength of medium, salt type, base nature and reaction temperature, allows a better control of the final characteristics of nanoparticles (size, shape and composition). The experimental challenge in the synthesis by co-precipitation is the control of the particle size to obtain a narrow particle size distribution. As-obtained particles tend to be rather polydisperse. To improve the uniformity and stability of SPION, modifications of the standard co-precipitation approach have been investigated by the use of organic additives as stabilization or reducing agents. Addition of polymers or polyelectrolytes to the iron chloride solution during co-precipitation can tune the physical properties (size, shape and crystallinity) of the SPION.[29,30] These polymers (for example, poly (acrylic acid)[29] or polyethyleneglycol-g-poly(glycerol monoacrylate)[30]) can act as surface coatings after complete nucleation and growth. These coatings are referred to as *in situ* because they are present during nanoparticle synthesis. Unfortunately, this approach can limit the crystallinity of SPION, which may affect their magnetic susceptibility.

More recently, some synthesis techniques have used high-temperature decomposition methods and organic iron precursors.[31,32] Sun *et al.* reported high-temperature reaction of iron (III) acetylacetonate, $Fe(acac)_3$, in phenylether or dibenzylether in the presence of alcohol, oleic acid and oleylamine, to yield monodisperse hydrophobic NPs with tunable sizes of 4–20 nm.[32] This strategy is promoted by the use of the seed-mediated growth method. Nanoparticle size increases up to 20 nm via the addition of new quantity of iron precursor in the nanoparticle suspension without the modification of size standard deviation. Hyeon *et al.*[33] reported the production of monodisperse iron oxide nanoparticles by using thermal decomposition of iron pentacarbonyl ($Fe(CO)_5$) in a solution of octylether containing oleic acid to yield an iron oleate complex at low temperature. Then, the iron oleate solution was decomposed at high temperature (300°C) to obtain 11 nm monodisperse iron nanoparticles followed by a controlled oxidation with trimethylamine as a mild oxidant, in order to form iron oxide nanoparticles.

Park *et al.*[34] also developed a similar approach to produce monodisperse nanoparticles in which the nanoparticle size is increased by one nanometer between each step. They used iron chloride and sodium oleate to generate an iron oleate complex *in situ* which was then decomposed at temperature between 240°C and 320°C in different solvents, such as 1-hexadecane, octylether, 1-octadecene, 1-eicosene or trioctylamine. Jana *et al.* described a decomposition approach for the synthesis of size and shape controlled magnetic oxide nanocrystals based on the pyrolysis of metal fatty acid salts in non-aqueous solution.[35] The process has exploited a large panel of fatty acids (such as decanoic acid, lauric acid, myristic acid, palmitic acid, oleic acid or stearic acid), hydrocarbon solvents (octadecene, n-eicosane, tetracosane, or a mixture of octadecene and tetracosane) and activation agents (primary amines or alcohol). Nearly monodisperse iron oxide nanoparticles could be produced. This process allows a size control (size range of 3–50 nm) and a shape control (spherical or cubic) according to the variation of concentration and the length of fatty acids. The limitation of these synthesis approaches is that additional steps are required to remove the hydrophobic coating, or to modify the surface with an amphiphilic surfactant to render the nanosystems usable for biomedical applications. A very simple synthesis of water soluble magnetite nanoparticles was reported by Li.[36] Using $FeCl_3{\cdot}6H_2O$ as iron source and 2-pyrrolidone as coordinating solvent, water soluble Fe_3O_4 nanocrystals were prepared under reflux (245°C). The same team developed a one-pot synthesis of water soluble magnetite nanoparticles prepared under similar reaction conditions by the addition of α,ω-dicarbonyl terminated PEG as a surface capping agent.[37] Even if these new techniques yield more uniform nanoparticles with superior magnetic properties, the co-precipitation method continues to be most widely used for biomedical applications because of an easy implementation and less hazardous materials and procedures.

Microemulsion and inverse micelle syntheses have been employed to prepare shape and size controlled SPION. Particularly, water-in-oil (w/o) microemulsions are formed by well-defined nano-droplets of the aqueous phase, dispersed by the assembly of surfactant molecules in a continuous oil phase. Microemulsion cavities can be considered as reactors. Most of the used methods are based on the coprecipitation process of iron precursors in basic condition. Two general methods could be used for the formation of magnetite nanoparticles. The first process is made up of two different microemulsions where the first one contains the iron precursors and the second one contains the base. By the mixing of both water in oil microemulsion systems, the colloid microdroplets coalesce and finally a precipitate appears in the micelles. The second method is composed of a microemulsion containing the iron precursors in which the base is then added. This induces the beginning of the coprecipitation mechanism. Vidal-Vidal *et al.*[38] have reported the synthesis of monodisperse SPION by a "one pot" microemulsion method. The spherical shaped particles capped with a monolayer coating of oleylamine show a narrow size distribution of 3.5 nm. Okoli *et al.*[39] described a complex microemulsion system based on the mixing of two microemulsion systems. The first microemulsion is obtained by the mixing of iron precursors (iron (II) and (III) chlorides) with the surfactants (CTAB: cetyltrimethylammonium bromide), co-surfactant (butanol), water and oil phase (*n*-octane). The second mixture containing the precipitating agent (NH_3) is slowly added to the first microemulsion where the reaction occurs and produces the formation of iron oxide nanoparticles.

Masih and coworkers[40] proposed an easy microemulsion method where the organic surfactants molecules (igepal-CO 520 (polyoxyethylene-(5)-nonylphenylether)) act both as a stabilizer of the microemulsion and as a capping layer surrounding the final nanoparticles.

In comparison to the nanoparticles produced by Massart team procedure,[41] particles obtained by microemulsion technique were smaller in size and had higher saturation magnetization.[42] Although the work-up of the synthesis is simple and fast, the elimination of surfactant excess requires the use of robust purification methods. Moreover, the total yield of the reaction is quite low as compared to other methods. To produce a large quantity of nanoparticles, it is necessary to use large amounts of solvent and surfactants. Therefore, it is obvious that the scale-up of the process is difficult.

The microemulsion and thermal decomposition methods usually lead to complex process or require relatively high temperature. As an alternative way, hydrothermal synthesis includes various wet-chemical technologies of crystallizing substance in a sealed reactor or autoclave systems at high temperature aqueous solution (130–250°C) and high vapor pressure (0.3–4 MPa). Several authors reported the synthesis of

SPION by hydrothermal method[43–45] with or without the presence of specific surfactants. Wang *et al.*[46] reported a one-step hydrothermal process to prepare highly crystalline Fe_3O_4 particles without surfactant. On the contrary, Zheng *et al.*[47] described a hydrothermal route for preparing Fe_3O_4 nanoparticles with a diameter of about 27 nm in the presence of sodium bis (2-ethylhexyl) sulfosuccinate (AOT) as surfactant.

Ge *et al.*[48] described a hydrothermal synthesis in which the nanoparticles were formed from the oxidation of ferrous chloride in basic aqueous solution (NH_4OH) under a high temperature (134°C) and a high pressure (2 bars). By the variation of experimental parameters such as iron precursor concentration, the particle diameter can be tuned from 15 nm to 31 nm. Although nearly monodisperse iron oxide nanoparticles can be formed, this synthetic strategy needs the use of extreme experimental conditions (high temperature and high pressure).

The sonochemical method has also been used to generate SPION.[49] The chemical effects of ultrasound from acoustic cavitation are the formation, growth and implosive collapse of bubbles in solution. The implosive collapse of the bubble generates a localized hotspot with transient temperatures of 5000 K, pressures of 1,800 atm, and cooling rates in excess of 1,010 K/s.[50] SPION can be simply synthesized by sonication of iron (II) acetate in water under an argon atmosphere. Vijayakumar *et al.*[51] reported a sonochemical synthetic route to prepare SPION with a size of 10 nm. These nanoparticles are superparamagnetic but their magnetization is very low. More recently, Pinkas *et al.*[52] developed a sonochemical synthetic method for preparing amorphous particles by sonolysis of $Fe(acac)_3$ under Ar with a small amount of water. The organic content and the surface area of the SPION can be controlled with an amount of water in the reaction mixture.

During the SPION synthesis, the polyols can be also used as capping agents for the control of particle growth and for the limitation of the agglomeration phenomena. Joseyphus *et al.*[53] studied the polyol influence on nanoparticle formation. Several parameters govern the production of particles such as the type of polyols, the iron (II) chloride precursor concentration, the hydroxide sodium concentration and reaction temperature. Zhang *et al.*[54] reported a thermolysis of iron (III) acetylacetonate in PEG associated with other polymer as poly(vinylpyrrolidone) (PVP) or poly(ethylene imine) (PEI). The nanoparticle size could be tuned in the range of 4.1–14.9 nm by the variation of experimental factors such as the reaction temperature, the reaction time and the PVP or PEI portions. This work demonstrated that the nanoparticles coated with PEG/PVP or PEG/PEI exhibit a much better stability in aqueous media than the PEG coated-nanoparticles. Bridot *et al.*[55] suggested the synthesis of iron oxide cores by the polyol method, which consists of the precipitation of metal oxide in high boiling point alcohol. Adding solid NaOH to iron chloride salts dissolved in diethyleneglycol (DEG) produces a black precipitate of agglomerated SPION that can be washed and suspended in acidic media as previously described,[56] then the iron oxide nanoparticles are stabilized by triethoxysilanepropyl succinic anhydride (TEPSA). In comparison to other methods, this approach presents several advantages. Indeed, this process allows the formation of non-agglomerated nanoparticles with well-defined shape and size. Due to its high boiling point, the polyol can be used as a solvent as well as a reducing agent and a surfactant. Although the polyol method offers a multitude of advantages, the scale-up does not allow the formation of uniform particles in term of size.

The above cited synthetic methods have some advantages and disadvantages for preparing SPION. In terms of size and morphology control of NP, thermal decomposition and hydrothermal synthetic ways seem the optimal method. To obtain hydrophilic biocompatible SPION, co-precipitation often is employed, but this method shows low control of the particle shape, broad distributions of sizes and some nanoparticle aggregations.

2. Coating and Stabilization of Magnetic Iron Oxide Nanoparticles

After synthesis, unmodified SPION are stable in high and low pH suspensions, but their *in vivo* use needs a specific coating. Surface modification and functionalization play critical roles in the development of any nanoparticle platform for biomedical applications. These surface coatings, small organic molecules or polymers, have to (i) protect against iron oxide agglomeration, (ii) provide reactive chemical functions for the conjugation of drug molecules or targeting ligands and (iii) limit non-specific cell interactions.

In the literature, the main coating agents are polymers (synthetic or naturals), small organic molecules, silica shell and biological molecules. A common strategy used for the surface modification is the formation of a silica shell. To proceed, alkoxysilane molecules or tetraethyl orthosilicate (TEOS) are generally used.[57] The advantage is that the silane groups can be covalently bound onto nanoparticle surface through the reaction between the hydroxyl groups present on iron oxide surface and the alkoxysilane functions (–Si–O–R where R is commonly methyl or ethyl group).[58] The cross-linking events induce the formation of a silica layer around the particles.[59] A large choice of terminal functional groups (alcohol, amine, epoxy, thiol and carboxylate)[60–62] can be used in order to protect iron oxide nanoparticles.

In the same way, coating agents with precious metal (such as gold) also are an effective protection to avoid the surface oxidation and to reduce nanoparticle agglomeration in aqueous solution.[63,64]

Small organic molecules are frequently used to stabilize the magnetic nanoparticles. The chemical functions used generally are carboxylates, phosphates and sulfates due to their high affinity for iron oxide surface. These strong interactions result from an ionic interaction between the acidic functions of the coating agents and the hydroxyl groups of nanoparticles. The most used carboxylic acids are citric and dimercaptosuccinic acids.[65,66] These polyacids form a stable colloidal suspension resulting from the high coordination on metal surface. Unfortunately, the ionic bonds between the carboxylic functions and the iron oxide surface are labile and can be easily broken by the elevation of temperature or by carboxylic compounds presenting a much higher affinity with the surface. Phosphate and phosphonate derivatives are also promising stabilizing candidates. Their absorption on metal surface is very stable and is able to form a strong interaction in aqueous solution.[67,68] In some works, bisphosphonate compounds were preferred in order to anchor double functions on the metal surface, involving the strengthening of the nanoparticle stability.[69,70]

The stabilization performed by biological molecules is not a common method. Some examples describe the surface covering with proteins such as avidin[71] or human serum albumin (HSA).[72,73] This process allows the formation of stable and biocompatible magnetic fluids.

Polymer coating offers the ability to obtain a biocompatible and biodegradable surface and to improve the blood circulation times depending on the polymer nature.[74,75] These polymers can be natural[76] or synthetic.[74,77]

Thanks to its interesting characteristics such as biocompatibility and biodegradability, one of the most natural polymers is dextran.[78] This polysaccharide can be strongly absorbed on nanoparticle surface, due to a strong interaction with hydrogen bonds formed between the hydroxyl groups present on the polymer chains and the surface of iron oxide cores.[79,80] Several preclinical MRI contrast agents have been elaborated with a dextran coating or its derivatives (carboxydextran and carboxymethyl).[81]

Typically, conventional dextran coatings are based on the cross linking of the polymer after the nanoparticle attachment using epichlohydrin.[82,83] The system has demonstrated a high circulation half-life in blood with no acute toxicity. However, other strategies were developed. Duguet *et al.*[84,85] reported the modification of the dextran structure by silane molecules. This strategy allows the covalent grafting on the surface. Although dextran is the favorite natural polymer, other polymers can be used such as chitosan,[86–88] gelatin,[89] alginate[90] and pullulan[91] as stabilizing agents. Another natural and biodegradable polymer is polylactic acid that can be used for the preparation of stable colloid suspension with typical hydrodynamic diameters ranging between 10 and 180 nm.[92,93]

Among the synthetic polymers, PEG is widely used due its properties such as the improvement of blood circulation time, hydrophilicity and biocompatibility. The process is commonly called PEGylation. It can also be coupled with other polymer to increase the hydrophilic properties. Two approaches are currently used to coat nanoparticles and consist in the addition of surfactants during the synthetic process or post-synthesis. Other polymers and copolymers which have been used to coat magnetic nanoparticles are polyvinyl alcohol (PVA),[94] polystyrene (PS),[95] PVP,[96] poly(acrylic acid) (PAA),[97] poly(ethylenimine) (PEI),[98–100] PAA-chitosan,[101] PEG,[102,103] dextran,[104] phospholipids.[105]

Polymeric coatings have been engineered to enhance SPION pharmacokinetics and tailored drug loading and release behaviors. Different polymers have been investigated where SPION coating was achieved via several approaches including *in situ* coating, post-synthesis adsorption or post-synthesis grafting. The two first coating methods (*in situ* and post synthesis modifications) with polymers (polysaccharides or copolymers) lead to coatings that uniformly encapsulate cores and in the third one (end grafted polymers), PEG (for example) is anchored to the nanoparticle surface by the polymer end groups, forming brush like extensions. Phospholipids form shell around the SPION core and the structure presents hydrophobic regions which can be used for drug encapsulation and delivery.

3. Drug Delivery Systems

The treatment of malignant tumors is a real challenge. The selective delivery of therapeutic agents into a tumor enhances the antitumor efficacy and decreases toxicity in normal tissues.[106–108] Drug delivery involves an easy concept: a small platform is used to deliver the appropriate amount of drug to a desired location inside the body. Moreover, using this technique allows regulation of the drug amount and of the delivery duration.

Nanoparticle-drug systems can accumulate to higher concentrations in certain solid tumors than free drugs via the enhanced permeability and retention (EPR) effect. In addition, actively tumor-targeted nanoparticles may further increase the local concentration of drug or change the intracellular biodistribution within the tumor via receptor-mediated internalization. For drug delivery systems, two main properties are required: firstly, the drug targeting to the desired region must reduce the side effects and secondly, the controlled release of the drug must avoid the classical overdoses. Numerous systems can be used such as micelles,[109,110] liposomes,[111] polymersomes,[112,113] nanoparticles,[114,115] dendrimers[116,117] or polymers.[118] All these systems are based on the same principle.

The drug is entrapped, attached, adsorbed, or encapsulated into or onto nano-matrices. Superparamagnetic nanoparticles are considered as an efficient nanovector since after their injection, the hybrid compounds can be transported by blood circulation and be concentrated in the tumor region by applying magnetic field on the specific target sites. Moreover, MRI can be used to validate the localization of magnetic drug delivery systems.

Therapeutic entities, such as small drugs, peptides, proteins or nucleic acids, can be incorporated in the SPION through loading on the surface layer or trapping within the nanoparticles themselves. When delivered to the target site, the loaded drugs are usually released by (i) diffusion, (ii) vehicle rupture or dissolution, (iii) pH-sensitive dissociation. Such delivery carriers have many advantages, including water-soluble, low toxic or non-toxic, biocompatible and biodegradable, long blood retention time and capacity for further modification. These therapeutic nanoparticle conjugations enable the simultaneous estimation of tissue drug levels and monitoring of therapeutic response.[119,120]

The drug is generally coupled on nanoparticle surface by covalent or ionic bonds. To release the drug in these specific sites, the link between the magnetic core and the drug must be cleaved. The link cleavage can be ensured by different external stimuli such as pH modification, temperature change or enzymatic cleavage.

Conventional anti-cancer agents such as doxorubicin (DOX) have been conjugated with tumor-targeted IO nanoparticles to achieve effective delivery. Recently Yang *et al.*[121] described folate receptor (FA) targeted SPION to deliver DOX to tumor cells (Figure 1). SPION were encapsulated in the multifunctional polymer vesicles in aqueous solution, the hydrophilic PEG bearing the FA targeting ligand located in outer layers, while the short hydrophilic PEG bearing the acrylate groups located in inner layers. DOX was conjugated onto the hydrophobic polyglutamate polymer segments via an acid-cleavable hydrazone bond and could be released at low pH value. FA-conjugated SPIO/DOX-loaded vesicles showed higher cellular

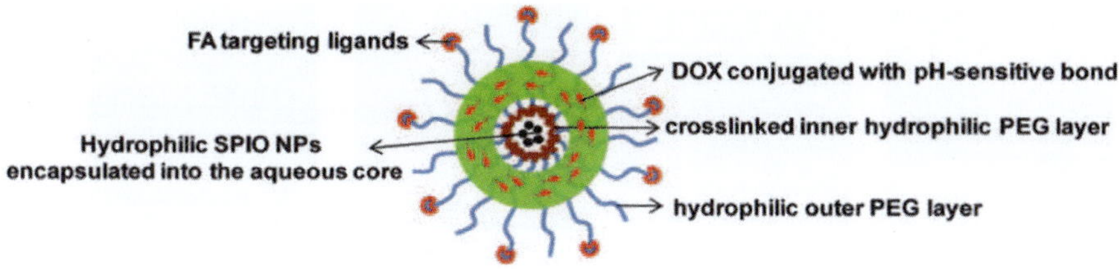

Fig. 1: Scheme of the amphiphilic triblock copolymers and the preparation process of the SPIO/DOX-loaded vesicles with cross-linked inner hydrophilic PEG layers. Reproduced with permission from Ref. 121.

uptake and cytotoxicity compared with FA-free vesicles due to FA-mediated endocytosis.

RNA interference (RNAi) is a promising molecular therapeutic tool due to its high specificity but small interfering RNA (siRNA) cannot reach the target tissue with a sufficient concentration due to RNase degradation. SPION have been used for delivering siRNA and monitoring their efficacy of therapy. Kumar *et al.*[122] synthesized a novel tumor targeted nano-system which consists of peptides (EPPT) that specifically target the antigen uMUC-1, SPION, NIR dye (Cy 5.5) and siRNA that targets the tumor-specific anti-apoptotic gene BIRC5. Systemic delivery to mice bearing human breast adenocarcinoma tumors showed significant increase of R_2 relaxation rate in the tumor, which remained significantly higher than the pre-injection values over time, suggesting that the concentration of nano-drug within the tumor tissue could be maintained. This confirmed and highlighted the feasibility to follow the accumulation and retention of drug-SPION *in vivo* by MRI. The efficacy of this system in the breast tumors was evaluated and showed a five-fold increase in the fraction of apoptotic nuclei in tumors.

Yang *et al.* prepared multifunctional magneto-polymeric nanohybrids (MMPN) modified with antibodies to target breast cancer and followed the treatment by MRI.[123] To obtain these systems, they encapsulated both magnetic hydrophobic nanoparticles and anticancer drug like DOX in an amphiphilic block copolymer. The *in vivo* drug release is observed thanks to the polymer degradation. MRI

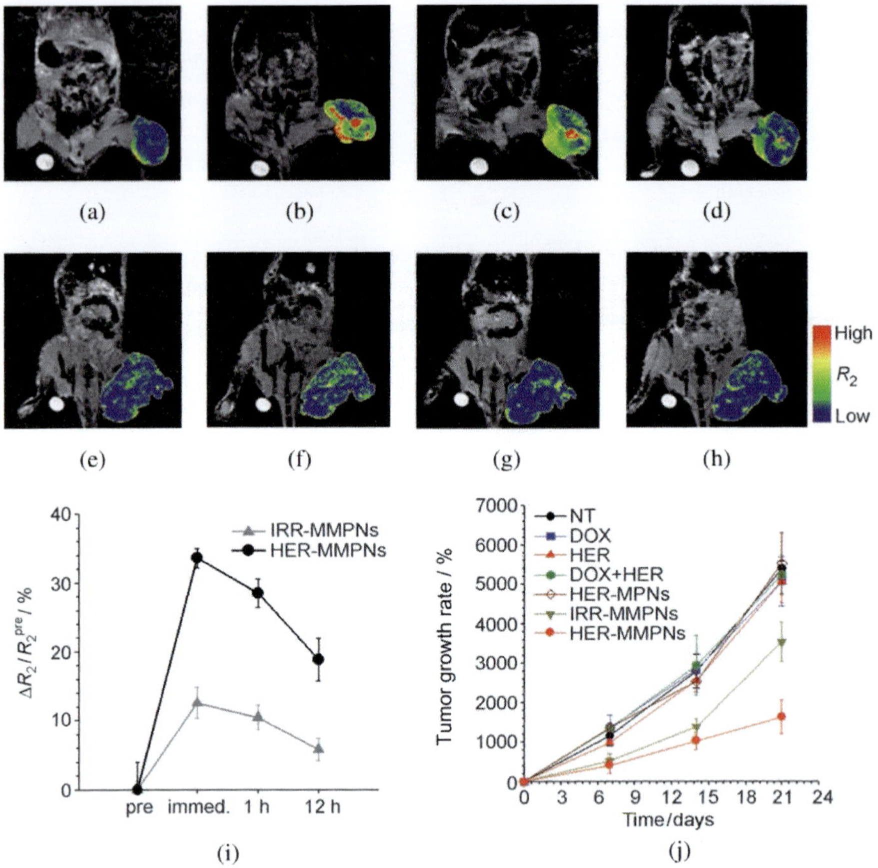

Fig. 2: MR images and color maps of the tumor region of cancer-targeting events of HER–MMPNs (a–d) and IRR–MMPNs (e–h) in NIH3T6.7 cells implanted in mice at various time intervals: (a), (e) pre-injection; (b), (f) immediately; (c), (g) 1 h; (d), (h) 12 h after injection of the MMPNs. (i) DR2/R2 pre-graph vs time before and after injection of MMPNs. (j) Comparative therapeutic-efficacy study in an *in vivo* model. Reproduced with permission from Ref. 123.

studies were performed on mice implanted in their proximal thigh region with NIH3T6.7 cell lines. Two kinds of MMPN were injected as contrast agents: HER–MMPN (nanoparticles conjugated with anti-herceptin antibody) and IRR-MMPN (nanoparticles conjugated with human IgG). The results are shown in Figure 2. HER–MMPN and IRR–MMPN induced tumor growth inhibition as compared with

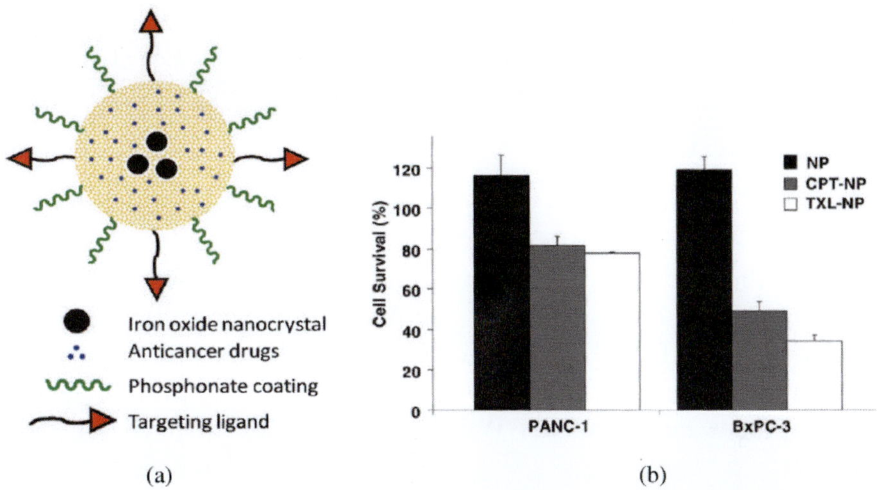

Fig. 3: Specific multifunctional mesoporous silica with encapsulated iron oxide nanoparticles and anticancer drugs (a); cell growth inhibition results showing therapeutic effect of drug (CPT= camptothecin and TXL= paclitaxel)-loaded nanosystèmes on two different pancreatic cancer cells (PANC-1 and BxPC-3). Drug free control nanoparticles were tested and were non- toxic. Reproduced with permission from Ref. 124.

control group (DOX, HER, DOX + HER or HER – MPN (HER conjugated with a non-drug loaded magnetic nanoparticles)). This article demonstrates the ability to design novel nanodrugs for diagnosis and treatment of different cancers.

Another example of drug delivery and imaging applications has been described by Liong *et al.*[124] The multifunctional nano-platform is based on fluorescent mesoporous silica nanoparticles where superparamagnetic iron oxide nano-objects and anticancer drugs (camptothecin or paclitaxel) are encapsulated (Figure 3). Surface conjugation with folic acid allows to increase the uptake into cells that overexpress FA and thus the drug delivery to cancer cells.

4. Conclusions

SPION are very promising for theranostic agents involving drug delivery and MR imaging. Numerous applications have already been described in literature and highlight the advantages of combining imaging and therapy (for example, see review in Refs. 125–128).

Acknowledgments

The ARC (research contract AUWB-2010 — 10/15-UMONS-5), the FNRS, ENCITE program, the COST TD1004 (Theranostics imaging and therapy: an action to develop novel nanosized systems for imaging-guided drug delivery), the Walloon Region (first spin-off program), the UIAP VII program and the Center for Microscopy and Molecular Imaging (CMMI, supported by the European Regional Development Fund and the Walloon Region) are thanked for their support.

References

1. V. P. Torchilin, *Adv. Drug Del. Rev.*, 58, 1532 (2006).
2. C. Sun, J. S. H. Lee, M. Q. Zhang, *Adv. Drug Del. Rev.*, 1252 (2008).
3. J. R. McCarthy, R. Weissleder, *Adv. Drug Del. Rev.*, 60, 1241 (2008).
4. S. Laurent, D. Forge, M. Port, A. Roch, C. Robic, L. V. Elst, R. N. Muller, *Chem. Rev.* 2064 (2008).
5. N. Lewinski, V. Colvin, R. Drezek, *Small,* 26 (2008).
6. A. K. Gupta, R. R. Naregalkar, V. D. Vaidya, M. Gupta, *Nanomedicine,* 23 (2007).
7. R. D. K. Misra, *Mater. Sci. Technol.*, 1011 (2008).
8. C. Corot, P. Robert, J. M. Idee, M. Port, *Adv. Drug Del. Rev.,* 1471 (2006).
9. J. D. G. Duran, J. L. Arias, V. Gallardo, A. V. Delgado, *J. Pharm. Sci.,* 2948 (2008).
10. A. Solanki, J. D. Kim, K. B. Lee, *Nanomedicine,* 567 (2008).
11. B. Thiesen, A. Jordan, *Int. J. Hyperthermia,* 467 (2008).
12. P. Decuzzi, M. Ferrari, *Biomater.,* 5307 (2006).
13. P. Decuzzi, F. Causa, M. Ferrari, P. A. Netti, *Ann. Biomed. Eng.,* 633 (2006).
14. H. S. Choi, W. Liu, P. Misra, E. Tanaka, J. P. Zimmer, B. I. Ipe, M. G. Bawendi, J. V. Frangioni, *Nat. Biotech.*, 1165 (2007).

15. W. C. Zamboni, *Oncologist,* 248 (2008).
16. S. M. Moghimi, A. C. Hunter, J. C. Murray, *Pharmacol. Rev.,* 283 (2001).
17. T. Banerjee, S. Mitra, A. K. Singh, R. K. Sharma, A. Maitra, *Int. J. Pharm.,* 93 (2002).
18. S. M. Moghimi, *Adv. Drug Del. Rev.,* 103 (1995).
19. Y. E. L. Koo, G. R. Reddy, M. Bhojani, R. Schneider, M. A. Philbert, A. Rehemtulla, B. D. Ross, R. Kopelman, *Adv. Drug Del. Rev.,* 1556 (2006).
20. Z. Liu, W. B. Cai, L. N. He, N. Nakayama, K. Chen, X.M. Sun, X. Y. Chen, H. J. Dai, *Nature Nanotech.*, 47 (2007).
21. J. M. Harris, R. B. Chess, *Nature Rev. Drug Disc.*, 214 (2003).
22. M. A. Willard, L. K. Kurihara, E. E. Carpenter, S. Calvin, V. G. Harris, *Int. Mater. Rev.*, 125 (2004).
23. A. H. Lu, E. L. Salabas, F. Schuth, *Angew. Chemie. Int. Ed.* 1222 (2007).
24. R. Massart, *IEEE Trans. Magn.*, 1247 (1981).
25. T. Sugimoto, E. Matijević, *J. Colloid Interface Sci.,* 227 (1980).
26. L. Babes, B. Denizot, G. Tanguy, J. J. Le Jeune, P. Jallet, *J. Colloid Interface Sci.,* 474 (1999).
27. O. Karaagac, H. Kockar, J. *Supercond. Nov. Magn.*, 2777 (2012).
28. C. Pereira, A. M. Pereira, C. Fernandes, M. Rocha, R. Mendes, M. Paz Fernandez-Garcia, A. Guedes, P. B. Tavares, J. M. Greneche, J. P. raujo, C. Freire, *Chem. Mater.*, 1496 (2012).
29. S. Si, A. Kotal, T. K. Mandal, S. Giri, H. Nakamura, T. Kohara, *Chem. Mater.,* 3489 (2004).
30. S. R. Wan, J. S. Huang, H. S. Yan, K. L. Liu, J. *Mater. Chem.*, 298 (2006).
31. J. H. Lee, Y. M. Huh, Y. Jun, J. Seo, J. Jang, H. T. Song, S. Kim, E. J. Cho, H. G. Yoon, J. S. Suh, J. Cheon, *Nat. Med.*, 95 (2007).
32. S. H. Sun, H. Zeng, *J. Am. Chem. Soc.,* 8204 (2002).
33. T. Hyeon, S. S. Lee, J. Park, Y. Chung, H. B. Na, *J. Am. Chem. Soc.,* 12798 (2001).
34. J. Park, K. An, Y. Hwang, J. G. Park, H. J. Noh, J. Y. Kim, J. H. Park, N. M. Hwang, T. Hyeon, *Nat. Mater.,* 891 (2004).
35. N. R. Jana, Y. Chen, X. Peng, *Chem. Mater,* 3931 (2004).

36. Z. Li, Q. Sun, M. Gao, *Angew. Chem. Int Ed.*, 123 (2005).
37. F. Q. Hu, L. Wei, Z. Zhou, Y. L. Ran, Z. Li, M. Y. Gao, *Adv. Mater.*, 2553 (2006).
38. J. Vidal-Vidal, J. Rivas, M. A. Lo´pez-Quintela, *Colloid. Surf.*, A 44 (2006).
39. C. Okoli, M. Boutonnet, L. Mariey, S. Järås, G. K. Rajarao, *J. Chem. Technol. Biotechnol.* 1386 (2011).
40. M. Darbandi, F. Stromberg, J. Landers, N. Reckers, B. Sanyai, W. Keune, H. Wende, *J. Phys. D: Appl. Phys.*, 195001 (2012).
41. F. A. Tourinho, R. Franck, R. Massart, *J. Mater. Sci.*, 3249 (1990).
42. A. B. Chin, I. I. Yaacob, *J. Mater. Process. Technol.* 235 (2007).
43. X. Hu, J. C. Yu, J. Gong, *J. Phys. Chem. C*, 11180 (2007).
44. S. Giria, S. Samantab, S. Majic, S. Gangulic, A. Bhaumikb, *J. Magn. Magn. Mater.* 296 (2005).
45. X. Liu, G. Qiu, A. Yan, Z. Wang, X. Li, J. *Alloy Compd.*, 216 (2007).
46. J. Wang, J. Sun, Q. Sun, Q. Chen, *Mater. Res. Bull.*, 1113 (2003).
47. Y. Zheng, Y. Cheng, F. Bao, Y. Wang, *Mater. Res. Bull.*, 525 (2006).
48. S. Ge, X. Shi, K. Sun, C. Li, J. R. Baker, M. M. Banaszak Holl, B. G. Orr, *J. Phys. Chem. C*, 13593 (2009).
49. J. H. Bang, K. S. Suslick, *J. Am. Chem. Soc.*, 2242 (2007).
50. K. S. Suslick, *Sci.*, 1439 (1990).
51. R. Vijayakumar, Y. Koltypin, I. Felner, A. Gedanken, *Mater. Sci. Eng.*, 101 (2000).
52. J. Pinkas, V. Reichlova, R. Zboril, Z. Moravec, P. Bezdicka, J. Matejkova, *Ultrason. Sonochem.*, 257 (2008)
53. R. J. Joseyphus, D. Kodama, T. Matsumoto, Y. Sato, B. Jeyadevan, K. Tohji, *J. Magn. Magn. Mater.*, 2393 (2007).
54. B. Zhang, Z. Tu, F. Zhao, J. Wang, *Appl. Surface Sci.*, 375 (2013).
55. J.-L. Bridot, D. Stanicki, S. Laurent, S. Boutry, Y. Gossuin, P. Leclère, R. Lazzaroni, L. Vander Elst, R. N. Muller, *Contrast Med. Mol. Imaging*, 466 (2013).
56. D. Forge, A. Roch, S. Laurent, H. Tellez, Y. Gossuin, F. Renaux, L. Vander Elst, R. N. Muller. *J. Phys. Chem. C*, 19178 (2008).
57. A. G. Roca, R. Costo, A. F. Rebolledo, S. Veintemillas-Verdaguer, P. Tartaj, T. Gonzalez-Carreno, M. P. Morales, C. J. Sema, *J. Phys. D: Appl. Phys.*, 224002 (2009).

58. H. Lee, M. K. Yu, S. Park, S. Moon, J. J. Min, Y. Y. Jeong, H. W. Kang, S. Jon, *J. Am. Chem. Soc.*, 12739 (2007).
59. R. De Palma, S. Peeters, M. J. Van Bael, H. Van den Rul, K. Bonroy, W. Laureyn, J. Mullens, G. Borghs, G. Maes, *Chem. Mater.*, 1821 (2007).
60. N. Kohler, G. E. Fryxell, M. Zhang, *J. Am. Chem. Soc.*, 7206 (2004).
61. E. K. U. Larsen, T. Nielsen, T. Wittenborn, H. Birkedal, T. Vorup-Jensen, M. H. Jakobsen, L. Ostergaard, M. R. Horsman, F. Besenbacher, K. A. Howard, J. Kjems, *ACS Nano*, 1947 (2009).
62. T. Ninjbadgar, D. F. Brougham, *Adv. Funct. Mater.*, 4769 (2011).
63. E. E. Carpenter, C. Sangregorio, C. J. O'Connor, *IEEE Trans. Magn.*, 3496 (1999).
64. H. Maleki, A. Simchi, M. Imani, B. F. O. Costa, *J. Magn. Magn. Mater.*, 3997 (2012).
65. L. Maurizi, H. Bisht, F. Bouyer, N. Millot, *Langmuir*, 8857 (2009).
66. N. Miguel-Sancho, O. Bomatí-Miguel, G. Colom, J. P. Salvador, M. P. Marco, *Chem. Mater.*, 2795 (2011).
67. H. Benbenishty-Shamir, R. Gilert, I. Gotman, E. Y. Gutmanas, C. N. Sukenik, *Langmuir*, 12082 (2011).
68. T. J. Daou, J. M. Greneche, G. Pourroy, S. Buathong, A. Derory, C. Ulhaq-Bouillet, B. Donnio, D. Guillon, S. Begin-Colin, *Chem. Mater.*, 5869 (2008).
69. A. Karimi, B. Denizot, C. Passirani, F. Hindré, J. Roux, P. Legras, J. J. Lejeune, *Eur. J. Pharm. Sci.*, 101 (2013).
70. Y. Lalatonne, C. Paris, J. M. Serfaty, P. Weinmann, M. Lecouvey, L. Motte, *Chem. Commun.*, 2553 (2008).
71. J. A. Park, J. J. Lee, I. S. Kim, B. H. Park, G. H. Lee, T. J. Kim, H. C. Ri, H. J. Kim, Y. Chang, *Colloids Surf. A*, 288 (2008).
72. Q. Quan, J. Xie, H. Gao, M. Yang, F. Zhang, G. Liu, X. Lin, A. Wang, H. S. Eden, S. Lee, G. Zhang, X. Chen, *Mol. Pharm.*, 1669 (2011).
73. J. Xie, J. Wang, G. Niu, J. Huang, K. Chen, X. Li, X. Chen, *Chem. Commun.*, 433 (2010).
74. C. Boyer, M. R. Whittaker, V. Bulmus, J. Liu, T. P. Davis, *NPG Asia Materials*, 23 (2010).
75. D. Forge, A. Roch, S. Laurent, H. Tellez, Y. Gossuin, L. Vander Elst, R. N. Muller, *J. Phys. Chem. C*, 19178 (2008).

76. A. M. G. C. Dias, A. Hussain, A. S. Marcos, A. C. A. Roque, *Biotechnology Advances*, 142 (2011).
77. M. Chanana, Z. Mao, D. Wang, *J. Biomed. Nanotechnol.*, 652 (2009).
78. L. Yun Tack, W. Kyoungja, C. Kyu-Sil, *IEEE Transactions Nanotechnol.*, 111 (2008).
79. M. C. Bautista, O. Bomati-Miguel, M. del Puerto Morales, C. J. Serna, S. Veintemillas-Verdaguer, *J. Magn. Magn. Mater.*, 20 (2005).
80. S. L. Easo, P. V. Mohanan, *Carbohyd. Polym.*, 726 (2013).
81. J. E. Rosen, L. Chan, D. B. Shieh, F. X. Gu, *Nanomedicine: NBM*, 275 (2012).
82. L. Josephson, C. H. Tung, A. Moore, R. Weissleder, *Bioconjug. Chem.*, 186 (1999).
83. J. R. McCarthy, R. Weissleder, *Adv. Drug Del. Rev.*, 1241 (2008).
84. J. Deng, J. He, J. S. Zheng, S. Terakawa, H. Huang, L. C. Fang, Y. Li, P. Cheng, L. L. Jiang, *Particul. Sci. Tech.*, 241 (2012).
85. E. Duguet, S. Vasseur, S. Mornet, G. Goglio, A. Demourgues, J. Portier, F. Grsset, P. Veverka, E. Pollert, *Bull. Mater. Sci.*, 581 (2006).
86. S. Chaleawlert-Umpon, V. Mayen, K. Manotham, N. Pimpha, *J. Biomater. Sci.*, 1515 (2010).
87. A. Szpak, G. Kania, T. Skórka, W. Tokarz, S. Zapotoczny, M. Nowakowska, *J. Nanopart. Res.*, 1 (2012).
88. Z. T. Tsai, J. F. Wang, H. Y. Kuo, C. R. Shen, J. J. Wang, T. C. Yen, *J. Magn. Magn. Mater.*, 208 (2010).
89. B. Gaihre, M. S. Khil, D. R. Lee, H. Y. Kim, *Int. J. Pharm.*, 180 (2009).
90. M. L. Ma, X. R. Qi, Y. Maitani, T. Nagai, *Int. J. Pharm.*, 177 (2007).
91. F. Gao, Y. Cai, J. Zhou, X. Xie, W. Ouyang, Y. Zhang, X. Wang, X. Zhang, X. Wang, L. Zhao, J. Tang, *Nano Res.*, 23 (2010).
92. F. Y. Cheng, S. P. Wang, C. H. Su, T .L. Tsai, P. C. Wu, D. B. Shieh, J. H. Chen, P. C. Hsieh, C. S. Yeh, *Biomaterials*, 2104 (2008).
93. S.-J. Lee, J.-R. Jeong, S.-C. Shin, J.-C., Kim, Y.-H. Chang, Y.-M. Chang, J.-D. Kim, *J. Magn. Magn. Mater.*, 2432 (2004).
94. L. Zhou, B. He, F. Zhang, *ACS Appl. Mater. Inter.*, 192 (2011).
95. A. Garcia, A. Tercjak, N. E. Zafeiropoulos, M. Stamm, I. Mondragon, *J. Polymer Sci. Part A: Polym. Chem.*, 4744 (2007).

96. S.-J. Bae, J.-A. Park, J.-J. Lee, G.-H. Lee, T.-J. Kim, D.-S. Yoo, Y. Chang, *Curr. Appl. Phys.*, 19 (2009).
97. Y. Y. Xu, M. Zhou, H. J. Geng, J. J. Hao, Q. Q. Ou, S. D. Qi, H. I. Chen, X. G. Chen, *Appl. Sur. Sci.*, 3897 (2012).
98. A. Masotti, A. Pitta, G. Ortaggi, M. Corti, C. Innocenti, A. Lascialfari, *Magn. Reson. Mater. Phys., Bio., Med.*, 77 (2009).
99. S. C. McBain, U. Griesenbach, S. Xenariou, A. Keramane, C. D. Batich, E. Alton, J. Dobson, *Nanotechnol.*, 19 (2008).
100. I. K. Park, C. P. Ng, J. Wang, B. Chu, C. Yuan, S. Zhang, S. H. Pun, *Biomaterials*, 724 (2008).
101. Y. Ge, S. Zhang, S. He, Y. Zhang, N. Gu, *J. Nanosci. Nanotechnol*, 1287 (2009).
102. K. Herve, L. Douziech-Eyrolles, E. Munnier, S. Cohen-Jonathan, M. Souce, H. Marchais, P. Limelette, F. Warmont, M. L. Saboungi, P. Dubois, I. Chourpa, *Nanotechnol.*, 19 (2008).
103. J. Y. Park, P. Daksha, G. H. Lee, S. Woo, Y. M. Chang, *Nanotechnol.*, 19 (2008).
104. T. Shen, R. Weissleder, M. Papisov, A. Bogdanov, T. J. Brady, *Magn. Reson. Med.*, 599 (1993).
105. V. Plassat, M. S. Martina, G. Barratt, C. Menager, S. Lesieur, *Int. J. Pharm.*, 118 (2007).
106. Y. Bae, T. A. Diezi, A. Zhao, G. S. Kwon, *J. Control Release*, 324 (2007).
107. J. Gang, S. -B. Park, W. Hyung, E. H. Choi, J. Wen, H. -S. Kim, Y. -G. Shul, S. Haam, S. Young Song, *J Drug Target*, 445 (2007).
108. J. H. Lee, Y. M. Huh, Y. W. Jun, J. W. Seo, J. T. Janq, H. T. Song, S. Kim, E. J. Cho, H. G. Yoon, J. S. Suh, J. Cheon, *Nat. Med.*, 95 (2007).
109. A. L. Glover, J. B. Bennett, J. S. Pritchett, S. M. Nikles, D. E. Nikles, J. A. Nikles, C. S. Brazel, *IEEE Trans. Magn.*, 231 (2013).
110. M. Talelli, C. J. F. Rijcken, T. Lammers, P. R. Seevinck, G. Storm, C. F. van Nostrum, W. E. Hennink, *Langmuir*, 2060 (2009).
111. W. T. Al-Jamal, K. Kostarelos, *Nanomed.* 85 (2007).
112. H. De Oliveira, J. Thevenot, S. Lecommandoux, *Nanomed. Nanobiotechnol.*, 525 (2012).

113. Z. Y. Qiao, R. Ji, X. N. Huang, F. S. Du, R. Zhang, D. H. Liang, Z. C. Li, *Biomacromol.*, 1555 (2013).
114. B. Chertok, B. A. Moffat, A. E. David, F. Yu, C. Bergemann, B. D. Ross, V. C. Yang, *Biomater.*, 487 (2008).
115. L. Yang, Z. Cao, H. K. Sajja, H. Mao, L. Wang, H. Huaying, H. Xu, T. Jiang, W. C. Wood, S. Nie, Y. A. Wang, *J. Biomed. Nanotechnol.*, 439 (2008).
116. Y. Chang, X. Meng, Y. Zhao, K. Li, B. Zhao, M. Zhu, Y. Li, X. Chen, J. Wang, *J. Colloid Interface Sci.*, 403 (2011).
117. S. H. Wang, X. Shi, M. Van Antwerp, Z. Cao, S. D. Swanson, X. Bi, J. R. Baker, *Adv. Funct. Mater.*, 3043 (2007).
118. J. K. Oh, J. M. Park, *Progr. Polymer Sci.*, 168 (2011).
119. G. M. Lanza, P. Winter, S. Caruthers, A. Schmeider, K. Crowder, A. Morawski, H. Zhang, M. J. Schott, S. A. Wickline, *Curr. Pharm. Biotechnol.*, 495 (2004).
120. M. Atri, *J. Clin. Oncol.*, 3299 (2006).
121. X. Yang, J. J. Grailer, I. J. Rowland, A. Javadi, S. A. Hurley, V. Z. Matson, D. A. Steeber, S. Gong, *ACS Nano*, 6805 (2010).
122. M. Kumar, M. Yigit, G. Dai, A. Moore, Z. Medarova, *Cancer Res.*, 7553 (2010).
123. J. Yang, C.-H. Lee, H. J. Ko, J.-S. Suh, H.-G. Yoon, K. Lee, Y.-M. Huh, S. Haam, *Angew. Chem. Int. Ed.* 46, 8836–8839 (2007).
124. M. Liong, J. Lu, M. Kovochich, T. Xia, S. G. Ruehm, A. E. Nel, F. Tamanoi, J. I. Zink, *ACS Nano* 889 (2008).
125. S. S. Kelkar, T. M. Reineke, *Bioconjug. Chem.*, 1879 (2011).
126. B. T. Luk, L. Zhang, *ACS Appl. Mater. Interfaces*, under press, 6, 21859 (2014).
127. S. Svenson, *Mol. Pharmaceutics*, 848 (2013).
128. F. Danhier, A. Le Breton, V. Préat, *Mol. Pharmaceutics*, 2961 (2012).

CHAPTER 4

MRI T1 WEIGHTED THERANOSTIC NANODEVICES

Lucie Sancey, François Lux, Géraldine Le Duc, Sabin Carme and Olivier Tillement*

Institute Light & Matter UMR5306 Team FENNEC, Lyon University
2, rue V. Grignard, 69622 Villeurbanne, France
**Olivier.tillement@univ-lyon1.fr*

Radiotherapy is the most commonly used non-surgical cancer therapy. To improve its efficacy, new generation of therapeutic agents that sensitize cells to ionizing radiation arises. Among them, nanodevices containing high atomic number (Z) atoms such as gadolinium (Gd) also possess contrast properties as T1 Gd-MRI that would allow monitoring of the radiosensitizing nanodevices within the tumor region. Such radiosensitizing and imaging nanodevices are called *theranostic* nanodevices. The example of the AGuIX®, a polysiloxane-Gd-based nanoparticle will be taken to demonstrate the importance of such imaging-guided radiosensitizing approach.

1. Introduction

At the time of personalized medicine, the development of indiscriminant cytotoxic agents to combat disease becomes rare. Non-targeted drugs in development mainly regroup *smart-drugs*, i.e., drugs that are furtive, non-toxic for healthy tissue, detectable, activatable, and rapidly eliminated through the organism.[1,2]

Theranostic nanodevices might fulfill these characteristics; they provide scientists and clinicians with information to enhance imaging modalities, with direct access to patient characteristics, i.e., selection of patients that might respond to treatment, monitoring of treatment efficacy and treatment optimization, as well as the therapeutic approach itself.

The basis for the administration of a theranostic nanodevices is to reach a favorable theranostic outcome with minimal adverse effects. For any administration routes, various biobarriers should be cross. When referring to any systemically injected nanodevice, the biobarriers can be the stability of the nanodevice — in presence of enzymes, diluted condition, or variation of pH — or the capacity to reach the tumor, i.e., distribution in the body, extravasation from the blood, and interaction with the cells or subcellular compartments.[3] Fortunately, the tumor vessels present an impaired endothelial barrier, with enlarged fenestrations that allow systemically injected nanodevices to escape from the blood stream to reach the tumor. This phenomenon is called EPR effect or enhanced permeability and retention effect.[4,5] Thanks to the EPR effect, the untargeted nanodevices with size <200 nm that reach the tumor might extravasated and be entrapped for long time due to the weak drainage of the tumor, allowing its imaging and treatment during this time. Moreover, this approach allows targeting the primary tumor and its metastases (>3 mm for vascularization), independently of their localization and their mutational status.

Different classes of theranostic nanodevices are in preclinical development or have already reached the clinic. They included particles designed for drug delivery approach, which act as a Trojan horse that cargoes highly cytotoxic agents and/or lipophilic compounds to the tumor site,[6] and smart activatable particles, controlled by specific stimuli including pH,[7] temperature,[8] redox potential,[9] enzyme, light,[10] ultrasounds,[11] voltage or X-rays.[12–14]

Independently of the nanodevice properties, the development of personalized medicine is concomitant to the development of companion diagnostic test, i.e., specific assay that will status on the effectiveness of a given treatment for a given patient. The idea is to tailor medical treatment to the individual characteristics of each patient, selecting patients that might benefit from the treatment, and excluding the predicted non-responding patients who would only suffer from adverse effects. These companion tests contribute to a better treatment for patients but are also of great economic interest as they could limit the use of expensive drugs that would not be efficient. If many of the Food and Drug Administration (FDA) approved companion diagnostic tests are based on genomics or histology/immunochemistry,[15] they could also be correlated to specific imaging, which mainly included nuclear imaging (PET or SPECT) or magnetic resonance imaging (MRI). As example, FerriScan®, a R2-MRI companion diagnostic, measures liver iron concentration and indicated which patients might need the deferasirox treatment, an oral iron chelator.[16]

A promising nanodevice regroups all these properties of a smart-nanodevice: the AGuIX®, a Gd-based nanoparticle developed by the team of Prof O. Tillement, ILM-UMR5306, Lyon.[17,18] AGuIX® is a furtive 3-nm size nanoparticle of 9 kDa, non-toxic for healthy tissue, and rapidly eliminated through the renal route after systemic injection.[19,20] Moreover, and due to the presence of Gd (average chemical composition of particle: $Gd_{10}Si_{30}C_{200}N_{50}O_{150}H_x$), the AGuIX® are detectable during MRI T1 acquisition,[21–24] and can be activated by X-rays when they reach the tumor.[12–14,17,25,26] These characteristics confer to the nanodevice a powerful imaged-guided radiosensitizing property (Figure 1): after systemic injection, the nanodevices are imaged using MRI, this later allows to adjust the radiotherapy in terms of localization (delineation of tumor volume if appropriate), delay between administration and radiotherapy, or fractionation planning.

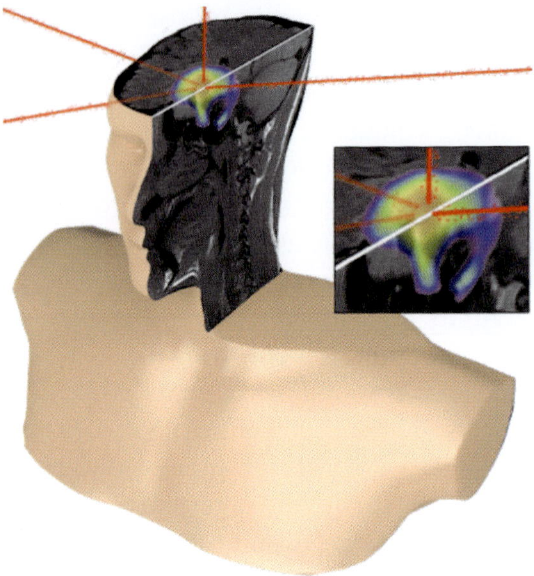

Fig. 1: A schematic illustration of guided and enhanced radiotherapy with theranostic AGuIX® nanoparticles.[14]

2. T1 Gd-MRI and Radiotherapy

From all the imaging techniques available in routine practice, MRI and contrast enhancement T1-weigthed after gadolinium (Gd) injection (T1 Gd-MRI) in particular, has been recognized as the gold standard method for the identification of the size, number, characterization and location of the tumor lesions.[27] When applied to radiotherapy, MRI is a key companion to treatment.[28] Before the radiation, MRI allows the precise localization of the tumor sites, which permits the definition of the target for treatment planning. During or just after the treatment, early assessment for response and early prediction for radiation toxicity might be observed by MRI, leading when necessary to re-optimization for radiation treatment based upon normal tissue toxicity and tumor response. Moreover, T1 Gd-MRI, obtained after systemic administration of paramagnetic contrast agent such as Gd-based agents, enhances the native contrast between different tissues.

T1 Gd-MRI is particularly useful for small lesions, and adjustment of the delineation of the tumor volume, especially for lesions close to vital or sensitive organ.[28] If MRI offers improved soft tissue contrast, the spatial accuracy might be optimized when coupled to computed tomography (CT), which allows the CT-based dose calculation.

The use of T1 Gd-MRI increases mainly in prostate cancer as MRI allows a better delineation of the prostate and rectal volume as compared to CT, as well as for Head & Neck, liver, lung, and breast tumors.[29–32] Concerning the brain tumor, primary and metastasis, MRI becomes unavoidable. In particular for unique lesion or few number (3–5 maximum) of small metastases (<30 mm), MRI is coupled to radiosurgery in a technique called stereotactic radiosurgery (SRS). This minimally invasive method might treat inaccessible lesions, in contrast to surgical resection, by precise delineation of the lesion borders, reducing radiation in the surrounding healthy tissue.[33–35]

Unfortunately, SRS might not be offered to patients with many (more than 3–5) or very large brain lesions. These patients are currently treated by Temozolomide® a chemotherapeutic agent and whole-brain radiotherapy (WBRT); unluckily, this treatment only allows a median survival of several months, depending of the pathology. In this case, the addition of a radiosensitizing drug to the WBRT, such as theranostic nanodevices containing Gd before the radiation treatment might offer patients a new perspective.

3. The Theranostic AGuIX® Nanodevice

With the aim of developing a theranostic nanodevice, Gd-based nanodevices made of a polysiloxane inorganic matrix surrounded by covalently grafted Gd chelates, was synthesized and named AGuIX® for Activation Guided by Irradiation by X-rays (Figure 2). The ultrasmall size of the nanodevices, 3 nm of hydrodynamic diameter, was selected to favor systemic distribution and renal elimination. The properties of the nanodevices will be summarized for imaging and therapy improvement.

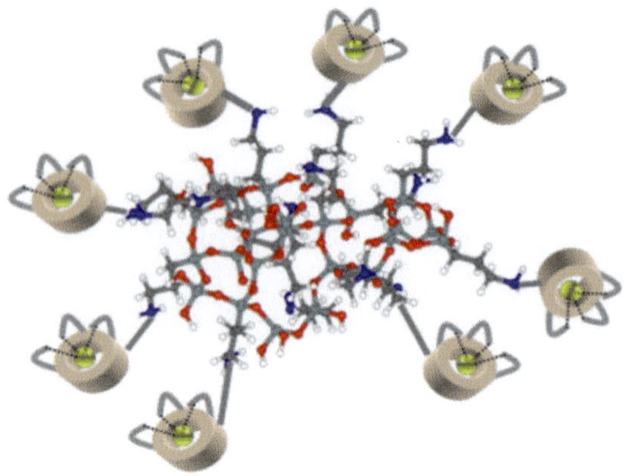

Fig. 2: A schematic illustration of AGuIX® nanoparticles. Green atoms are Gd chelated by DOTA. The polysiloxane matrix is composed mainly of silicon in grey and oxygen in red. The nanoparticles display a high Gd content (15 wt.%), a 3 nm size, a mass of about 9 kDa and the following chemical formula: $Gd_{10}Si_{30}C_{200}N_{50}O_{150}H_x$.[14]

3.1. *Imaging properties*

Due to the presence of Gd, the AGuIX® possess contrast enhancement properties for T1 MRI. After systemic administration, the ultrasmall nanodevices distributed in the body, as shown in the Figure 3(a) obtained few seconds after systemic administration in monkey, and reached the kidneys since the first blood passages. Without any brain lesion or damage, the nanodevice cannot cross the blood–brain barrier (BBB); but in presence of brain tumor or metastases, the AGuIX® reached the tumor and accumulated through EPR effect for several hours, depending of the tumor properties (Figures 3(b)–3(c)).

Such T1 Gd-MRI enhancement has been reported in various tumor types including brain tumor and metastases, lung tumors (after systemic or airway administration), hepatic tumors, as well as various types of sub-cutaneous tumors in rodents.[21,36] Due to its chemical composition, the nanodevice is also a multimodal imaging compound. Indeed, instead of a Gd atom, other atoms might be chelated such as the radioactive PET $^{64}Cu/^{68}Ga$, or SPECT ^{111}In nuclides. Such combination of positive T1 contrast and nuclear labeling might

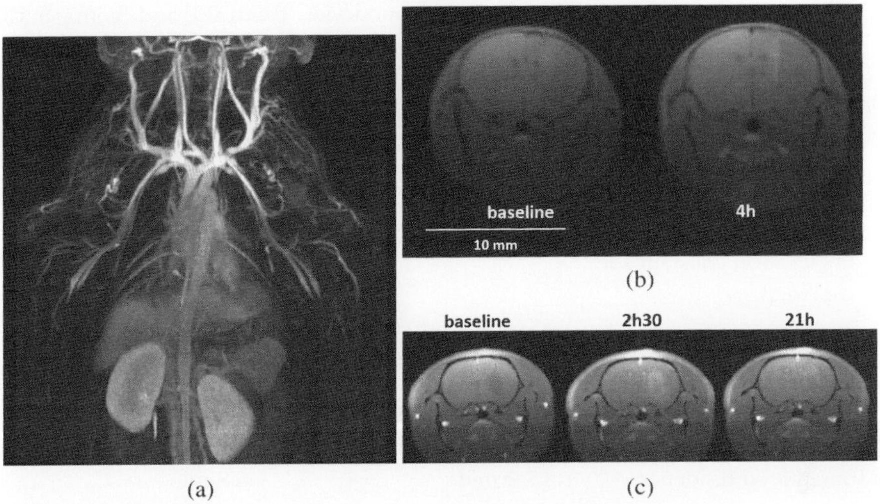

Fig. 3: MRI examples obtained from (a) healthy Cynomolgus monkey, (b) mouse-bearing melanoma metastasis or (c) rat-bearing 9L glioma.

be very interesting for dual or multimodal imaging, combining the resolution of MRI and the sensitivity of nuclear imaging.

In summary, T1 Gd-MRI experiments have demonstrated that AGuIX® enhances contrast imaging much more efficiently than commercial molecular contrast agent DOTAREM® (see Table 1), owing their higher relaxivity properties and residence time in the body. The accumulation in both the primary tumor and metastases by EPR effect will help to define precisely the targeted volume, adjust the treatment planning, and assess the response.

3.2. *Radiosensitizer effect*

High atomic number Gd ($Z = 64$) and gold ($Z = 79$)-containing compounds might be used for theranostic approach due to their strong X-ray absorption coefficients which improved contrast over a wide energy range as compared to soft tissues. Hainfeld and colleagues have been the first to demonstrate the potential of gold nanodevices for efficient high-Z radioenhancement using 250 kVp X-ray therapy.[38,39]

Table 1. Properties of the theranostic nanodevice AGuIX® and commercial DOTAREM® contrast agent.

Characteristic	AGuIX®	DOTAREM®
Hydrodynamic diameter	<3 nm	≈ 1 nm
Molecular weight	8700 $g \cdot mol^{-1}$	560 $g \cdot mol^{-1}$
Number of Gd atoms	10	1
Complexation constant for Gd ($\log\beta_{110}$)	24.78	25.58
Longitudinal relaxivity (r1)	11.4 $mmol^{-1} \cdot s^{-1}$ at 1.4T 6 $mmol^{-1} \cdot s^{-1}$ at 7T	10.6 $mmol^{-1} \cdot s^{-1}$ at 1.5T 3 $mmol^{-1} \cdot s^{-1}$ at 7T
Transverse relaxivity (r2)	12.99 $mmol^{-1} \cdot s^{-1}$ at 1.4T	10.3 $mmol^{-1} \cdot s^{-1}$ at 1.5T[37]
Mouse blood residence time	13.2 min	6.8 min
Elimination	Renal	Renal
MRI signal enhancement	73.9 ± 4.5	23.5 ± 5.6
MRI contrast to noise	8.3 ± 1.3	2.9 ± 2.0
Radiosensitizing property	Yes	No
Clinical use	Not yet (Phase I planned for end of 2015).	Approved

To explain this phenomenon, the predictive models of sensitization based on mass energy absorption coefficient of high-Z elements and soft tissue (water) take into account two major effects. At energies <150 keV, the photoelectric effect prevails and is significantly higher for high-Z element as compared to soft tissue, leading to the radioenhancement. At higher energies such as 6 MeV range used for radiotherapy, the Compton interaction preponderates and was predicted to be similar for soft tissues and high-Z elements.[40,41]

If the radiosensitization observed at these high energies was first attributed to biological mechanisms such as oxidative stress or alteration of cell cycle, recent modeling demonstrated that high-Z element-containing nanoparticles submitted to ionizing radiation induce local but very intense nano-sized ionization. For example, McMahon *et al.* reported that at the vicinity of gold nanoparticle (≈100 nm), energy deposition was equivalent to hundreds of Gray or even more.[42] Such predictive model has recently been obtained with AGuIX® nanodevices by this team. They demonstrated that the clustering of Gd atoms within the nanodevice leads to heterogeneous ionizing radiation after X-ray exposure with very high local radioenhancement (Figure 4).

If the physical events that appear during radiation in presence of high-Z containing nanodevices are still incompletely determined, the radioenhancement is a biological fact.

3.3. *Radiosensitizing nanodevice*

Seventeen international teams have demonstrated the potential of the AGuIX® as radiosensitizer *in vitro*, using various range of energies (from kilo to million of electron volts of photon as well as fast ions) and various radioresistant cell lines using very small concentration of nanodevices.[14] To make a long story short, the main result obtained was that in presence of the nanodevice and radiotherapeutic treatment performed with conventional X-ray exposure, the biological effect observed was similar to the one obtained without the nanodevices using fast ions. This strong efficacy was related to complex and irreversible DNA damage at the vicinity of the nanodevice. To better understand this phenomenon, examples are shown in Figure 5 on four radioresistant cell lines after photon (a–c) or carbon (d) exposure in presence of the particles.[14,25,26,43] Moreover, it was interesting to note that the presence of AGuIX® during carbon radiation also leads to a radioenhancement of the treatment, giving a very promising perspective (Figure 5(d)).

3.3.1. *In vivo studies*

One peculiarity of the AGuIX® is the possibility of various administration methods, which might be the systemic route, intra-tumoral if applied, or by the airways for lung treatment.

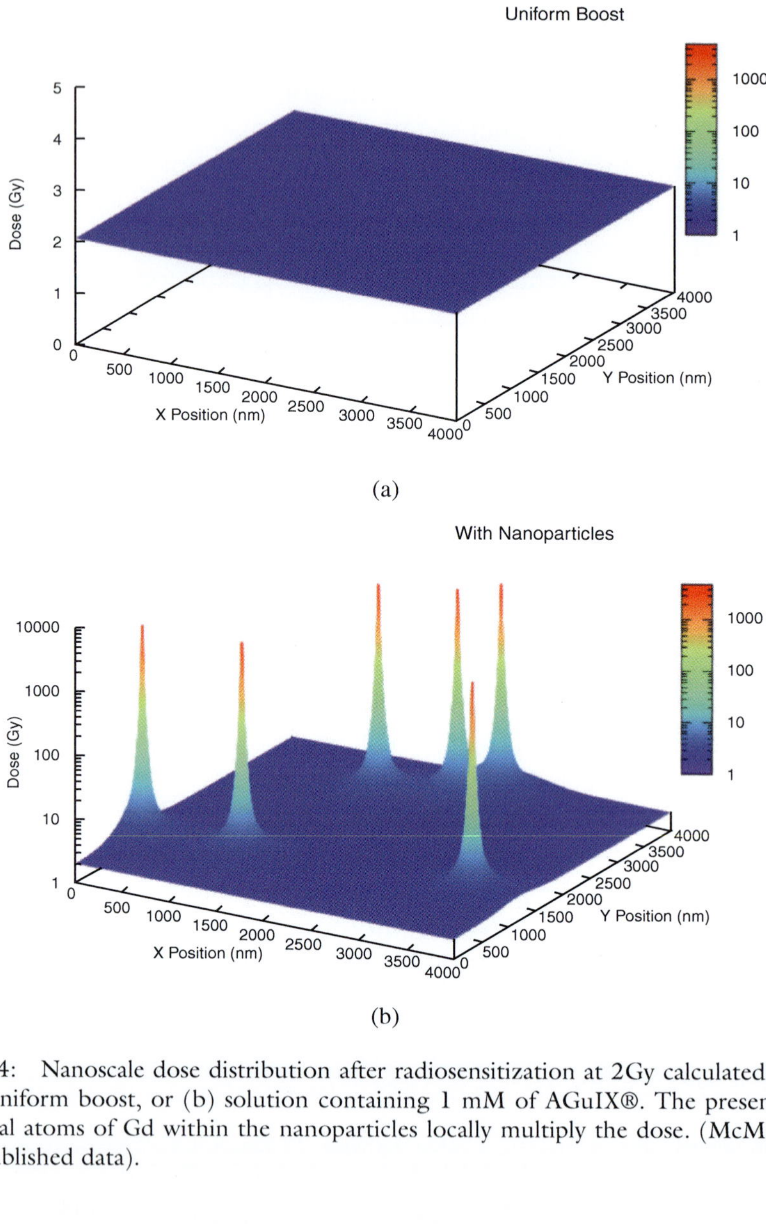

Fig. 4: Nanoscale dose distribution after radiosensitization at 2Gy calculated from (a) uniform boost, or (b) solution containing 1 mM of AGuIX®. The presence of several atoms of Gd within the nanoparticles locally multiply the dose. (McMahon, unpublished data).

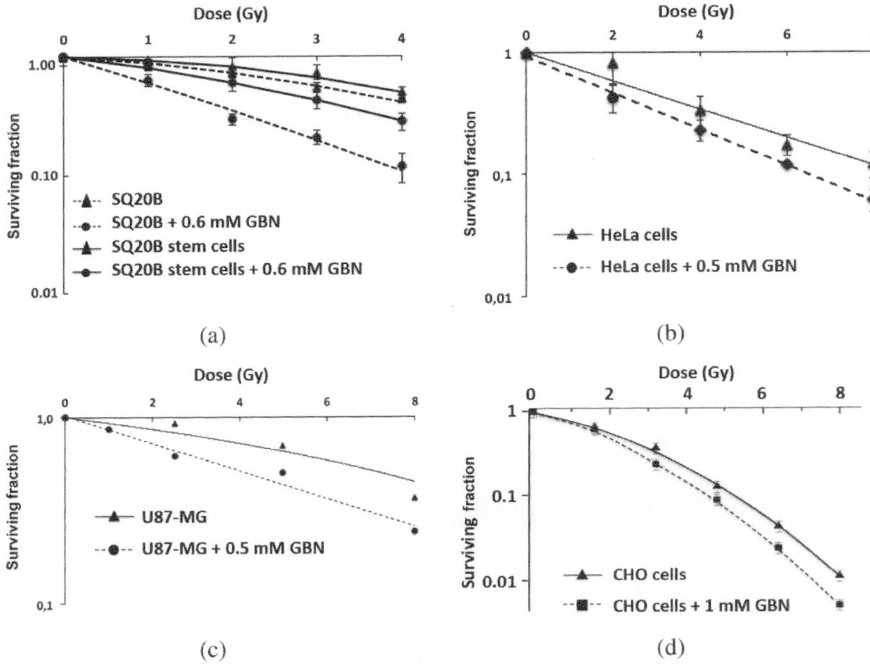

Fig. 5: Example of biological effect *in vitro* on radioresistant cell lines: (a) head and neck SQ20B, (b) cervix HeLa cells, (c) glioma U87-MG cells and (d) Hamster CHO cells. Under photon exposure (a–c), the biological effect obtained in presence of the AGuIX® (circles) was enhanced as compared to irradiation alone (triangles) and similar to the one observed without AGuIX® using heavy ions (d).[14,25,26,43]

Systemic administration appears as the most appropriate route in particular for multiple metastatic lesions or non-accessible tumors. Accumulated by EPR effect, the theranostic nanodevice might be followed using MRI before treatment, in order to treat the patient at the opportune moment, when the nanodevice escape from the blood stream and the healthy tissue while remaining in the tumor region. Different analysis of the tumor and healthy surrounding tissue indicated that only a few amount of Gd (<10 μmol/g of tissue) in the tumor was necessary to obtain the radioenhancement effect. This observation indicated that intra-tumor and airways administration would require fewest amount of nanodevice as compared to the systemic route.

Table 2. Examples of median survival time (MeST) and increase in life span (ILS % vs IR alone) obtained for rats-bearing 9L gliosarcoma treated by microbeam radiotherapy (MRT, AGuIX® 56 μmol, I.V.) or mice-bearing H358 lung tumors treated by photon radiation (1 μmol, airways).

Group		MeST (days)	ILS (% vs IR)
9L-Rats[13, 14]	Untreated	19/22	NA
	Irradiation (IR)	45/47	—
	Dotarem® + IR (20 min)	38	−17.4
	AGuIX® + IR (20 min)	90/102.5	+ 95.6/122.8
	AGuIX® + IR (24 h)	95.5	107.6
H358-mice[12]	Untreated	77	NA
	Irradiation (IR)	83	—
	AGuIX® + IR (24 h)	112	34.9

Following the nanodevice's systemic injection, the various experiments demonstrated that radiation treatment might be performed from few minutes to 24 h post administration at least (see Table 2). This large time frame might allow performing several irradiations following a unique administration and adjusting the treatment and fractionation schedule. These two points are the parameters that will need to be optimized for personalized treatment. Moreover, depending on the characteristics of the tumor, the time between administration of the nanodevice and radiation therapy might also be adjusted using individualized imaging data. At last, the amount of nanodevice injected to patient might be another adjustable variable. If the modern guidelines are usually based on the patient weight or body surface, the tumor size, EPR properties (defined using MR imaging), localization or aggressiveness might also be taken into account for better-personalized medicine. Currently, the amount of AGuIX® used for treatment is similar to the amount of molecular contrast agent used for MRI investigation. When compared to human, the data obtained on rodents and non-human primates correspond to a human equivalent dose (HED) of 100 $mg \cdot kg^{-1}$ for weekly injection.

4. Conclusions and Outlook

The theranostic nanodevice AGuIX® is an ultra-small particle (<3 nm size), which might be administrated through systemic, intra-tumor and airway's route. Followed by T1 MRI, the nanodevice presents a renal elimination and a non-specific accumulation in tumors through EPR effect. Furthermore, due to the presence of Gd, a high-Z element, the nanodevice possesses strong radiosensitizing properties, as gold, hafnium or platinum-containing compounds. The radioenhancement properties have been demonstrated using various cell lines, various injection modes and various radiations from kiloelectron to million electron volts for photons as well as fast ions. These properties correspond to the clinical reality: huge variation of tumor characteristics intra-patient and inter-patients that might be treated using 6 MeV or fast ions radiation.

The biological consequences of the radioenhancement are cell membrane and complex and irreversible DNA damages induced at the vicinity of the nanodevices after electronic activation and Auger cascades in a similar way to other high-Z nanoparticles (gold and platinum).

The on-going regular pre-clinical investigations performed on rodents and non-human primates are highly favorable to the next first-in-human administration. In collaboration with the radiotherapy department (CHU of Grenoble), the first clinical phase I trial will include patients with multiple brain metastases and is planned for end of 2015.

Acknowledgments

This work was supported by the COST action TD1004 "theranostics imaging and therapy: an action to develop novel nanosized systems for imaging-guided drug delivery" as well as the LABEX PRIMES (ANR-11-LABX-0063). We would like to express our gratitude to French program ANR-12-RPIB-0010 Multimage, ANR TheraGuIma, and ANR-12-P2N-0009-Gd-Lung. We would like to thank those who provided preprints or unpublished data that were used in this article.

References

1. J. H. Sakamoto, A. L. van de Ven, B. Godin, E. Blanco, R. E. Serda, A. Grattoni, A. Ziemys, A. Bouamrani, T. Hu, S. I. Ranganathan, E. de Rosa, J. O. Martinez, C. A. Smid, R. M. Buchanan, S. Y. Lee, S. Srinivasan, M. Landry, A. Meyn, E. Tasciotti, X. Liu, P. Decuzzi, M. Ferrari, *Pharmacol. Res.*, 57 (2010).
2. I. S. Vizirianakis, in *Handbook of Personalized Medicine: Advances in Nanotechnology, Drug Delivery, and Therapy* (2014). Pan Stanford. ISBN9789814411196.
3. M. Ferrari, *Trends Biotechnol.*, 181 (2010).
4. H. Maeda, *Adv. Enzyme Reg.*, 189 (2001).
5. H. Maeda, *Ther. Deliv.*, 627 (2014).
6. E. Tasciotti, X. Liu, R. Bhavane, K. Plant, A. D. Leonard, B. K. Price, M. M. Cheng, P. Decuzzi, J. M. Tour, F. Robertson, M. Ferrari, *Nat. Nano.*, 151 (2008).
7. F. Muhammad, M. Guo, W. Qi, F. Sun, A. Wang, Y. Guo, G. Zhu, *JACS,* 8778 (2011).
8. B. S. Tian, C. Yang, C. *J Nanosc. Nanotechnol.*, 1871 (2011).
9. R. Cheng, F. Meng, C. Deng, H. A. Klok, Z. Zhong, *Biomater.*, 3647 (2013).
10. M. P. Melancon, M. Zhou, C. Li, *Acc. Chem. Res.*, 947 (2011).
11. Q. L. Zhou, Z. Y. Chen, Y. X. Wang, F. Yang, Y. Lin, Y. Y. Liao, *Biomed Res. Int.,* 963891 (2014).
12. S. Dufort, A. Bianchi, M. Henry, F. Lux, G. Le Duc, V. Josserand, C. Louis, P. Perriat, Y. Cremillieux, O. Tillement, J. L. Coll, *Small,* 215 (2014).
13. G. Le Duc, I. Miladi, C. Alric, P. Mowat, E. Brauer-Krisch, A. Bouchet, E. Khalil, C. Billotey, M. Janier, F. Lux, T. Epicier, P. Perriat, S. Roux, O. Tillement, *ACS Nano*, 9566 (2011).
14. L. Sancey, F. Lux, S. Kotb, S. Roux, S. Dufort, A. Bianchi, Y. Cremillieux, P. Fries, J. L. Coll, C. Rodriguez-Lafrasse, M. Janier, M. Dutreix, M. Barberi-Heyob, F. Boschetti, F. Denat, C. Louis, E. Porcel, S. Lacombe, G. Le Duc, E. Deutsch, J. L. Perfettini, A. Detappe, C. Verry, R. Berbeco, K. T. Butterworth, S. J. McMahon, K. M. Prise, P. Perriat, O. Tillement, *Brit. J. Radiol.*, 20140134 (2014).

15. S. Anderson, K. J. Bloom, D. U. Vallera, J. Rueschoff, C. Meldrum, R. Schilling, B. Kovach, J. R. Lee, P. Ochoa, R. Langland, H. Halait, H. J. Lawrence, M. C. Dugan, *Arc. Pathol. Lab. Med.*, 1385 (2012).
16. T. G. St Pierre, A. El-Beshlawy, M. Elalfy, A. Al Jefri, K. Al Zir, S. Daar, D. Habr, U. Kriemler-Krahn, A. Taher, *Magnetic Reson. Med.*, 2215 (2014).
17. F. Lux, A. Mignot, P. Mowat, C. Louis, S. Dufort, C. Bernhard, F. Denat, F. Boschetti, C. Brunet, R. Antoine, P. Dugourd, S. Laurent, L. Vander Elst, R. Muller, L. Sancey, V. Josserand, J. L. Coll, V. Stupar, E. Barbier, C. Remy, A. Broisat, C. Ghezzi, G. Le Duc, S. Roux, P. Perriat, O. Tillement, *Angew. Chem.*, 12299 (2011).
18. A. Mignot, C. Truillet, F. Lux, L. Sancey, C. Louis, F. Denat, F. Boschetti, L. Bocher, A. Gloter, O. Stephan, R. Antoine, P. Dugourd, D. Luneau, G. Novitchi, L. C. Figueiredo, P. C. de Morais, L. Bonneviot, B. Albela, F. Ribot, L. Van Lokeren, I. Dechamps-Olivier, F. Chuburu, G. Lemercier, C. Villiers, P. N. Marche, G. Le Duc, S. Roux, O. Tillement, P. Perriat, *Chem.*, 6122 (2013).
19. A. Bianchi, S. Dufort, F. Lux, A. Courtois, O. Tillement, J. L. Coll, Y. Cremillieux, *Magma*, 303 (2014).
20. D. Kryza, J. Taleb, M. Janier, L. Marmuse, I. Miladi, P. Bonazza, C. Louis, P. Perriat, S. Roux, O. Tillement, C. Billotey, *Bioconj. Chem.*, 1145 (2011).
21. A. Bianchi, S. Dufort, P. Y. Fortin, F. Lux, G. Raffard, N. Tassali, O. Tillement, J. L. Coll, Y. Cremillieux, *NMR Biomed.*, 971 (2014).
22. I. Miladi, G. Duc, D. Kryza, A. Berniard, P. Mowat, S. Roux, J. Taleb, P. Bonazza, P. Perriat, F. Lux, O. Tillement, C. Billotey, M. Janier, *J. Biomaterials Appl.*, 385 (2013).
23. W. Rima, L. Sancey, M. T. Aloy, E. Armandy, G. B. Alcantara, T. Epicier, A. Malchere, L. Joly-Pottuz, P. Mowat, F. Lux, O. Tillement, B. Burdin, A. Rivoire, C. Boule, I. Anselme-Bertrand, J. Pourchez, M. Cottier, S. Roux, C. Rodriguez-Lafrasse, P. Perriat, *Biomater.*, 181 (2013).
24. C. Aspord, D. Laurin, M. Janier, C. A. Mandon, C. Thivolet, C. Villiers, P. Mowat, A. M. Madec, O. Tillement, P. Perriat, C. Louis, F. Berard, P. N. Marche, J. Plumas, C. Billotey, *Nanoscale*, 11409 (2013).
25. M. Luchette, H. Korideck, M. Makrigiorgos, O. Tillement, R. Berbeco, *Nanomed.* 1751, (2014).

26. E. Porcel, O. Tillement, F. Lux, P. Mowat, N. Usami, K. Kobayashi, Y. Furusawa, C. Le Sech, S. Li, S. Lacombe, *Nanomed.*, 1601 (2014).
27. F. Dhermain. *Chin. J. Cancer,* 16 (2014).
28. K. S. Subedi, T. Takahashi, T. Yamano, J. Saitoh, K. Nishimura, Y. Suzuki, T. Ohno, T. Nakano, *J. Radia. Res.*, 135 (2013).
29. R. Alvarado, J. T. Booth, R. M. Bromley, H. B. Gustafsson, *J. Appl. Clin. Med. Phys.*, 4085 (2013).
30. L. I. Cervino, J. Du, S. B. Jiang, *Phys. Med. Biol.,* 3773 (2011).
31. P. Metcalfe, G. P. Liney, L. Holloway, A. Walker, M. Barton, G. Delaney, S. Vinod, W. Tome, *Technol. Cancer Res. Treat.*, 429 (2013).
32. M. Pinkawa, F. Schoth, D. Bohmer, G. Hatiboglu, A. Sharabi, D. Song, M. J. Eble, *Exp. Rev. Anticancer Ther.,* 75 (2013).
33. G. Bowden, H. Kano, Z. J. Tempel, E. Caparosa, E. Monaco, A. Niranjan, J. Flickinger, J. D. Luketich, L. D. Lunsford, *J. Neuro-Oncol.,* 141 (2014).
34. C. C. Lee, C. P. Yen, Z. Xu, D. Schlesinger, J. Sheehan, *J. Neurosurg.*, 52 (2014).
35. T. R. Smith, R. R. Lall, R. R. Lall, I. J. Abecassis, O. M. Arnaout, M. H. Marymont, K. R. Swanson, J. P. Chandler, *J. Neurosurg.*, 1 (2014).
36. P. Fries, J. N. Morelli, F. Lux, O. Tillement, G. Schneider, A. Buecker, *Nanomed. Nanobiotechnol.*, 559 (2014).
37. S. Yu, S. Choi, S. KiM, E. Goo, Y. Ji, B. Choe, *Curr. Appl. Phys.*, 857 (2013).
38. J. F. Hainfeld, D. N. Slatkin, T. M. Focella, H. M. Smilowitz, *Brit. J. Radiol.*, 248 (2006).
39. J. F. Hainfeld, D. N. Slatkin, H. M. Smilowitz, *Phys. Med. Biol.*, N309 (2004).
40. K. T. Butterworth, S. J. McMahon, F. J. Currell, K. M. Prise, *Nanoscale,* 4830 (2012).
41. K. T. Butterworth, J. A. Wyer, M. Brennan-Fournet, C. J. Latimer, M. B. Shah, F. J. Currell, D. G. Hirst, *Radiat. Res.,* 381 (2008).
42. S. J. McMahon, W. B. Hyland, M. F. Muir, J. A. Coulter, S. Jain, K. T. Butterworth, G. Schettino, G. R. Dickson, A. R. Hounsell, J. M. O'Sullivan, K. Prise, D. G. Hirst, F. J. Currell, *Radiother. Oncol.,* 412 (2011).
43. I. Miladi, M. T. Aloy, E. Armandy, P. Mowat, D. Kryza, N. Magne, O. Tillement, F. Lux, C. Billotey, M. Janier, C. Rodriguez-Lafrasse, *Nanomed.,* 247 (2014).

CHAPTER 5

OPTICAL IMAGING AND CHEMOTHERAPY

Guillaume Bort, Simona Mura and Patrick Couvreur*

Institut Galien Paris-Sud,
UMR 8612, CNRS, Univ. Paris-Sud,
Université Paris-Saclay, Faculté de Pharmacie,
5 rue JB Clément, 92296 Châtenay-Malabry, France
**patrick.couvreur@u-psud.fr*

Nanoscale drug delivery systems which combine in a single tool imaging and therapeutic functions, (i.e., nanotheranostics) have attracted a great deal of interest due to the possibility to monitor in real-time both distribution/drug release and the effectiveness of the treatment thus, allowing an immediate adjustment of the therapeutic protocol. Among the various modalities, this chapter will focus on the optical imaging combined to the delivery of anticancer drugs and the main achievement obtained in this field will be discussed. Nanotheranostics displaying multi-imaging properties will be also presented.

1. Introduction

A great deal of attention is currently focused on the emerging field of "personalized medicine", which holds the promises of enabling (i) detection and monitoring over time of an individual patient's disease and (ii) on-demand tuning of the therapeutic treatments. In this context, a large variety of theranostic nanosystems ("*nanotheranostics*"), which integrate therapeutic and imaging functions in the same tool, have been designed in the last decade to achieve a better understanding on the mechanism and efficiency of drug release as well as for monitoring in real-time the treatment efficacy.[1] Among the numerous approaches, nanotheranostics which combine therapeutic molecules and molecules or particles detectable by optical imaging aroused high interest and have been widely explored. Indeed, optical imaging is one of the most promising imaging modality due to its high sensitivity, high spatiotemporal resolution for both *in vivo* and *in vitro* imaging, and relatively low cost. Investigation of processes at the cellular and molecular levels is also possible. Many theranostic systems require the use of ultraviolet (UV) excitation to be activated or detected. However, while UV light showed great possibility for controlling/monitoring systems *in vitro*, the *in vivo* application is severely limited by the low penetration depth (due to strong light absorption and scattering of soft tissues) and induction of high cellular damage. On the other hand, near-infrared (NIR) light (700–950 nm) exhibits low tissue absorbance, leading to deeper penetration in living tissues (3 cm in thick animal tissues and up to 10 cm in less attenuating organs such as breast)[2,3] and displays lower damaging potential. For this reason the development of activating/monitoring nanotheranostics based on NIR light is more attractive. Metal containing probes, such as semiconductor quantum dots (QDs), lanthanides (Ln) or gold, are playing a major role in this field.[4–6]

While the first developed systems were used only to confirm the presence of the drug carrier at the targeted site, further sophistication of the technology enabled to monitor and quantify the *in situ* drug release. Finally, recently designed stimuli-sensitive nanotheranostics offer a way for a precise "on-demand" control of the drug release. In this chapter, examples of the most important achievements realized with nanotheranostics combining non-invasive optical imaging and cancer chemotherapy are discussed.

2. Fluorescent Drug-Containing Nanotheranostics

Fluorescent drugs enable easy tracking of drug-loaded nanocarriers without addition of any complementary fluorescent tag. Doxorubicin (Dox), an anthracycline antibiotic inducing cell death mainly by intercalating DNA,[7] is the most commonly used anticancer drug displaying fluorescent properties. Due to the auto-quenching of Dox fluorescence, the drug release from a carrier can be detected by monitoring the variation of the fluorescence signal over time. Such shift can also confirm the effectiveness of a specific stimulus to trigger the drug release. For instance, the strong increase of the fluorescent signal observed after exposure of poly(ethylene glycol)-*b*-poly(γ-benzyl L-glutamate) (PEG-SS-PBLG) micelles, bearing dox through a disulfide bond, to glutathione (GSH) concentration higher than 1 mM, confirmed the bioreductible character of the system and the possibility to trigger Dox release.[8]

However, although easy to detect, several parameters have to be taken into account when the fluorescence signal is used to quantify the Dox. Indeed, the Dox concentration itself, the local microenvironment and the interaction with cellular components may influence Dox fluorescence intensity by changing its quantum efficiency. For instance, Dox fluorescence is dramatically quenched upon intercalation between the DNA base pairs, thus measured signal intensity do not represent the Dox concentration and might not correlate with the drug therapeutic efficacy.[9,10] Nevertheless, precise Dox quantification in tumor tissue could be achieved by application of Monte Carlo-based models of light-tissue interaction[11] or other approaches such as the forward-adjoint fluorescence model.[12] Besides Dox, mitoxantrone[10] and camptothecin (Cpt)[13] could also be detected due to their intrinsic fluorescence.

3. Fluorescently Labelled Nanotheranostics

In the absence of fluorescent drug molecules, nanocarrier distribution and/or drug release can be monitored by designing fluorescently-tagged systems. Various NIR dyes such as indocyanine green (ICG), Cyanine5.5 (Cy5.5), lipophilic 3,3'-dioctadecyloxacarbocyanine perchlorate (DiO) are commonly employed. The dye can be either physically encapsulated or covalently linked to the building material. In both case, quantification of dye loading is required for complete and reliable characterization of the system. When biodegradable polymers are used, low-destructive methods such as combination of spectroscopic and microscopic techniques (e.g., steady-state fluorescence, anisotropy and emission and anisotropy lifetime decay profiles) are recommended to avoid inaccurate dye loading assessment due to the degradation of the polymer itself.[14]

Physical encapsulation of the amphiphilic ICG into cytochrome *c*-loaded nanoparticles (NPs) made of a water-soluble hyperbranched poly-hydroxyl polymer was proposed to track them *in vitro* and easily quantify their uptake by MCF7 and A549 cells by NIR fluorescence (NIRF). In addition, the dye enabled to assess the role of receptor-mediated internalization when these NPs were functionalized with folic acid (FA).[15] Co-loading of Cy5.5 and paclitaxel (Ptx) into chitosan-based NPs, known for their stability in serum, deformability (compared to the polystyrene beads) and rapid uptake in tumor cells was also reported.[16] *In vivo* whole-body NIRF imaging in early-stage SCC7 (murine squamous cell carcinoma cells) tumor-bearing mice showed a higher tumor accumulation of these NPs compared to rigid polystyrene beads. Fluorescence intensity was proportional to NP accumulation and tumor size, thus the kinetic of dye accumulation enabled to monitor the therapeutic response and optimize the treatment protocol. Highest tumor accumulation was achieved between 1 and 3 days post-injection and persisted for up to 10 days while a considerably low uptake was observed in the liver and spleen. The optimized therapeutic protocol derived from NIRF imaging data (20 mg Ptx/kg body weight, administered using 4 injections every 3 days) led to efficient antitumor activity significantly enhancing animal survival and minimizing the severe toxicity associated with free Ptx. Encapsulation of hydrophobic dyes and drug molecules into aminoacid-based NPs was also reported.[17,18]

Formulation of nanotheranostics using chemically modified materials was chosen by other groups in order to avoid any possible misinterpretation of the imaging results as consequence of fluorescent dye desorption and/or release. For example, dye-labelled lipids were introduced in the liposomal formulation when fluorescent RGD-functionalized Dox-loaded liposomes were prepared by the thin film hydration method, mixing DSPC, cholesterol, DOPE, DSPE-mPEG2000, DSPE-cRGDfK and BODIPY-modified DOPE. Compared to the free drug (1 mg·Kg^{-1}, intravenously injected), these liposomes showed 15-fold increase in antimetastatic activity in clinically relevant pancreatic (murine R40P) and renal (human SN12C-RFP) cell orthotopic models of spontaneous metastasis, whereas no weight loss was observed.[19] The presence of BODIPY-DOPE in the liposome membrane allowed *in vivo* tracking and observation by intravital microscopy of liposomes binding to the tumor neovasculature. Similarly, fluorescent-labelled Dox-loaded liposomes functionalized with a tumor cells-binding peptide (CSNIDARAC) were easily prepared by inserting the Cy7.5-modified-DOPE in the lipid bilayer.[20] Significant tumor accumulation was observed by non-invasive *in vivo* imaging, 2 h after intravenous injection of the functionalized liposomes in H460 lung tumor-bearing mice (2 mg Dox/kg body weight). The higher tumor accumulation of these liposomes compared to the non-functionalized counterpart resulted in a higher inhibition of tumor growth.

With the aim to combine imaging with a spatiotemporal controlled delivery of drugs, stimuli-responsive nanotheranostics were also designed. pH-sensitive sugar-functionalized Dox-loaded fluorescent micelles were prepared blending poly(*N*-isopropyl acrylamide-*co*-methacryl acid)-*g*-poly(D,L-lactide), mPEG-PLA, galactosamine-PEG-PLA and FITC-PEG-PLA.[21] A significant release of Dox (70% in 140 h) was measured in PBS at pH 5.0, leading to dramatic cytotoxicity on HepG2 human hepatocellular carcinoma cells. Dox and FITC fluorescent signals were used to monitor, by confocal laser scanning microscopy (CLSM), intracellular distribution in HeLa cells of both micelles and released drug. In another study, both empty and Dox-loaded NPs were prepared with Cy5.5-labeled glycol chitosan modified with different degrees of hydrophobic *N*-acetyl histidine, which endowed the NPs with pH-responsiveness.[22] Non-invasive *in vivo* imaging was used to monitor NP biodistribution and tumor targeting efficiency which was strongly influenced by the presence of *N*-acetyl histidine and Dox in the NP. Indeed, Dox loading showed to affect the physicochemical properties of the chitosan NPs resulting in different biodistribution profiles between empty and Dox-loaded NPs due to the stabilization effect of the Dox in the core of the chitosan NPs provided by hydrophobic interactions. A higher tumor accumulation was observed with empty NPs containing the highest amount of *N*-acetyl histidine (7.8 wt.%), whereas, for Dox-loaded ones the highest accumulation was reached in presence of only 3.3 wt.% of *N*-acetyl histidine. Interestingly, similar biodistribution profiles were obtained with both optical and scintigraphic (^{131}I-labelled NPs) imaging. The most important targeting ability was then associated with a significant anticancer efficacy in HT29 tumor bearing mice.

Examples of responsive nanocarriers in which stimuli tuned both drug release and fluorescence emission were also reported. For instance, Satchi-Fainaro *et al.* conjugated both Cy5 and Ptx to *N*-(2-hydroxypropyl) methacrylamide (HMPA) copolymer through a GFLG linker sensitive to cathepsin B, a lysosomal cysteine protease overexpressed in several tumor types.[23] Resulting NPs were non-fluorescent due to the self-quenching effect of Cy5. However, in the presence of cathepsin B, the cleavage of the linker led to Ptx and Cy5 release, concomitant with the emission of a fluorescence signal. After NP intravenous injection in 4T1 tumor-bearing mice, *in vivo* fluorescence imaging confirmed the linker cleavage in tumors. A disulphide bond was used to design a NIR prodrug by linkage of dicyanomethylene-4*H*-pyrane (DCM), a NIR fluorophore, to Cpt (DCM–SS–CPT) and the conjugate was then encapsulated into PEG–PLA micelles.[24] Drug release and simultaneous NIRF emission were observed *in vitro* after reductive cleavage of the disulfide bond (GSH 2.5 mM). Then, *in vivo* drug release in the reductive cytosolic conditions was monitored by NIRF and these redox responsive NPs displayed a higher antitumor activity compared to the free drug in human breast cancer BCap-37 tumor xenograph model.

Fluorescent ruthenium(II) polypyridyl complexes have been used as light-sensitive mesoporous silica nanoparticles (MPSNPs) capping system and fluorescent reporters of ruthenium interaction with its target.[25] Upon visible light irradiation, the replacement of the monodentale ligand, which anchored the complex to the NP pores with a water molecule, led to the release of a non-fluorescent aqua ruthenium (II) complex. Fluorescence was then recovered after interaction with DNA due to the absence of water in such closely packed molecular superstructure. When Ptx was loaded in the pores, irradiation triggered the concomitant release of the two drugs.

3.1. *Combination of optical with other imaging modalities*

Combination of more than one imaging modality in a single nanotheranostic has been investigated by several groups. For instance, Li *et al.* described liposomes made of DSPC/cholesterol/Gd-DOTA-DSPE/DOTA-DSPE, fluorescently labeled by insertion of the IRDye-DSPE in the bilayer and loaded with Dox.[26] The Gd-DOTA-DSPE component endowed the liposome with magnetic resonance imaging (MRI) contrast enhancement properties, whereas the DOTA-DSPE enabled surface radiolabeling with ^{64}Cu for positron emission tomography (PET) imaging. Single-photon emission computed tomography (SPECT) imaging could also be realized by loading ^{99m}Tc. Intratumoral injection of these multifunctional liposomes in a squamous cell carcinoma of head and neck xenograft model in rats was monitored by magnetic resonance (MR), NIRF, SPECT or PET imaging. MR images (T_1 or T_2-weighted) provided a 3D high-resolution microdistribution of the liposomes in the tumor, whereas optical imaging was used for detecting the locoregional retention and systemic distribution at superficial areas of the body, and nuclear images accurately measured the quantitative biodistribution of administrated radioactivity *in vivo*. Nevertheless, despite the Dox encapsulation, no proof of the therapeutic efficacy was provided and the use of this nanodevice as theranostic system still needs to be demonstrated.

MRI and optical imaging were also combined in peptide-functionalized Pluronic® L-121 polymersomes loaded with Cpt (0.4 wt.%) and superparamagnetic iron oxide NPs (SPIONs, 6 nm) and surface decorated with a fluorescent dye.[27] Compared to the free Cpt, drug-loaded polymersomes showed enhanced cytotoxic activity against prostate cancer cells (PC-3). Specific cell binding and internalization were confirmed by flow cytometry and confocal microscopy. In addition, their high transverse relaxivity (r_2 = 394 $s^{-1}\cdot mM^{-1}$) enabled to generate significant T_2-weighted MRI contrast.

Association of optical and ^{19}F MRI detection was also proposed with celecoxib-loaded perfluoro poly (ethylene glycol) ether nanoemulsion decorated with NIR fluorescent dyes (Cellvue® NIR815 or Cellvue® Burgundy).[28] The nanoemulsion droplets suppressed the cyclooxygenase-2 (COX-2) activity in macrophages and could potentially be used *in vivo* to track macrophage tumor infiltration.

4. Mesoporous Silica-Based Nanotheranostics

Mesoporous Silica NPs (MSNPs) have robust and well-defined structures with excellent biocompatibility and biodegradability thanks to the absence of heavy elements and toxic degradation products. These particles can be easily modified by tuning their surface properties and their porosity thus enabling to achieve high host molecule payloads.[29] MSNPs having intrinsic NIR photoluminescence, attributed to quantum confinement effect, were firstly applied by Sailor *et al.* for *in vivo* monitoring of both (i) accumulation in tumor, liver and spleen and (ii) degradation to soluble silicic acid.[30] Electrostatic interactions between Dox and the negatively charged porous SiO_2 surface allowed preparing drug-loaded MSNPs which exhibited a similar or slightly greater cytotoxicity compared to the free drug *in vitro* on MDA-MB-435 human breast carcinoma cells. The *in vivo* biodistribution study of MSNPs performed by whole-body fluorescence imaging showed that a dextran coating was efficient to slow down the degradation of the particles.

More recently, luminescent MSNPs were prepared by calcination which led to the generation of emitting carbon dots (CDs) in the particle matrix.[31] c(RGDyK) functionalized MPSNs were injected intravenously in U87MG tumor-bearing mice and distribution as well as tumor accumulation were monitored by *in vivo* whole body fluorescence imaging. Despite the fact that Dox was loaded in these NPs (70 wt.%), no proof of the antitumor activity of such NPs was provided.

Another kind of MSNPs with unique NIR-to-Vis upconverting luminescence imaging properties (excitation at 980 nm) and high drug loading of water-insoluble drugs was prepared by embedding Si nanocrystals in the mesoporous wall of the NPs and encapsulating graphite-like carbon in the mesopores.[13] CTP was loaded into the pores of the same MSNPs, whose surface was then modified with PEG chains and hyaluronic acid (HA) for selective targeting of the CD44 receptors overexpressed on several cancer cells. Important cytotoxicity was observed *in vitro* on CD44 expressing MDA-MB-468 breast cancer cells and NIR-to-Vis luminescence imaging enabled to simultaneously monitor the NP uptake.

MR, optical and drug delivery properties were combined in rod-like nanostructures (length 200 ± 23 nm; diameter: 85 ± 8 nm) composed of a large hollow core and a double layered shell (inner magnetic shell and mesoporous outer shell) coated with rhodamine B (Rho B), and loaded with docetaxel or Cpt.[32] Drug loaded NPs exhibited greater cytotoxicity compared to the free drug *in vitro* on HeLa cancer cells and the fluorescent properties enabled to monitor and quantify uptake by flow cytometry and confocal microscopy. In addition, due to their high transverse relaxivity (r_2 = 124.3 $mM^{-1} \cdot s^{-1}$, 3 T), it was possible to follow by MRI the NP biodistribution after intravenous injection in mice (2.5 mg Fe/kg body weight).

5. Semiconductor QDs-Based Nanotheranostics

Semiconductor QDs exhibit unique optical and electronic properties due to quantum-confined structures. They have tunable fluorescence emission from visible to IR wavelengths controlled by their size (1–10 nm) and composition, broad absorption with narrow photoluminescence spectra, large absorption coefficients, high quantum yield and good photostability.[33] Due to these properties they have been successfully used as traceable probes in several nanotheranostics.[4] Although their intrinsic toxicity (especially when containing Cd and Pb) has limited clinical translation,[34] recent developments claimed the preparation of biocompatible QD formulations adapted for *in vivo* applications.[4] But this would deserve a more convincing demonstration.

As example, CdSe/ZnS core-shell QD490 were conjugated with A10 RNA aptamers, recognizing the extracellular domain of the prostate specific membrane antigen (PSMA), and Dox was loaded in the double-stranded stem of the A10 aptamer (intercalation into the GC sequences).[35] This assembly resulted in a reversible self-quenching system based on a Bi-FRET mechanism (i.e., donor–acceptor Förster resonance energy transfer (FRET) model between QD and Dox and donor–quencher model FRET between Dox and aptamer) which led to a recovery of Dox fluorescence only when Dox was released. Cellular uptake of the QDs through PSMA binding and Dox release (either by physical dissociation or degradation of the aptamer) was observed after incubation within LNCaP prostate cancer cells. Cytotoxic activity of QDs was equivalent to the free drug.

Mucin1 (MUC1) aptamer specific for mutated MUC1 mucin, overexpressed in many cancer cells, was used by Minko *et al.* for the functionalization of QDs to which Dox was conjugated *via* a pH-sensitive acyl hydrazone bond;[36] Fluorescence of conjugated Dox was quenched due to a FRET process between the QD and the drug, and then recovered after its release (35% in 5 h at pH 5.0). Functionalized Dox-loaded QD displayed higher cytotoxicity compared to the free drug and to their non-functionalized counterpart in multidrug resistant A2780-AD human ovarian cancer cells *in vitro*. Greater accumulation in the tumor was also observed after systemic administration in mice model of A2780-AD tumor xenograft (Figure 1).

QD were also associated with lipid-based formulations, and encapsulated in the hydrophobic core of DSPE–PEG micelles[37] or inserted in the bilayer of liposomes with different properties (i.e., cationic, PEGylated or deformable).[38] When these formulations were loaded with Cpt or irinotecan, the highest cytotoxicity (*in vitro* on B16F10 cells) and greater *in vivo* tumor accumulation were observed

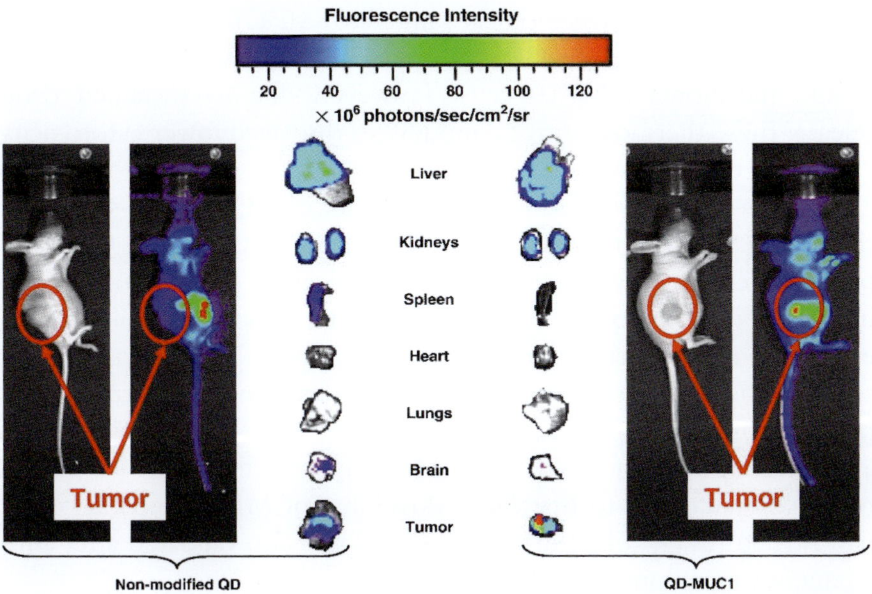

Fig. 1: Organ and tumor content of non-modified QDs and aptamer-targeted QD (QD–MUC1). Multidrug resistant A2780/AD cells were injected subcutaneously into the flanks of nude mice. The distribution of QD and QD–MUC1 in the whole animal was observed in real-time 24 h after intravenous injection using the IVIS imaging system. Immediately after mice were sacrificed and *ex vivo* imaging was performed on excised organs. Reprinted with permission from Ref. 36. Copyright 2011 Elsevier B.V.

with the cationic formulations (intratumoral injection).[38] Interestingly, encapsulation in liposomes enabled to increase the tumor accumulation of Cpt but not that of irinotecan, as compared to free drugs.

To prepare theranostic thermosensitive nanogels, Bi_2O_3 QDs were immobilized inside PVA nanogels encapsulating temozolomide (TMZ) as therapeutic agent (DNA alkylating prodrug).[39] Such nanogels undergo a reversible temperature-triggered volume phase transition which led to (i) a modification of the physicochemical microenvironment of the QDs and a variation of the fluorescence signal and (ii) a controlled release of TMZ (7% at 37°C vs 19% at 40°C for 24 h). Such responsiveness was exhibited in response to variation of temperature over a physiological range (37–40°C). Fluorescence and dark field imaging allowed to monitor the uptake of nanogels by mouse melanoma B16F10 cells. However, due to sustained drug release, these thermosensitive nanodevices displayed lower cytotoxicity compared to the free drug.

Another strategy relied on the localization of QD at the surface of the drug carrier. For instance, layers of negatively charged QDs and positively charged poly(allylamine hydrochloride) (PAH) polyelectrolytes were used to coat Dox-loaded magnetic mesoporous silica-based ellipsoidal nanostructures $Fe_3O_4@SiO_2@mSiO_2$.[40] Thanks to the presence of the silica, no quenching of QD fluorescence occurred. It was possible to observe the intracellular localization of the nanostructures after incubation with MCF7 cells, when higher cytotoxicity was monitored comparatively to free Dox. Possibility of MRI detection of the nanostructures ($r_2 = 143$ $mM^{-1}\cdot s^{-1}$ at 3 T) was also validated after subcutaneous injection into mouse.

6. Lanthanide-Doped Upconversion Nanotheranostics

Lanthanide (Ln)-doped upconversion nanoparticles (UCNPs) have received considerable attention in bio-imaging application due to their significant advantages over other optical imaging systems. UCNPs are constituted of a host material (or host lattice) (such as $NaYF_4$, Y_2O_3 or G_2O_3) which is doped with one or more Ln ions (dopant or activator ions) (e.g., Er^{3+} (green light) or Tm^{3+} (blue light)).[41] UCNPs convert long wavelength radiation (NIR) to shorter wavelength light (visible/UV) through sequential NIR photon absorption or non-radiative energy transfer from a sensitizer (such as Yb^{3+}) to the Ln ion. Emission profiles of UCNPs are tailored by energy level transitions of the Ln ions.

NIR light sensitivity allows fluorescence imaging in relatively deep tissues (~3 cm) with a high signal-to-noise ratio, due to the low tissue scattering and absorption at these wavelengths. Additionally, UCNPs exhibit exceptional photostability, narrow emission peaks, long emission life time, tuneable emissions and large anti-stokes shifts compared to the conventional organic fluorescent dyes. Interestingly, UCNPs show lower cytotoxicity than QD[42–44] and their luminescence signal is several orders of magnitude much stronger. PEGylation was proposed to increase the UCNP biocompatibility.[45] Theranostic Ln-doped down conversion NPs (converting high energy photons — UV light — to low energy photons — visible or NIR light) were also reported but they display limited biological applications due to the low penetration of UV photons.[46–49]

For instance, intense green light was emitted under 980 nm NIR irradiation of $Yb(OH)CO_3@YbPO_4:Er^{3+}$ Dox-loaded UCNPs and the signal progressively increased with the drug release which reduced the quenching effect mediated by the encapsulated drug.[50] Incubation of HeLa cells with these NPs was monitored by fluorescence imaging, revealing their uptake which resulted in greater cytotoxicity compared to the free drug. Anticancer molecules other than the Dox were also loaded in UCNPs. The anionic drug fluorouracil (5FU) was intercalated among layers of positively charged MgAl-layered double hydroxide nanosheets deposited on the surface of $Y_2O_3:Er^{3+}$, $Yb^{3+}@SiO_2$ nanospheres.[51] Luminescent properties were validated and a higher cytotoxicity on MCF-7 cells was obtained compared to the free drug, possibly due to the positively charged surface of the UCNPs. In another study, CisPt(IV) and Rho B were conjugated to mPEG-*b*-PCL-*b*-PLL and then loaded in oleic acid-stabilized UCNPs.[52] These UCNPs@Pt-RhoB were efficiently internalized in HeLa cells and the loaded platinium Pt(IV) prodrug was reduced to the active Pt(II), leading to higher apoptosis compared to both the free drug and the polymer prodrug. Antitumor activity was also confirmed *in vivo* on SKOV-3 ovarian carcinoma bearing mice. The proof of concept of their optical detection was, however, only provided in *C. elegans.* Since *trans*-Pt(IV) prodrugs could be activated by UV, blue and green light, such an approach could represent an efficient strategy to decrease Pt(II) toxicity in healthy tissues.[53–55]

High stability, good dispersion in biological media and unique porous structure were achieved preparing UCNPs by one step synthesis using nucleotide-Ln ion supramolecular networks as precursors, rather than the conventional method (i.e., transfer from organic solvent).[56] Different nucleotides (i.e., GMP, AMP, UMP, CMP) were used and the charged phosphate played an essential role in the preparation of porous UCNPs in which Dox was loaded. The theranostic features of such NPs were confirmed *in vitro* in A549 lung carcinoma cells. Other modifications of the preparation method included (i) the replacement of the source of fluoride host material ($NaBF_4$ vs HF)[57] and (ii) electron beam irradiation of the solid particles,[58] in order to achieve a more environmentally friendly or one-step synthesis, respectively. Dox was loaded in the resulting NPs which maintained their upconversion properties enabling to monitor the cell uptake.

In other systems, the UCNPs were used as a mediator to absorb the NIR photons and convert them into high energy photons (from the UV to the NIR region) used to trigger drug release[59,60] or to promote cell targeting.[61] For instance, Dox-loaded PEGylated $NaYF_4$Yb, Tm@SiO_2 UCNPs were functionalized with caged FA using the *o*-nitrobenzylphotolabile group.[61] Caged-FA-PEGylated UCNPs@SiO_2-Dox were intravenously injected into mice bearing HeLa tumors and the tumor region was irradiated (1 h, 980 nm, 1.8 $W \cdot cm^{-2}$). Monitoring of the upconversion NIR emission confirmed that NIR irradiation was required for on-demand tumor targeting and UCNPs were found to accumulate at the tumor site during the first 5 h after injection. Moreover, tumor growth was significantly inhibited using irradiated caged FA-PEGylated UCNPs@SiO2-Dox NPs as compared to the free drug, the irradiated non-targeted UCNP and the non-irradiated caged-FA UCNP.

***Combination of upconversion luminescence (UCL) with other imaging modalities*:** Alkali ion doped CaF_2:Yb^{3+}, Er^{3+} UCNPs were reported for UCL/computed tomography (CT) imaging.[62] Ln-doped CaF_2 UCNPs are more biocompatible than the $NaYF_4$-based counterparts due to the high stability and non-hygroscopic behavior of CaF_2. These UCNPs display excellent NIR to visible upconversion ability and the presence of alkali ions in the fluoride crystal lattice influences the Yb^{3+}–Er^{3+} distance, thus tuning the energy transfer and the Ln emission. For instance, a CaF_2 shell was used to enhance the emission properties of CaF_2:Yb^{3+}, Er^{3+}, Cs^{+}@ CaF_2 UCNPs which were then coated with oleic acid and α-CD to obtain a hydrophilic system. Uncharged Dox was loaded in the hydrophobic oleic acid layer and quickly released in acidic conditions as a result of Dox protonation and weakening of hydrophobic interactions. Dox-loaded UCNPs showed higher cytotoxicity compared to the free drug *in vitro* in A549 and HeLa cells. Interestingly, when these UCNPs were injected in the foot, backside and thin muscle of mouse (up to 5 mm depth), the green UCL emission under 980 nm NIR laser could be observed by naked eyes from the three regions. Due to the high degree of X-ray absorption of Yb, these NPs displayed higher sensitivity as CT contrast agent than the commercial iopromide 300.

MRI contrast properties were also combined to UCL by using the $NaGdF_4$ as coating or core of different Dox loaded-UCNPs.[63–66] As example, Dox loaded $NaYF_4$:Tm/Yb@$NaGdF_4$ core/hollow mesoporous silica shell UCNPs were prepared and quenching of UCNPs emissions at 450 nm and 477 nm was observed due to luminescence resonance energy transfer (LRET) between the donor UCNPs and the acceptor Dox.[64] In addition, the reduced probability of water molecules to bind to the Gd^{3+} ions led to a significant drop in the longitudinal relaxation r_1 value (from 12.29 $mM^{-1}\cdot s^{-1}$ to 2.96 $mM^{-1}\cdot s^{-1}$ at 3 T). Dox release upon 980 nm light excitation led to the recovery of both UCL and MR signals, which showed excellent linear relationship with the amount of released drug, allowing for quantitative measurements. Imaging features were validated in HeLa cells and in Zebrafish embryos after UCNPs injection in heart ventricles (51% enhancement in the T_1-MR signal intensity) (Figure 2). Analogue signal recovery was observed when Dox was replaced by CisPt, and monitored *in vivo* by MRI in walker-256 tumor-bearing rats (Figure 2). Despite the theranostic potential of this system, its therapeutic ability is not yet demonstrated and still needs further investigation.

Lin *et al.* used PEG coated $NaYF_4$:Yb^{3+}/Tm^{3+}@$NaGdF_4$/Yb^{3+} UCNPs (65 nm) to convert the NIR light (980 nm) into UV (290–370 nm) and activate a dicarboxyl light-sensitive *trans*-Pt(IV) prodrug

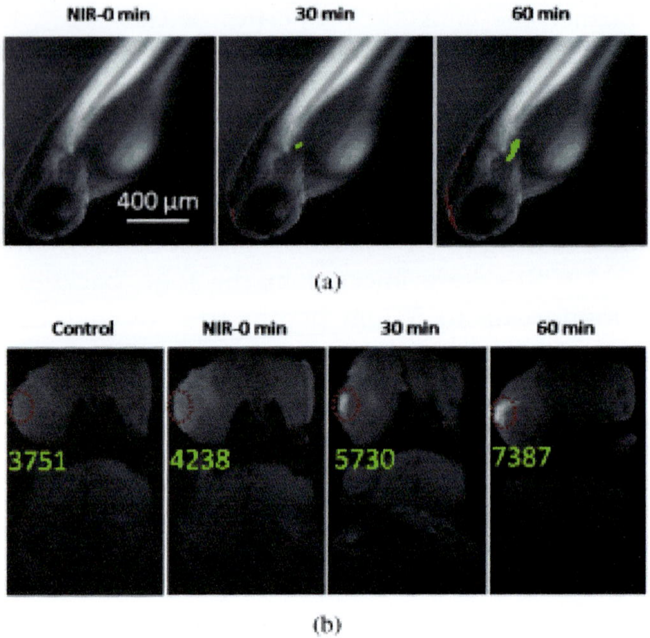

Fig. 2: (a) CLSM images of zebrafish, (green and red correspond to UCNP and Dox signals respectively). (b) T_1-MR images of a walker-256 tumor-bearing Sprague Dawley rat injected with CisPt–UCNPs before and after NIR exposure for different time durations. Red circles indicate the tumor area where CisPt–UCNPs were injected. Green values indicate T_1-MR signal intensities before and after NIR exposure. The power density of NIR light employed was 1.5 $W \cdot cm^{-2}$. Reprinted with permission from Ref. 64. Copyright 2014 WILEY-VCH Verlag GmbH & Co. KGaA, Weinheim.

trans, trans, trans-[$Pt(N_3)_2(NH_3)(py)(O_2CCH_2CH_2COOH)_2$] (DPP) covalently conjugated on the surface of the UCNP–PEG (26 mg Pt/UCNP-DPP-PEG g).[67] Although very complex, this system combines drug delivery with UCL, MR (Gd^{3+} ions) and CT (Gd^{3+} and Yb^{3+}) imaging properties, which allows precise monitoring of NPs after intratumoral and intravenous injection. (Figure 3). UCNP–DPP–PEG (0.65 mgPt/kg body weight) intratumorally injected displayed a significant inhibition of tumor growth in H22 hepatic tumor-bearing mice after irradiation at 980 nm, while only reduced anticancer activity was observed when irradiated at 365 nm, due to the lower tissue

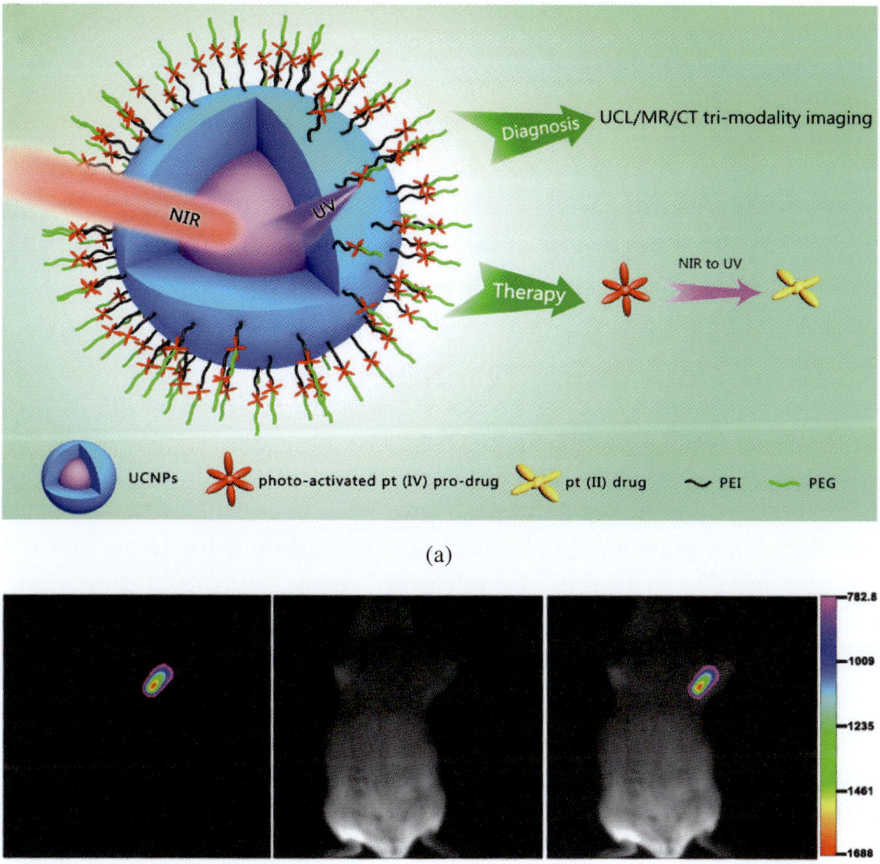

(a)

(b) (c) (d)

Fig. 3: (a). Schematic illustration of UCNP–DPP–PEG NPs (b–d). *In vivo* UCL imaging of a tumor-bearing Balb/c mouse after injection of UCNPs at the tumor site: UCL (b), bright field (c), and overlay images (d). Adapted with permission from Ref. 67. Copyright 2013 American Chemical Society.

penetration of UV light. Other trimodal imaging particles loaded with Dox *via* a pH sensitive hydrazone bond were also reported.[68]

UCL and magnetic properties (allowing magnetic guidance by an external magnetic field) were exhibited by Fe_3O_4@$mSiO_2$@α-$NaYF_4$:Yb^{3+}, Er^{3+} nanorattles, consisting of a silica-coated magnetite inner core coated with hollow mesoporous silica and layers of

Yb^{3+}/Er^{3+}-doped cubic α-$NaYF_4$.[69] Application of the magnetic field increased cell accumulation and cytotoxicity of Dox-loaded nanorattles *in vitro* in human hepatoma cells (QGY-7703) as compared to without magnetic field; enhanced tumor accumulation *in vivo* in H22 tumor-bearing mice was also observed after monitoring by UCL whole-body imaging. Such increased tumor accumulation resulted in higher tumor suppression (96%) compared to nanorattles without magnetic guidance (53%) and to the free drug (35%).

7. Gold Containing Nanotheranostics

Gold NPs exhibit tunable localized surface plasmon resonance (SPR), which allows to achieve deep-tissue imaging in the light-transparent NIR biological window (700–950 nm) and/or localized temperature increase. This photothermal effect can be exploited for hyperthermal therapy and/or to trigger the release of drugs from gold-containing drug delivery systems. In addition, gold-based systems can act as imaging agents in combination with various fluorophores. Such approach could be used to detect variation of the fluorophore/gold distance, on the basis of the fluorescence quenching effect of gold, and therefore provide useful information on nanocarrier biodistribution and related drug delivery efficiency.[70]

Various approaches have been adopted to prepare gold containing nanotheranostics. For instance, PEG–PLGA–Au half shell NPs were developed to simultaneously actuate chemotherapy (Dox loading) and hyperthermia upon NIR irradiation.[71] Synergistic effect was observed in A431 human epidermoid carcinoma tumor-bearing mice after NIR irradiation (2.56 $W\cdot cm^{-2}$ for 10 min, generating an intratumoral temperature increase to 50–70°C). This protocol led to a complete destruction of the tumor 7 days after intravenous injection of the NPs whose tumor accumulation was monitored by *in vivo* whole body NIR imaging. Complete gold coating of Dox-loaded PLGA NPs and liposomes was also proposed.[72,73]

As an alternative strategy, bovine serum albumin (BSA) stabilized gold clusters were encapsulated into polymer NPs composed of mPEG-PLGA and ε-polylysine.[74] Further, NPs labelling with FITC enabled to monitor their tumor accumulation in B16-F10 melanoma bearing mice by *in vivo* two-color imaging. Co-loading of Dox (hydrophilic core), Ptx (hydrophobic layer) and surviving siRNA (external surface), targeting different essential metabolic pathways of tumor cells, resulted in a significant therapeutic efficacy. Interestingly, the surviving siRNA being released before the other two drugs, induced a sensitization effect playing a crucial role to obtain the strong antitumor activity.

Another original system consisted in amphiphilic gold NPs coated with BGLA Raman reporters and mixed polymer brushes of hydrophilic PEG and pH sensitive hydrophobic chains (Figure 4(a)).[75] These amphiphilic gold NPs were self-assembled into plasmonic vesicles adapted for tumor-targeted drug delivery and monitoring of cargo release by plasmonic imaging and Raman spectroscopy. The vesicles were functionalized with the antiHER2 antibody and loaded with Dox which was released at pH 5 in late endosomes/lysosomes, due to the transition of hydrophobic brushes to hydrophilic ones, further triggering vesicles disassembly. Raman spectroscopy, dark field and fluorescence imaging allowed to independently track assembled/disassembled vesicles and Dox release, thus permitting to precisely monitor the fate of the plasmonic vesicles when incubated with HER2-positive SKBR-3 breast cancer cells. Vesicle cellular binding, vesicle disassembly, drug release in the cytosol and penetration in the nucleus were clearly visualized. (Figure 4(b)). To be noted that Dox-loaded targeted vesicles exhibited higher cytotoxicity compared to the non-targeted ones, with a five-fold reduction of the IC_{50} (0.31 μg/mL).

In another study, hybrid nanogels composed of a silver–gold NP core, a shell made of thermo-responsive non-linear PEG-based hydrogel and HA chains as targeting ligands, were loaded with TMZ.[76] Temperature variations induced reversible swelling and shrinking of the gel providing modification of the physicochemical environment and of the mesh size in the gel network which affected the fluorescence of the silver–gold core and regulated the drug release. In addition, a synergistic effect of chemo and photothermal therapy was observed *in vitro* on B16F10 mouse melanoma cells upon NIR irradiation.

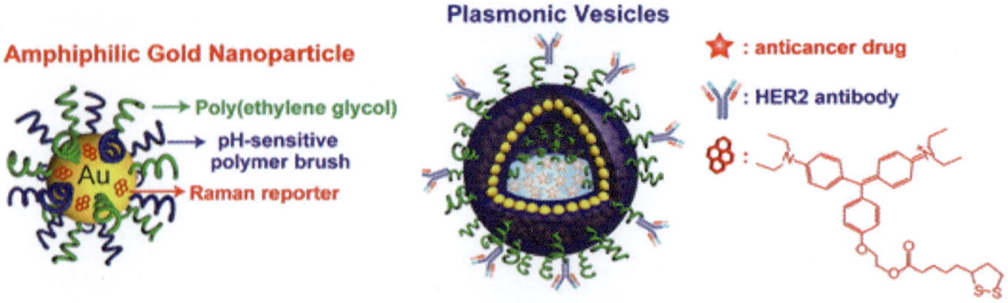

(a)

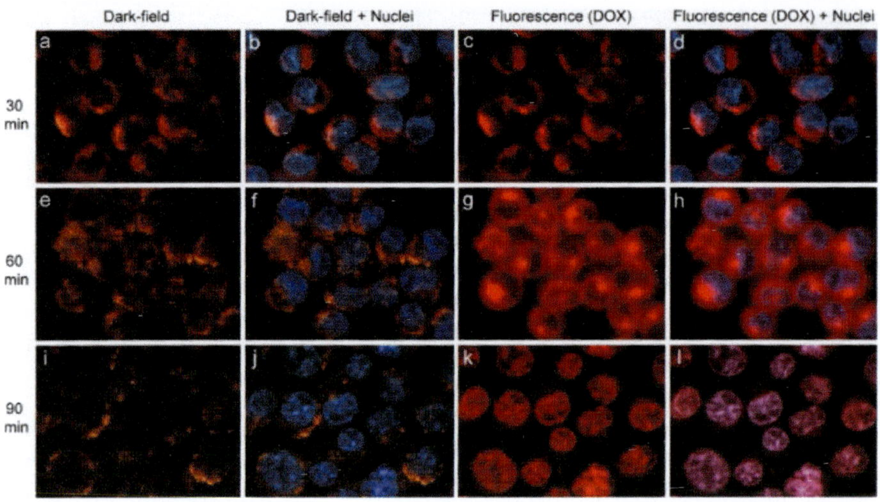

(b)

Fig. 4: (a) Schematic illustration of the amphiphilic gold NP and assembled plasmonic vesicle. (b) Dark-field, fluorescence and the overlaid images of SKBR-3 cells labeled with Dox-loaded pH-sensitive plasmonic vesicles after 30, 60 and 90 min incubation; Dox has a red fluorescence, and cell nuclei were counterstained with Hoechst 3342 exhibiting blue fluorescence. Adapted with permission from Ref. 75. Copyright 2012 American Chemical Society.

As an alternative to the loading of gold NPs into a supramolecular nanodevice, direct modification of the gold surface was proposed. For instance, spherical gold NPs were functionalized with PEG chains, biotin molecules and Rho B-linked β-cyclodextrins (β-CD) used as Ptx pocket.[77] Reductive condition (10 mM GSH) promoted the release of Ptx (*via* ligand exchange) and Rho B, which was associated with the emission of a strong fluorescence signal previously quenched by the proximity to the gold surface. Ligand-mediated uptake and cytotoxicity of these NPs were monitored by flow cytometry and confocal microscopy in Hela cancer cells. Electrostatic interactions were also used to load Dox at the surface of amine and carboxylic acid-terminated GNRs.[78] Taking advantage of both GNR luminescence and Dox fluorescence, it was possible to monitor by multi-fluorescence lifetime imaging, GNR uptake (KB cancer cells), as well as drug release thanks to the reduced quenching effect of GNRs over Dox fluorescence. Surface of gold nanorods was also modified with a mesoporous silica layer[79] or with biofriendly C-dots.[80] In both cases, the porous nature of the coating allowed Dox loading and a combination of chemo and photothermal therapy was observed upon NIR irradiation. Imaging properties of these systems enabled their tracking *in vitro,* in different cell lines.

8. Iron Oxide-Based Nanotheranostics

Iron oxide nanoparticles (IONPs) have found wide clinical application as MRI contrast agents, thanks to their high transverse relaxivity r_2, which leads to a pronounced negative contrast on T_2-weighted MR images (hypointensity). In addition, when exposed to an alternative magnetic field, they generate heat in the surrounding medium due to hysteresis loss and/or Néel relaxation. Therefore, they have been extensively used for selective increase of temperature in tumors, (i.e., hyperthermia).[81] Opportune modifications of IONPs also enable to combine imaging features (fluorescence and MR) and magnetic guidance.

For instance, USPIO NPs were coated with the hydrophilic biocompatible *N*-phosphonomethyliminodiacetic acid (PMIDA) and then amine-derivatized in order to introduce Rho B, FA (targeting ligand) and methotrexate (therapeutic agent) *via* amide, thiourea and pH-labile ester linkage, respectively.[82] *In vitro* experiments were performed on FA receptor expressing HeLa cells. NPs uptake as well as cytotoxicity, mediated by a faster intracellular drug release in acidic conditions, were assessed. In addition, NPs showed high transverse relaxivity ($r_2 = 295 \pm 7\ s^{-1}\cdot mM^{-1}$, 0.3 T), allowing their use as imaging contrast agents.

In another approach, lipophilic NIR dyes (dialkylcarbocyanine fluorophore, DiI or DiR) and drugs (Ptx) were loaded together within the hydrophobic pockets of poly(acylic acid) (PAA) at the surface of IONPs.[83] NPs surface was further functionalized with FA *via* copper-catalyzed azide–alkyne cycloaddition (click chemistry) for cancer cell targeting. NPs were stable in buffer at pH 7.4, while a fast drug release was observed in the presence of esterase or in acidic conditions (pH 4.0). Cytotoxicity of the NPs was demonstrated on the lung carcinoma A549 cell line. Simultaneous MR ($r_2 = 202\ s^{-1}\cdot mM^{-1}$, 0.47 T) and fluorescence imaging of NP uptake in folate-receptor expressing A549 cells was performed.

IONPs coating with phosphonic acid terminated poly(4-*O*-acryloyl benzaldehyde-*b*-oligoethylene glycol-acrylate) block copolymers provided both a hydrophilic, biocompatible layer at the IONP surface and functional groups for conjugation of Dox *via* pH sensitive Schiff base/imine bonds (IONP@P(HBA)-*b*-P(OEGA) + Dox).[84] Dox intracellular release and localization were precisely monitored in H1299 lung and MCF-7 breast cancer cells using fluorescence lifetime imaging microscopy (FLIM) coupled with Phasor plot analysis (Figure 5). Such technique detects changes in Dox fluorescence lifetime on the basis of its microenvironment, thus allowing to follow accumulation in the different intracellular compartments. Cell uptake of Dox-loaded IONPs in multicellular 3D tumor spheroids was also investigated by multiphoton excitation microscopy and increase of cytotoxicity comparatively to the free drug was observed. In addition, transverse relaxation of the IONPs was enhanced by 70% after Dox release ($r_2 = 223\ s^{-1}\cdot mM^{-1}$ and $386\ s^{-1}\cdot mM^{-1}$ at 9.4 T before and after Dox release, respectively), which suggests their potential application for monitoring drug release by MRI.

Surface modification of IONPs was also realized using (i) the Rotavirus capsid surface protein VP4,[85] (ii) self-assembled DNA biopolymer,[86] or (iii) gold.[87] The latter where further functionalized and combined in a system with five different functions: Cancer cell targeting, MR and optical imaging, photothermal and chemotherapy. Derivatization of gold surface with carboxylic terminated PEG chains

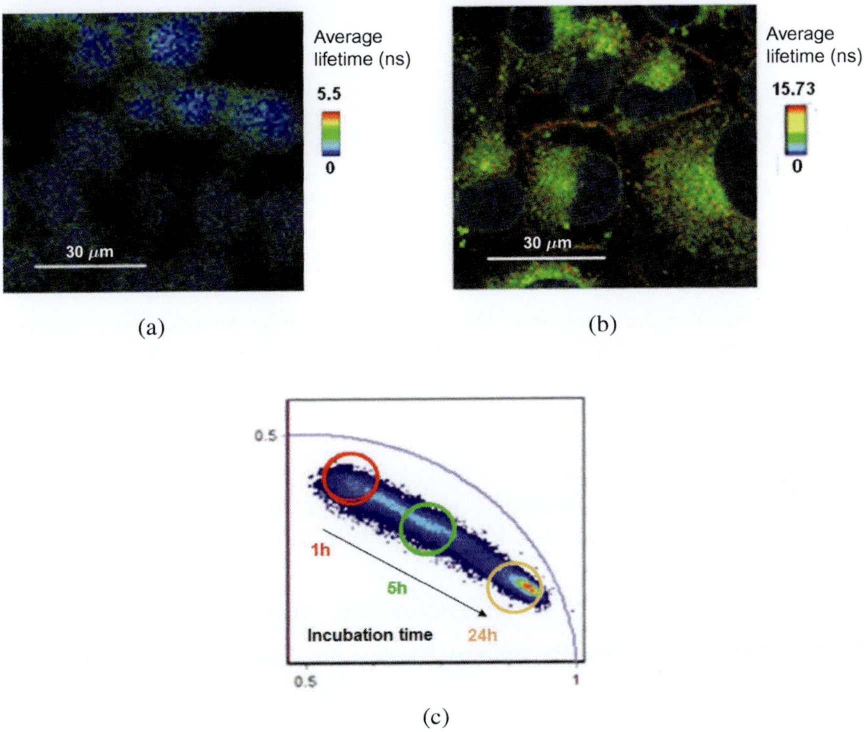

Fig. 5: (a-b) FLIM images showing cell uptake of native Dox (a) and IONP@P(HBA)-*b*-P(OEGA) + Dox (b) using H1299 cells after 5 h of incubation. (c) Phasor plot derived from the FLIM images at different incubation times with IONP@P (HBA)-*b*-P(OEGA) + Dox. Red region of interest (ROI) corresponds to the signal after 1 h of incubation; green ROI and orange ROI correspond to the signals after 5 h and 24 h, respectively. Each ROI corresponds to different lifetimes of Dox in the cells corresponding to different amounts of Dox released from IONP@P(HBA)-*b*-P(OEGA) + Dox. Adapted with permission from Ref. 84. Copyright2013 American Chemical Society.

and a capture probe (5′-(GCT) 7 -T 10 -SH-3′) allowed both the hybridization with the dye-modified sgc8 aptamer and the Dox loading *via* intercalation into the GC base pairs and electrostatic interaction with the carboxyl groups (Figure 6).[87] Fluorescence imaging was used to monitor NPs cell uptake and Dox release. Drug release was promoted by NIR irradiation, leading to degradation of nucleotides and dehybridization of aptamer mediated by the localized increase of

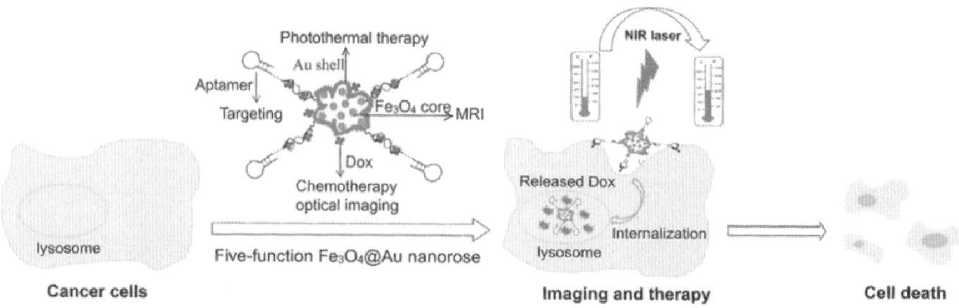

Fig. 6: Schematic representation of five-function Fe_3O_4@Au nanorose for cancer cell targeting, MRI, optical imaging, photothermal and chemotherapy. Reprinted with permission from Ref. 87. Copyright 2013 WILEY-VCH Verlag GmbH & Co. KGaA, Weinheim.

temperature, which also enabled to combine chemotherapy and photothermal therapy. Cytotoxicity on CCRF–CEM cells indeed increased upon laser irradiation. The magnetic core allowed to monitor cell uptake also by MRI T_2 measurement.

9. Radioluminescent Nanotheranostics

As previously discussed, the *in vivo* application of optical imaging is hindered by the tissue auto-fluorescence, light adsorption and scattering. Although better tissue penetration is obtained by NIR light irradiation, the detection of fluorescent probes is still limited to few centimeters and the resolution is very low. In this context, X-ray excited optical luminescence (XEOL) approaches were introduced recently to address these issues. These imaging modalities are based on the selective excitation and optical detection of X-ray excitable phosphor NPs, which emit NIR light when excited by X-ray photons. Thus, unprecedented high imaging resolution could be successfully achieved in deep tissues due to the very low background provided by this new technique.[88–90]

For instance, Anker *et al.* used XEOL to monitor drug delivery and biodistribution of a drug nanocarrier *in vivo*.[91] Practically, spindle-shaped monodispersed silica nanocapsules (length of 420 ± 20 nm and width of 130 ± 15 nm,) were loaded with Dox (5 wt.%) and coated with X-ray scintillator Gd_2O_2S:Tb or Gd_2O_2S:Eu and pH sensitive PSS/PAH multilayers. The X-ray absorption by the Gd_2O_2S host lattice produced electron-hole pairs which excited the Tb^{3+} or Eu^{3+} centers, leading to the emission of visible or NIR light. The quenching effect of loaded Dox on specific emission wavelengths enabled to detect Dox release *in vitro* by monitoring the increase of X-ray luminescence intensity; faster release was observed at pH 5.0 compared to pH 7.4. *In vivo* tracking of Gd_2O_2S:Eu-coated nanocapsules was performed by monitoring luminescence after irradiation with a miniature X-ray source. The presence of the PSS/PAH layers led to a slower liver and spleen accumulation compared to the same but non-coated NPs. Interestingly, the presence of Gd^{3+} ions made these nanocapsules adapted for MRI (r_2 ~50 $mM^{-1}\cdot s^{-1}$). Similarly, metroxantrone-loaded core shell NPs composed of Gd_2O_2S:Eu and Yt^{3+}, Tm^{3+} were designed to combine the advantages of UCL, MR and radioluminescence imaging, which allowed submillimeter resolution through thick deep tissues (> 1 cm).[92]

Despite the great interest of these systems as imaging and drug delivery tools, their real theranostic potential still remains to be demonstrated, as no proof of their therapeutic activity has been described yet.

10. Miscellaneous

PEI–PLA copolymers were used to prepare Ptx-loaded (5.11 wt.%) luminescent polymer dots (PDs) which possess ultrabright and multicolor fluorescent properties.[93] pH-dependent variation of the PD structure rigidity was found to influence the fluorescence signal. Antitumor efficacy was assessed after intravenous injection of the PDs in MCF-7 tumor-bearing mice (compared to free Ptx) and *ex vivo* fluorescence confirmed the tumor accumulation.

High water solubility, easy surface modification, biocompatibility, good cell permeability, high photostability and excitation-dependent multicolor emission make carbon dots (CDs) particularly attractive for the design of nanotheranostics.[94] CD surface-modified with a Pt(IV) complex were intratumorally injected (2 injections spaced by 24 hs) in

H22 hepatocarcinoma-bearing mice and tracked by *in vivo* fluorescence. Significant antitumor activity was observed, with a 82.4% reduction of tumor volume in 72 h.[95]

11. Conclusion

Optically detectable nanotheranostics enabling sustained drug release were extensively studied in the last decades. A large variety of sophisticated nanoplatforms were proposed for providing and monitoring a therapeutic effect in real-time in order to adjust the treatment on-demand. However, in spite of the large variety of approaches proposed until now, challenges still remain to be overcome such as the improvement of detection in deep tissues, the direct monitoring of the therapeutic effect or the on-demand control of therapeutic action. To be noted that most of the studies were performed *in vitro* cell culture experiments. Even if the proof of concept of few of the described systems has been already done in preclinical animal models, administration was generally performed intratumorally, instead of intravenously which is the route of administration used in the clinical routine. Finally, the toxicological issues are generally not investigated following the usual guidelines for drug development. There is, therefore, plenty of room for further research on nanodevices for optical imaging and therapy.

List of Abbreviations

2-(4-(bis(4-(diethylamino)phenyl)(hydroxy)methyl)phenoxy)ethyl 5-(1,2-dithiolan-3-yl)pentanoate (BGLA), 6-(((4,4-difluoro-5-(2-thienyl)-4-bora-3a,4a-diaza-s-indacene-3-yl)styryloxy)acetyl) aminohexanoic acid (BODIPY), bovine serum albumin (BSA), carbon dot (CD), β-cyclodextrin (β-CD), confocal laser scanning microscopy (CLSM),cyclooxygenase-2 (COX-2), camptothecin (Cpt), computed tomography (CT), Cyanine5.5 (Cy5.5), dicyanomethylene-4*H*-pyrane (DCM), 3,3'-dioctadecyloxacarbocyanine perchlorate (DiO), dioleoylphosphatidylethanolamine (DOPE), 1,4,7,10-tetraazacyclododecane-1,4,7,10-tetraacetic acid (DOTA), Doxorubicin (Dox), *trans,*

trans, trans-[$Pt(N_3)_2(NH_3)(py)(O_2CCH_2CH_2COOH)_2$] (DPP), distearoylphosphatidylcholine (DSPC), distearoylphosphatidylethanolamine (DSPE), folic acid (FA), fluorescein isothiocyanate (FITC), fluorescence lifetime imaging microscopy (FLIM), Förster resonance energy transfer (FRET), glutathione (GSH), hyaluronic acid (HA), *N*-(2-hydroxypropyl) methacrylamide (HMPA), indocyanine green (ICG), iron oxide nanoparticle (IONP), lanthanide (Ln), luminescence resonance energy transfer (LRET), methoxy poly(ethylene glycol) (mPEG), mesoporous silica nanoparticle (MPSN), magnetic resonance (MR), nuclear magnetic resonance imaging (MRI), Mucin1 (MUC1), near-infrared (NIR), NIR fluorescence (NIRF), nanoparticle (NP), poly(acylic acid) (PAA), poly(allylamine hydrochloride) (PAH), poly(γ-benzyl L-glutamate) (PBLG), L-α-phosphatidylcholine (PC), polymer dot (PD), poly(ethylene glycol) (PEG), poly(ethylene imine) (PEI), positron emission tomography (PET), egg L-α-phosphatidyl-DL-glycerol (PG), poly(D, L-lactide) (PLA), *N*-phosphonomethyliminodiacetic acid (PMIDA), prostate specific membrane antigen (PSMA), poly(sodium 4-styrenesulfonate) (PSS), paclitaxel (Ptx), semiconductor quantum dot (QD), rhodamine B (Rho B), region of interest (ROI), single-photon emission computed tomography (SPECT), superparamagnetic iron oxide nanoparticle (SPION), surface plasmon resonance (SPR), temozolomide (TMZ), upconversion luminescence (UCL), lanthanide-doped upconversion nanoparticle (UCNP), ultrasmall superparamagnetic iron oxide (USPIO), ultraviolet (UV), X-ray excited optical luminescence (XEOL).

References

1. M. S. Muthu, D. T. Leong, L. Mei, S.-S. Feng, *Theranostics*, 660 (2014).
2. G. Chen, J. Shen, T. Y. Ohulchanskyy, N. J. Patel, A. Kutikov, Z. Li, J. Song, R. K. Pandey, H. Agren, P. N. Prasad, G. Han, *ACS Nano*, 8280 (2012).
3. S. Srinivasan, B. W. Pogue, S. Jiang, H. Dehghani, C. Kogel, S. Soho, J. J. Gibson, T. D. Tosteson, S. P. Poplack, K. D. Paulsen, *Proc. Natl. Acad. Sci. U. S. A.*, 12349 (2003).

4. K.-T. Yong, Y. Wang, I. Roy, H. Rui, M. T. Swihart, W.-C. Law, S. K. Kwak, L. Ye, J. Liu, S. D. Mahajan, J. L. Reynolds, *Theranostics*, 681 (2012).
5. J. Shen, L. Zhao, G. Han, *Adv. Drug Deliv. Rev.*, 744 (2013).
6. Y. Jin, *Acc. Chem. Res.*, 138 (2014).
7. S. R. Rajski, R. M. Williams, *Chem. Rev.*, 2723 (1998).
8. T. Thambi, H.-Y. Yoon, K.-M. Kim, I.-C. Kwon, C.-K. Yoo, J.-H. Park, *Bioconjug. Chem.*, 1924 (2011).
9. P. Mohan, N. Rapoport, *Mol. Pharmaceutics*, 1959 (2010).
10. J. R. Mourant, T. M. Johnson, G. Los, I. J. Bigio, *Phys. Med. Biol.*, 1397 (1999).
11. G. M. Palmer, R. J. Boruta, B. L. Viglianti, L. Lan, I. Spasojevic, M. W. Dewhirst, *J. Control. Release*, 457 (2010).
12. T. M. Baran, T. H. Foster, *Lasers Surg. Med.*, 542 (2013).
13. Q. He, M. Ma, C. Wei, J. Shi, *Biomater.*, 4392 (2012).
14. T. P. Gustafson, Y. H. Lim, J. A. Flores, G. S. Heo, F. Zhang, S. Zhang, S. Samarajeewa, J. E. Raymond, K. L. Wooley, *Langmuir*, 631 (2014).
15. S. Santra, C. Kaittanis, J. M. Perez, *Mol. Pharmaceutics*, 1209 (2010).
16. K. Kim, J. H. Kim, H. Park, Y.-S. Kim, K. Park, H. Nam, S. Lee, J. H. Park, R.-W. Park, I.-S. Kim, K. Choi, S. Y. Kim, K. Park, I. C. Kwon, *J. Control. Release*, 219 (2010).
17. S. Santra, J. M. Perez, *Biomacromolecules*, 3917 (2011).
18. J. Y. Lee, D.-Y. Choi, M. Y. Cho, K. E. Park, S.-H. Lee, S. Hun Cho, K. S. Hong, Y. T. Lim, *Small*, 901 (2014).
19. E. A. Murphy, B. K. Majeti, L. A. Barnes, M. Makale, S. M. Weis, K. Lutu-Fuga, W. Wrasidlo, D. A. Cheresh, *Proc. Natl. Acad. Sci. USA.*, 9343 (2008).
20. X. He, M.-H. Na, J.-S. Kim, G.-Y. Lee, J. Y. Park, A. S. Hoffman, J.-O. Nam, S.-E. Han, G. Y. Sim, Y.-K. Oh, I.-S. Kim, B.-H. Lee, *Mol. Pharmaceutics*, 430 (2011).
21. C.-K. Huang, C.-L. Lo, H.-H. Chen, G.-H. Hsiue, *Adv. Funct. Mater.*, 2291 (2007).
22. B. S. Lee, K. Park, S. Park, G. C. Kim, H. J. Kim, S. Lee, H. Kil, S. J. Oh, D. Chi, K. Kim, K. Choi, I. C. Kwon, S. Y. Kim, *J. Control. Release*, 253 (2010).
23. S. Ferber, H. Baabur-Cohen, R. Blau, Y. Epshtein, E. Kisin-Finfer, O. Redy, D. Shabat, R. Satchi-Fainaro, *Cancer Lett.*, 81 (2014).

24. X. Wu, X. Sun, Z. Guo, J. Tang, Y. Shen, T. D. James, H. Tian, W. Zhu, *J. Am. Chem. Soc.*, 3579 (2014).
25. M. Frasconi, Z. Liu, J. Lei, Y. Wu, E. Strekalova, D. Malin, M. W. Ambrogio, X. Chen, Y. Y. Botros, V. L. Cryns, J.-P. Sauvage, J. F. Stoddart, *J. Am. Chem. Soc.,* 11603 (2013).
26. S. Li, B. Goins, L. Zhang, A. Bao, *Bioconjug. Chem.*, 1322 (2012).
27. R. Bleul, R. Thiermann, G. U. Marten, M. J. House, T. G. S. Pierre, U. O. Haefeli, M. Maskos, *Nanoscale*, 11385 (2013).
28. S. K. Patel, Y. Zhang, J. A. Pollock, J. M. Janjic, *PLoS One*, e55802 (2013).
29. M. W. Ambrogio, C. R. Thomas, Y.-L. Zhao, J. I. Zink, J. F. Stoddart, *Acc. Chem. Res.,* 903 (2011).
30. J.-H. Park, L. Gu, G. von Maltzahn, E. Ruoslahti, S. N. Bhatia, M. J. Sailor, *Nat. Mater.*, 331 (2009).
31. H. Chen, Z. Zhen, W. Tang, T. Todd, Y.-J. Chuang, L. Wang, Z. Pan, J. Xie, *Theranostics*, 650 (2013).
32. H. Wu, S. Zhang, J. Zhang, G. Liu, J. Shi, L. Zhang, X. Cui, M. Ruan, Q. He, W. Bu, *Adv. Funct. Mater.*, 1850 (2011).
33. A. P. Alivisatos, *Science*, 933 (1996).
34. A. M. Derfus, W. C. W. Chan, S. N. Bhatia, *Nano Lett.*, 11 (2004).
35. V. Bagalkot, L. Zhang, E. Levy-Nissenbaum, S. Jon, P. W. Kantoff, R. Langer, O. C. Farokhzad, *Nano Lett.*, 3065 (2007).
36. R. Savla, O. Taratula, O. Garbuzenko, T. Minko, *J. Control. Release*, 16 (2011).
37. R. Kumar, A. Kulkarni, D. K. Nagesha, S. Sridhar, *Theranostics*, 714 (2012).
38. C.-J. Wen, C. T. Sung, I. A. Aljuffali, Y.-J. Huang, J.-Y. Fang, *Nanotechnol.*, 325101 (2013).
39. H. Zhu, Y. Li, R. Qiu, L. Shi, W. Wu, S. Zhou, *Biomater.*, 3058 (2012).
40. Y. Chen, H.-R. Chen, S.-J. Zhang, F. Chen, L.-X. Zhang, J.-M. Zhang, M. Zhu, H.-X. Wu, L.-M. Guo, J.-W. Feng, J.-L. Shi, *Adv. Funct. Mater.*, 270 (2011).
41. D. J. Naczynski, M. C. Tan, R. E. Riman, P. V. Moghe, *J. Mater. Chem. B*, 2958 (2014).
42. R. J. Palmer, J. L. Butenhoff, J. B. Stevens, *Environ. Res.*, 142 (1987).
43. A. M. Derfus, W. C. W. Chan, S. N. Bhatia, *Nano Lett.*, 11 (2003).

44. Y. Sun, W. Feng, P. Yang, C. Huang, F. Li, *Chem. Soc. Rev.*, 1509 (2015).
45. L. Dong, D. An, M. Gong, Y. Lu, H.-L. Gao, Y.-J. Xu, S.-H. Yu, *Small*, 3235 (2013).
46. X. Zhai, M. Yu, Z. Cheng, Z. Hou, P.-A. Ma, D. Yang, X. Kang, Y. Dai, D. Wang, J. Lin, *Dalton Trans.*, 12818 (2011).
47. Y. Dai, C. Zhang, Z. Cheng, P. A. Ma, C. Li, X. Kang, D. Yang, J. Lin, *Biomater.*, 2583 (2012).
48. X. Kang, D. Yang, P. a. Ma, Y. Dai, M. Shang, D. Geng, Z. Cheng, J. Lin, *Langmuir*, 1286 (2013).
49. Z. Xu, Y. Gao, S. Huang, P. A. Ma, J. Lin, J. Fang, *Dalton Trans.*, 4846 (2011).
50. Z. Xu, P. A. Ma, C. Li, Z. Hou, X. Zhai, S. Huang, J. Lin, *Biomaterials*, 4161 (2011).
51. C. Chen, L. K. Yee, H. Gong, Y. Zhang, R. Xu, *Nanoscale*, 4314 (2013).
52. P. A. Ma, H. Xiao, X. Li, C. Li, Y. Dai, Z. Cheng, X. Jing, J. Lin, *Adv. Mater.*, 4898 (2013).
53. N. J. Farrer, J. A. Woods, L. Salassa, Y. Zhao, K. S. Robinson, G. Clarkson, F. S. Mackay, P. J. Sadler, *Angew. Chem. Int. Ed.*, 8905 (2010).
54. F. S. Mackay, J. A. Woods, P. Heringova, J. Kasparkova, A. M. Pizarro, S. A. Moggach, S. Parsons, V. Brabec, P. J. Sadler, *Proc. Natl. Acad. Sci. U. S. A.*, 20743 (2007).
55. Y. Min, J. Li, F. Liu, E. K. L. Yeow, B. Xing, *Angew. Chem. Int. Ed.*, 1012 (2014).
56. L. Zhou, Z. Li, Z. Liu, M. Yin, J. Ren, X. Qu, *Nanoscale*, 1445 (2014).
57. D. Yang, X. Kang, P. A. Ma, Y. Dai, Z. Hou, Z. Cheng, C. Li , J. Lin, *Biomater.*, 1601 (2013).
58. D. Yang, Y. Dai, P. A. Ma, X. Kang, Z. Cheng, C. Li, J. Lin, *Chem. — Eur. J.*, 2685 (2013).
59. Y. Yang, B. Velmurugan, X. Liu, B. Xing, *Small*, 2937 (2013).
60. J. Liu, W. Bu, L. Pan, J. Shi, *Angew. Chem. Int. Ed.*, 4375 (2013).
61. Y.-H. Chien, Y.-L. Chou, S.-W. Wang, S.-T. Hung, M.-C. Liau, Y.-J. Chao, C.-H. Su, C.-S. Yeh, *ACS Nano*, 8516 (2013).
62. W. Yin, G. Tian, W. Ren, L. Yan, S. Jin, Z. Gu, L. Zhou, J. Li, Y. Zhao, *Dalton Trans.*, 3861 (2014).

63. J.-N. Liu, W. Bu, L.-M. Pan, S. Zhang, F. Chen, L. Zhou, K.-L. Zhao, W. Peng, J. Shi, *Biomater.*, 7282 (2012).
64. J. Liu, J. Bu, W. Bu, S. Zhang, L. Pan, W. Fan, F. Chen, L. Zhou, W. Peng, K. Zhao, J. Du, J. Shi, *Angew. Chem. Int. Ed.*, 4551 (2014).
65. Y.-Y. Chen, P.-A. Ma, D.-M. Yang, Y. Wu, Y.-L. Dai, C.-X. Li, J. Lin, *Chem. -Asian J.*, 506 (2014).
66. C. Li, D. Yang, P. a. Ma, Y. Chen, Y. Wu, Z. Hou, Y. Dai, J. Zhao, C. Sui, J. Lin, *Small*, 4150 (2013).
67. Y. Dai, H. Xiao, J. Liu, Q. Yuan, P. A. Ma, D. Yang, C. Li, Z. Cheng, Z. Hou, P. Yang, J. Lin, *J. Am. Chem. Soc.*, 18920 (2013).
68. D. Yang, Y. Dai, J. Liu, Y. Zhou, Y. Chen, C. Li, P. A. Ma, J. Lin, *Biomater.*, 2011 (2014).
69. F. Zhang, G. B. Braun, A. Pallaoro, Y. Zhang, Y. Shi, D. Cui, M. Moskovits, D. Zhao, G. D. Stucky, *Nano Lett.*, 61 (2012).
70. B. Dubertret, M. Calame, A. J. Libchaber, *Nat. Biotechnol.*, 365 (2001).
71. S.-M. Lee, H. Park, K.-H. Yoo, *Adv. Mater.*, 4049 (2010).
72. A. Topete, M. Alatorre-Meda, P. Iglesias, E. M. Villar-Alvarez, S. Barbosa, J. A. Costoya, P. Taboada, V. Mosquera, *ACS Nano*, 2725 (2014).
73. Y.-D. Jin, X.-H. Gao, J. *Am. Chem. Soc.*, 17774 (2009).
74. H. Wang, Y. Wu, R. Zhao, G. Nie, *Adv. Mater.*, 1616 (2013).
75. J. Song, J. Zhou, H. Duan, *J. Am. Chem. Soc.*, 13458 (2012).
76. W. Wu, J. Shen, P. Banerjee, S. Zhou, *Biomater.*, 7555 (2010).
77. D. N. Heo, D. H. Yang, H.-J. Moon, J. B. Lee, M. S. Bae, S. C. Lee, W. J. Lee, I.-C. Sun, I. K. Kwon, *Biomater.*, 856 (2012).
78. B. Book Newell, Y. Wang, J. Irudayaraj, *Eur. J. Med. Chem.*, 330 (2012).
79. Z. Zhang, L. Wang, J. Wang, X. Jiang, X. Li, Z. Hu, Y. Ji, X. Wu, C. *Chen, Adv. Mater.*, 1418 (2012).
80. S. Pandey, M. Thakur, A. Mewada, D. Anjarlekar, N. Mishra, M. Sharon, *J. Mater. Chem. B*, 4972 (2013).
81. A. J. Cole, V. C. Yang, A. E. David, *Trends Biotechnol.*, 323 (2011).
82. M. Das, D. Mishra, P. Dhak, S. Gupta, T. K. Maiti, A. Basak, P. Pramanik, *Small*, 2883 (2009).
83. S. Santra, C. Kaittanis, J. Grimm, J. M. Perez, *Small*, 1862 (2009).
84. J. S. Basuki, H. T. T. Duong, A. MacMillan, R. B. Erlich, L. Esser, M. C. Akerfeldt, R. M. Whan, M. Kavallaris, C. Boyer, T. P. Davis, *ACS Nano*, 10175 (2013).

85. W. Chen, Y. Cao, M. Liu, Q. Zhao, J. Huang, H. Zhang, Z. Deng, J. Dai, D. F. Williams, Z. Zhang, *Biomater.*, 7895 (2012).
86. J. Zheng, G. Zhu, Y. Li, C. Li, M. You, T. Chen, E. Song, R. Yang, W. Tan, *ACS Nano*, 6545 (2013).
87. C. Li, T. Chen, I. Ocsoy, G. Zhu, E. Yasun, M. You, C. Wu, J. Zheng, E. Song, C. Z. Huang, W. Tan, *Adv. Funct. Mater.*, 1772 (2014).
88. G. Pratx, C. M. Carpenter, C. Sun, R. P. Rao, L. Xing, *Opt. Lett.*, 3345 (2010).
89. G. Pratx, C. M. Carpenter, C. Sun, L. Xing, *IEEE Trans. Med. Imaging*, 1992 (2010).
90. C. M. Carpenter, G. Pratx, C. Sun, L. Xing, *Phys. Med. Biol.*, 3487 (2011).
91. H. Chen, T. Moore, B. Qi, D. C. Colvin, E. K. Jelen, D. A. Hitchcock, J. He, O. T. Mefford, J. C. Gore, F. Alexis, J. N. Anker, *ACS Nano*, 1178 (2013).
92. H. Chen, B. Qi, T. Moore, F. Wang, D. C. Colvin, L. D. Sanjeewa, J. C. Gore, S.-J. Hwu, O. T. Mefford, F. Alexis, J. N. Anker, *Small*, 3364 (2014).
93. Y. Sun, W. Cao, S. Li, S. Jin, K. Hu, L. Hu, Y. Huang, X. Gao, Y. Wu, X.-J. Liang, *Sci. Rep.*, 3036 (2013).
94. S. N. Baker, G. A. Baker, *Angew. Chem. Int. Ed.*, 6726 (2010).
95. M. Zheng, S. Liu, J. Li, D. Qu, H. Zhao, X. Guan, X. Hu, Z. Xie, X. Jing, Z. Sun, *Adv. Mater.*, 3554 (2014).

CHAPTER 6

PLASMONIC NANOPARTICLES-COATED MICROBUBBLES FOR THERANOSTIC APPLICATIONS

Mark A. Borden*, Jacob D. Dove and Todd W. Murray†

Department of Mechanical Engineering,
University of Colorado
Campus Box 427, 1111 Engineering Drive, Boulder,
CO 80309, USA
**mark.borden@colorado.edu*
†todd.murray@colorado.edu

Nanoparticles that exhibit surface plasmon resonance can be harnessed for photoacoustic imaging and photothermal therapy. Recent research by our group has shown that arraying plasmonic nanoparticles around spherical gas-filled microbubbles can enhance the collective nanoparticle response for these applications. For photoacoustic imaging, the acoustic emission can be coupled to the microbubble resonance frequency for enhanced detection by clinical ultrasound scanners. For photothermal therapy, the nanoparticle heating can be coupled to a mechanical response of the microbubble, possibly enabling new modes of tissue ablation and drug delivery. This chapter reviews how to construct plasmonic microbubbles, as well as theoretical and experimental observations of their photothermal–mechanical properties and potential theranostic applications.

1. Introduction

Surface plasmon resonance occurs when the frequency of incident photons matches the natural frequency of surface electrons. Metal nanoparticles can be engineered to display surface plasmon resonance at specific optical wavelengths by manipulating their size, shape and composition.[1] The surface plasmon resonance effect of these so-called "plasmonic nanoparticles" can be harnessed to capture light energy and convert it to heat. There has been extensive work on the use of plasmonic nanoparticles as photoacoustic or photothermal contrast agents, as well as the targeting of these particles to specific biomarkers by conjugating them with antibodies or proteins.[2–10]

Photoacoustic imaging is an emerging modality that combines ultrasound with light to image optical contrast with high spatial resolution within optically diffuse media, such as biological tissue.[11,12] In this technique, a pulsed laser source is used to irradiate a region of tissue. The light follows a tortuous path as it scatters and propagates through the tissue; a process analogous to thermal diffusion. Absorption of laser light by subsurface tissue constituents leads to local heating, thermal expansion and acoustic wave generation through the "thermoelastic effect". The strength of the acoustic signal generated in a given region of tissue is directly proportional to the amount of light that is absorbed. The acoustic signal is detected on the tissue surface using an ultrasound transducer. The measured signals are then processed to produce an image of the subsurface optical absorption profile.

Photoacoustic imaging can exploit the large difference that exists in optical absorption between different tissue types. Hemoglobin, for example, is a strong optical absorber and thus photoacoustic imaging excels at imaging the vasculature. Photoacoustic imaging at multiple wavelengths can provide additional information. Blood oxygenation, for example, can be measured by taking advantage of the differences in the optical absorption spectra of oxyhaemoglobin and deoxyhaemoglobin.[13] In addition to endogeneous contrast, photoacoustic imaging with exogeneous contrast agents can lead to image enhancement and the ability to selectively image preferred regions of tissue. In combination with targeting strategies, these agents also allow for imaging of cellular or molecular events. A wide variety of photoacoustic contrast agents have been employed for photoacoustic imaging including gold nanospheres, nanorods and nanoshells, various dyes including indocyanine green and methylene blue, and carbon nanotubes.[14]

Photoacoustic and ultrasound imaging provide complementary information, with the former allowing for the detection of differences in optical absorption within tissue and the latter allowing for differences in acoustic impedance to be observed. In the case of ultrasound imaging, microbubbles have been shown to be effective contrast agents due to their compressible gas core and harmonic oscillations.[15,16] Microbubbles are generally comprised of a phospholipid and/or polymer shell filled with air or insoluble gas, with typical sizes in the 1–10 μm diameter range. The primary role of the shell is to stabilize the bubbles against dissolution in the blood by reducing the surface tension and providing a barrier for gas diffusion.[17] Microbubbles have been widely used for imaging of blood flow and analysis of perfusion in tissue in clinical and pre-clinical settings. As with photoacoustic contrast agents, microbubbles can be designed to carry a payload for molecular imaging, therapy, or multimodality imaging.[18–20]

Contrast agents for multimodality imaging are often composite structures, built of components that each show a strong response to a different imaging field. For example, microbubbles have been loaded with iron oxide or gadolinium to create a single construct providing contrast enhancement in both ultrasound and magnetic resonance imaging.[21,22] Similarly, microbubbles loaded with an optically absorbing dye or light absorbing particles can offer additional contrast in optical or photoacoustic imaging.[23,24] We have recently developed a facile approach for the fabrication of gold nanosphere-templated microbubbles that allows for control of the nanosphere placement and loading density, as well as microbubble size.[25,26] These microbubbles show an exceptionally large photoacoustic response while retaining the ultrasound contrast echogenicity of unloaded microbubbles. This chapter provides an overview of the microbubble fabrication and characterization procedures. In addition, theoretical model calculations and experimental results demonstrating contrast enhanced ultrasound and photoacoustic imaging are given, along with an experimental approach allowing one to probe individual microbubble responses to pulsed optical illumination using light extinction. We conclude with a discussion of future applications of nanoparticle-loaded microbubbles for imaging and therapy.

2. Plasmonic Microbubble Fabrication

The microbubbles can be fabricated using standard commercially available phospholipids, such as 1,2-distearoyl-sn-glycero-3-phosphocholine (DSPC), 1,2-distearyol-sn-glycero-3-phosphoethanolamine-N-[methoxy(polyethylene glycol)2000] (DSPE–PEG2000) and 1,2-distearoyl-sn-glycerol-3-phospho-ethanolamine-N[biotinyl (polyethylene glycol)-2000] (DSPE–PEG2000-B).[25] It is best to use a gas core comprising a very low solubility species, such as perfluorobutane (PFB).[19]

Microbubbles coated with DSPC: DSPE–PEG2000:DSPE–PEG2000-B at various molar ratios can be fabricated using probe sonication and size isolation techniques to the desired diameter range using differential centrifugation.[27] Briefly, the lipid solutions are placed in a sonicator to fully disperse the lipid solution and heat it above the phospholipid main phase transition temperature (~55°C for DSPC).[28] The sonicator tip is then raised to the liquid–gas interface and PFB gas is allowed to fill the head space. The solution is then sonicated at high power for 10 s to generate lipid-encapsulated microbubbles. The microbubbles are sized and counted by standard particle sizing techniques, such as electrical impedance volumetric zone sensing with a Beckman–Coulter Multisizer III. Note that we have found single-particle light extinction sizing methods to be less accurate owing to non-linear scattering effects.[29]

Size-isolation is performed with a standard bucket-rotor centrifuge. For example, the polydisperse microbubble solution can be centrifuged at 300 relative centrifuge force (RCF) for 5 min to separate the microbubbles from free lipid particles in solution. The polydisperse microbubbles are then size-selected through a three-step centrifuge process. First, microbubbles >4 μm are collected by centrifugation at 90 RCF for one min. The resulting cake is then re-suspended and centrifuged at 70 RCF for 1 min. The infranatant is collected, removing >5 μm microbubbles, and then centrifuged at 90 RCF to concentrate the remaining size-isolated microbubbles.

Biotin–streptavidin provides a simple nanoparticle-to-microbubble conjugation strategy for proof-of-concept. Many types of streptavidin-tagged nanoparticles can be purchased commercially. Other conjugation chemistries, such as maleimide-thiol, can also be used to load the nanoparticles onto the microbubble.[30] In the following sections, we review studies on 4 μm size-selected, biotin-functionalized microbubbles conjugated to 5–7 nm streptavidin–gold spheres. The microbubbles and nanoparticles are mixed for 2 h at a 1:1 ratio of biotin:avidin, where in this case one nanoparticle contains one avidin. After conjugation, the plasmonic microbubbles can be dispersed in phosphate buffer saline (PBS) and allowed to separate from unconjugated nanoparticles through gravitational flotation.

Figure 1(a) outlines the synthesis scheme for plasmonic microbubbles. Lipid-encapsulated PFB microbubbles are synthesized and size-selected to 4–5 μm diameter. The microbubble surface is functionalized with biotin, which binds to the avidin-tagged gold nanoparticles. Biotin–avidin is a straightforward approach to systematically study the effects of nanoparticle loading density. 5 nm gold spheres provide only one avidin per nanoparticle, which prevents cross-linking and aggregation during conjugation.

Figure 1(b) shows a typical size distribution of plasmonic microbubbles. The median diameter in this case was 3.9 μm, with 96.6% of the population between diameters of 2 μm and 8 μm. This correlated well with dark field microscopy, as shown in Figure 1(c). Verification of gold nanoparticle binding to the microbubble shell can be done with inductively coupled plasma mass spectrometry (ICP–MS),

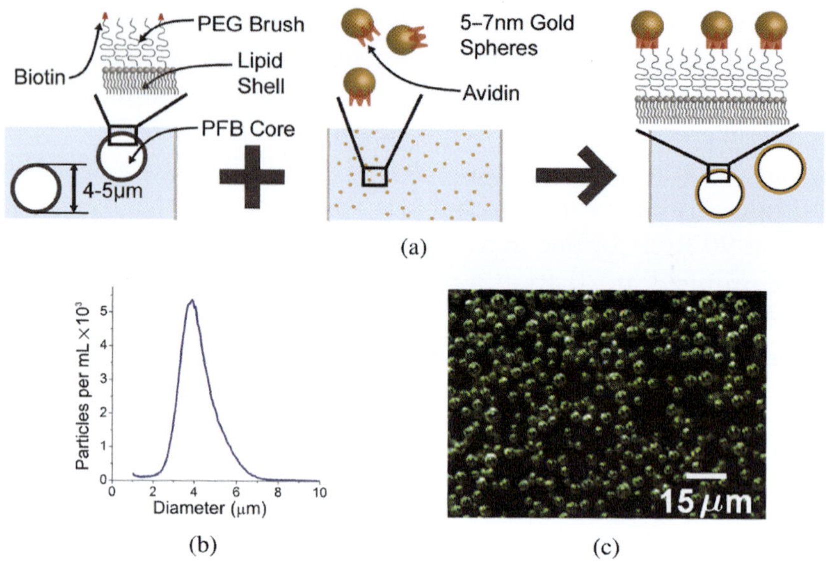

Fig. 1: (a) Schematic illustrating the conjugation scheme allowing for stoichiometric control over nanoparticle templating on microbubbles. (b) A typical size distribution measured after conjugation of nanoparticles to size-selected microbubbles with a 0.25% biotin mole fraction. (c) Dark field microscopy image of plasmonic microbubbles with a 0.25% biotin mole fraction. Taken from Dove *et al.*[25]

multi-photon luminescence microscopy and optical spectroscopy. For example, we estimate ~400,000 nanoparticles per 3-μm diameter microbubble.[25] The measured gold content increases linearly with biotin content up to saturation. It has been suggested that avidin contains two opposing faces, with two biotin binding pockets per face.[31] In our system, one avidin face was occupied by the gold nanosphere, while the other face exposed two free binding pockets to the biotin moieties on the microbubble surface.

3. Theory of Plasmonic Microbubble Oscillations

In this section, a model is presented where pulsed laser illumination causes a gold nanoparticle-coated microbubble to oscillate. There are three distinct physical processes that must occur in order for a pulsed laser source to drive a nanoparticle-coated bubble into oscillation. First, the optical pulse must be absorbed and converted into heat by the nanoparticle shell. Then the heat generated in the shell needs to diffuse into the gas core of the bubble. Lastly, the heated gas core must rapidly expand causing the bubble to oscillate once the laser pulse is terminated. Optical absorption by a nanoparticle is explained by Mie theory. The specific details of Mie theory have been omitted here as several reviews and texts have already covered the details.[32–34] Instead the focus is placed on pulsed laser heating of nanoparticles and nanoparticle-coated bubbles, and coupling the heated gas core into the dynamics of a bubble. First, pulsed laser heating of individual nanoparticles is examined. Then the model is expanded to a shelled bubble and the temperature rise in the gas core is calculated. Finally, the heated gas core is coupled into a modified Rayleigh–Plesset equation specific for lipid-shelled microbubbles.

3.1. *Photothermal response of a nanoparticle*

Nanoparticles efficiently convert the absorbed optical energy into heat, which then diffuses into the surrounding medium. Using linear heat transfer theory, a solution for the transient thermal field surrounding a nanoparticle can be obtained. The focus will be placed on spherical nanoparticles where an analytical solution exists. The heat equation for a gold nanosphere surrounded by a fluid can be represented in spherical coordinates (r, θ, φ) with angular symmetry and can be expressed as:

$$\frac{1}{r}\frac{\partial}{\partial r^2}\left(rT_L\right)=\frac{1}{\alpha_L}\frac{\partial T_L}{\partial t}, \tag{1}$$

$$\frac{1}{r}\frac{\partial}{\partial r^2}\left(rT_{NP}\right)-\frac{1}{\alpha_{NP}}\frac{\partial T_{NP}}{\partial t}=-\frac{Q(t)}{k_{NP}}. \tag{2}$$

Here, T is the temperature, α is the thermal diffusivity, k is the thermal conductivity and $Q(t)$ is the heating function. The subscripts, NP and L, represent the nanoparticle and the liquid, respectively. Because of the length and time scales involved in pulsed laser heating of nanoparticles, the heat transfer process is purely conductive and convection is neglected. This assumption is valid if the Grashof number is sufficiently small (Gr << 1). The Grashof number is a ratio of the buoyancy to viscous forces and scales by the 3rd power of the characteristic length. Using the nanoparticle radius (2.5 nm) as the characteristic length, the Grashof number is found to be << 1, allowing for convection to be neglected.

The heating function for pulsed laser illumination describes conversion of the optical absorption rate to the thermal power density (thermal energy per unit volume and time) within the nanoparticle. Because the quantum yield exhibited by metallic nanoparticles is very low (~10^{-6}) (i.e., the nanoparticle does not fluoresce), the conversion of optical absorption to heating can be assumed to be unity.[35] The form for the heating function can then be expressed as:

$$Q(t) = \frac{F_0 C_{abs}}{4/3\pi R_{NP}^3} g(t), \tag{3}$$

where F_0 is the fluence of the incident laser pulse, C_{abs} is the optical absorption coefficient calculated from Mie theory, R_{NP} is the radius of the nanoparticle, and $g(t)$ is the temporal profile of the pulsed laser having been normalized in time (i.e., the integrated temporal response represents unity). Here, $F_0 C_{abs}$ is the amount of optical energy the nanoparticle can absorb, which is distributed over the nanoparticle volume to give an absorbed energy density. The temporal profile of the pulsed laser can be described as:[36]

$$g(t) = 2\frac{t^3}{\tau_p^4} e^{-\left(\frac{t}{\tau_p}\right)^2}. \tag{4}$$

Here, τ_p is the pulse width. The boundary conditions at the gold–liquid interface are continuous temperature and heat flux and are expressed as:

$$T_L |_{r=R_{NP}} = T_{NP} |_{r=R_{NP}}, \tag{5}$$

$$k_L \frac{\partial T_L}{\partial r}\bigg|_{r=R_{NP}} = k_{NP} \frac{\partial T_{NP}}{\partial r}\bigg|_{r=R_{NP}}. \tag{6}$$

The temperature of the nanoparticle and liquid are initially equal to the ambient temperature (T_0) before the optical pulse arrives:

$$T_L\,|_{t=0} = T_{NP}\,|_{t=0} = T_0. \tag{7}$$

For convenience, the substitution, $\theta = T - T_0$, can be used such that the initial condition is $\theta = 0$ at $t = 0$. To solve Eqs. (1) and (2), integral transform techniques are used. Here, the Laplace transform is used to transform the time domain into the *s*-domain:

$$\frac{\partial}{\partial r^2}\left(r\tilde{\theta}_L\right) - r\left(\frac{s}{\alpha_L}\right)\tilde{\theta}_L = 0 \tag{8}$$

$$\frac{\partial^2}{\partial r^2}\left(r\tilde{\theta}_{NP}\right) - r\left(\frac{s}{\alpha_{NP}}\right)\tilde{\theta}_{NP} = -\frac{r\tilde{Q}(s)}{k_{NP}}, \tag{9}$$

where, the tilde marks the Laplace transformed temperature.
The functional form of the *q*-switched laser pulse provided in Eq. (4) does not have an explicit Laplace transform. Therefore, a slightly different functional form for the temporal profile of laser pulse will be used as described below:

$$\hat{g}(t) = \frac{5^7}{6!}\frac{t^6}{\tau^7}e^{-\left(\frac{5t}{\tau}\right)}. \tag{10}$$

The difference in pulse shape obtained using Eq. (10) instead of (4) is minor. The Laplace transform of the heating function can be expressed as:

$$\tilde{Q}(s) = \frac{5^7}{6!}\frac{F_0 C_{\text{abs}}}{4/3\pi R_{NP}^3}(5 + s\tau)^{-7}. \tag{11}$$

Applying the boundary conditions, Eqs. (5) and (6), to Eqs. (8) and (9) with the condition that as *r* approaches zero the temperature must be defined (i.e., not approach infinity), the transient thermal field in the surrounding liquid and inside the nanoparticle takes the form:

$$\tilde{\theta}_L(r,s) = \frac{\tilde{Q}(s)}{k_{NP} p_{NP}^2} \frac{R_{NP}}{r} \frac{\left[\sinh(p_{NP}R_{NP}) - p_{NP}R_{NP}\cosh(p_{NP}R_{NP})\right] e^{-p_L(r-R_{NP})}}{(1+p_L R_{NP}) M(s)}, \tag{12}$$

$$\tilde{\theta}_{NP}(r,s) = \frac{\tilde{Q}(s)}{k_{NP} p_{NP}^2}\left[1 + \frac{k_L}{k_p}\frac{R\sinh(p_{NP}r)}{rM(s)}\right], \tag{13}$$

where

$$M(s) = \frac{\sinh(p_{NP}R_{NP}) - p_{NP}R_{NP}\cosh(p_{NP}R_{NP})}{1 + p_L R_{NP}} - \frac{k_L}{k_{NP}}\sinh(p_{NP}R_{NP}), \tag{14}$$

$$p_{NP} = \sqrt{\frac{s}{\alpha_{NP}}}, \tag{15}$$

$$p_L = \sqrt{\frac{s}{\alpha_L}}. \tag{16}$$

The time domain solution can be obtained through a numerical Laplace inversion of Eqs. (12) and (13). Using this solution the optical heating provided by a nanoparticle can be examined and coupled to the oscillations of a nanoparticle-coated microbubble.

3.2. *Photothermal response of a nanoparticle-coated gas bubble*

The photothermal heating of a nanoparticle-coated bubble can now be considered. Here, it is assumed that the gold nanoparticles coat the bubble at a high surface density, such that the problem can be simplified to a thin shell of gold surrounding a bubble submersed in water. The equations governing heat diffusion are expressed as:

$$\frac{1}{r}\frac{\partial}{\partial r^2}\left(rT_g\right)=\frac{1}{\alpha_g}\frac{\partial T_g}{\partial t}, \tag{17}$$

$$\frac{1}{r}\frac{\partial}{\partial r^2}\left(rT_S\right)-\frac{1}{\alpha_{NP}}\frac{\partial T_S}{\partial t}=-\frac{Q(t)}{k_{NP}}, \tag{18}$$

$$\frac{1}{r}\frac{\partial}{\partial r^2}\left(rT_L\right)=\frac{1}{\alpha_L}\frac{\partial T_L}{\partial t}, \tag{19}$$

where the subscripts, g, S and L represent the gas, shell and liquid, respectively. The heating function $Q(t)$ now represents the thermal power distributed throughout the shell volume and can be represented as:

$$Q(t)=\frac{E_{\text{abs}}}{4\pi R_g^2 R_S}\hat{g}(t), \tag{20}$$

where R_g is the radius of the gas bubble, the shell thickness is equal the diameter of the nanoparticle (here it is assumed $R_{NP} << R_g$) and E_{abs} is the amount of absorbed optical energy. Assuming the nanoparticles coat the bubble with a surface density ρ_{Load}, the absorbed optical energy can be expressed as:

$$E_{\text{abs}} = F_0 C_{\text{abs}} \rho_{\text{Load}} 4\pi R_g^2. \tag{21}$$

Combing Eqs. (20) and (21) gives:

$$Q(t)=\frac{F_0 C_{\text{abs}} \rho_{\text{Load}}}{2R_{NP}}\hat{g}(t). \tag{22}$$

The heating function for a nanoparticle-templated microbubble is found to scale with nanoparticle loading density, ρ_{Load}, and is independent of bubble size.

The boundary conditions are the continuity of temperature and heat flux across the interfaces, and are expressed as:

$$T_g \big|_{r=R_g} = T_S \big|_{r=R_g}, \tag{23}$$

$$T_S \big|_{r=R_g+2R_{NP}} = T_L \big|_{r=R_g+2R_{NP}}, \tag{24}$$

$$k_g \left.\frac{\partial T_g}{\partial r}\right|_{r=R_g} = k_S \left.\frac{\partial T_S}{\partial r}\right|_{r=R_g}, \tag{25}$$

$$k_S \left.\frac{\partial T_S}{\partial r}\right|_{r=R_g+2R_{NP}} = k_L \left.\frac{\partial T_L}{\partial r}\right|_{r=R_g+2R_{NP}}. \tag{26}$$

The Laplace transform is used to solve Eqs. (17)–(19). The solutions for the transformed temperatures of the gas, shell and liquid can be expressed in the Laplace domain (using the substitution, $\theta = T - T_0$) as:

$$\tilde{\theta}_g(r,s) = \frac{1}{r} A_1 \sinh\left(p_g r\right), \tag{27}$$

$$\tilde{\theta}_S(r,s) = \frac{1}{r}\left[A_2 \sinh\left(p_S r\right) + A_3 \cosh\left(p_S r\right)\right] + \frac{\tilde{Q}(s)}{k_2 p_L^2}, \tag{28}$$

$$\tilde{\theta}_g(r,s) = \frac{1}{r} A_4 e^{-(p_L r)}, \tag{29}$$

$$p_S = \sqrt{\frac{s}{\alpha_{NP}}}, \tag{30}$$

$$p_g = \sqrt{\frac{s}{\alpha_g}}. \tag{31}$$

Applying the boundary conditions, Eqs. (23)–(26), to Eqs. (27)–(29), the unknowns, A_1, A_2, A_3 and A_4 can be found. The time domain solution for pulsed laser heating of a shelled bubble can be obtained through use of a numerical Laplace inversion. The maximum temperature rise was observed to occur at the gas–shell interface. Similar to a nanoparticle, heat dissipates into the surrounding medium immediately. Due to the order of magnitude difference in thermal diffusivities, heat can propagate into the gas core more quickly than in water.

The total thermal energy delivered to the gas can be calculated by considering the temperature gradient created in the gas core. Essentially, the presence of the heated shell creates a heat flux into the gas that can be expressed as:

$$q(t) = -k_g \left. \frac{\partial T_g(r,t)}{\partial r} \right|_{r=R_g}. \tag{32}$$

The total heat flux can be integrated over time to quantify the thermal energy delivered, W, to the gas core:

$$W(t) = \int_0^t 4\pi R_g^2 q(t)\, dt. \tag{33}$$

The heat flux follows the optical pulse profile, with the majority of heat delivered within the first few nanoseconds. At later times, heat transfer from the gas core occurs into the surrounding medium, which results in a negative heat flux. Note the initial heat flux into the bubble (heat generation) is orders of magnitude greater than the heat flux out of the bubble (cooling), but the timescales associated with cooling are orders of magnitude longer than the heating. Taking into account the heat capacity of the gas, the average temperature of the gas core, T_B, can be calculated:

$$T_B(t) = \frac{W(t)}{C_{p,g}} \left(\frac{BT_0}{P_{e,g} 4\pi R_g^3} \right), \tag{34}$$

where, $C_{p,g}$ is the specific heat of the gas, $P_{e,g}$ is the pressure of the gas core when the bubble is at rest, T_0 is the temperature of the gas core, and B is the ideal gas constant. It should be noted that this is a simplification that ignores the time scales associated with heat diffusion within the gas core (there is no dependence on r). However, the estimates for the thermal energy delivered to the gas core are still correct. This model gives a rough first approximation of the temperature rise in the gas core for a nanoparticle-coated bubble illuminated with a pulsed laser.

3.3. *Photothermal oscillations of a gas bubble*

3.3.1. *Modified rayleigh–plesset model for a heated bubble*

The dynamic response of the gas bubble to a pulsed laser will now be examined. As the gas core of the bubble heats up, the volume increases, thus driving bubble oscillation. The pressure of the gas core at equilibrium can be expressed as:

$$P_{g,e} = P_0 + \frac{2\sigma}{R_0}, \tag{35}$$

where, P_0 is the ambient hydrostatic pressure of the liquid, σ is the surface tension of the gas liquid interface and R_0 is the resting radius of the gas bubble (equal to R_g in the sections describing bubble heating). Eq. (35) is the Laplace equation which describes the increase in pressure due to a curved surface in tension. Assuming the gas obeys the ideal gas law, the pressure of the gas core during laser heating can be expressed as:

$$P_g(t) = \frac{nBT_g(t)}{V(t)}, \tag{36}$$

where, n is the number of moles of the gas, B is the ideal gas constant and V is the volume of the gas core. The use of the ideal gas law is only valid for timescales much slower than the heat diffusion through the gas core. Given the time and length scales associated with laser heating, the gas is not expected to behave ideally. However, to a first approximation the ideal gas law is used, and an average temperature increase in the gas can be calculated to estimate a pressure increase. Assuming the gas is not diffusing into or out of the core, this quantity can be related to the state of the bubble at equilibrium through the following expression:

$$P_g(t) = P_{g,e}\left(\frac{V_0}{V(t)}\right)\left(\frac{T(t)}{T_0}\right). \tag{37}$$

Combining Eqs. (37) and (35), the pressure of the liquid, P_L, just surrounding the bubble can be expressed as:

$$P_L(t) = P_{g,e}\left(\frac{R_0}{R}\right)^3\left(\frac{T(t)}{T_0}\right) - \frac{2\sigma}{R}. \tag{38}$$

Here, R has been introduced as the time dependent radius of the bubble. Combining the previous expressions, we have:

$$P_L(t) = \left(P_0 + \frac{2\sigma}{R_0}\right)\left(\frac{R_0}{R}\right)^3\left(\frac{T(t)}{T_0}\right) - \frac{2\sigma}{R}. \tag{39}$$

While the bubble is oscillating, there is a restoring force due to the shell elasticity. In addition, there are viscous losses in both the surrounding fluid and the shell. Balancing the normal stresses at the interface results in the following expression:[37]

$$P_g(t) - P_L(t) = 4\chi\left(\frac{1}{R_0} - \frac{1}{R}\right) + 4\mu\frac{\dot{R}}{R} + 4\kappa_s\frac{\dot{R}}{R^2}. \tag{40}$$

Here, the χ is the shell elasticity, μ is the viscosity of the liquid, κ_s is the viscosity in the shell and the dot represents a derivative with respect to time. The Rayleigh–Plesset equation models the dynamics of an oscillating spherical gas bubble and is described as:[38,39]

$$\frac{P_L(t) - P_0}{\rho_L} = \frac{3\dot{R}^2}{2} + R\ddot{R}, \tag{41}$$

where ρ_L is the density of the liquid. Combining the previous expressions, the dynamic response of a heated gas bubble is:

$$\frac{3\dot{R}^2}{2} + R\ddot{R} = \frac{1}{\rho_L}\left[\begin{array}{l}\left(P_0 + \frac{2\sigma}{R_0}\right)\left(\frac{R_0}{R}\right)^3\left(\frac{T(t)}{T_0}\right) - P_0 - 4\chi\left(\frac{1}{R_0} - \frac{1}{R}\right)\\ -4\mu\frac{\dot{R}}{R} - 4\kappa_s\frac{\dot{R}}{R^2}\end{array}\right]. \tag{42}$$

This equation can be solved using a finite-difference numerical approach. The initial conditions are:

$$R = R_0 \,|_{t=0}, \tag{43}$$

$$\dot{R} = 0 \,|_{t=0}\,. \tag{44}$$

Using the expression for the temperature of the gas bubble, the dynamic response of a bubble to a pulsed laser heating can be examined.

3.3.2. *Dynamic response of a pulsed laser heated bubble*

The transient response of a bubble due to pulsed laser heating is shown in Figure 2(a). Here, the ambient pressure was 1 atm (0.83 bar in Boulder, CO), ρ_L was 1,000 kg/m^3, μ was 8.9×10^{-4} Pa*s, χ was 1.0 N/m, κ_s was 5×10^{-9} kg/s, σ was assumed to be negligible and T_0 was 298 K. The heating, $T(t)$, is shown in Figure 2(b) and was calculated with an optical pulse width of 1 ns and a fluence of 1 mJ/cm^2. Here, the amplitude of the bubble oscillations are shown as radial displacement where 0 corresponds to the resting radius of the bubble. Initially, the bubble expands due to the heated gas core reaching the maximum radial displacement on the first oscillation. Due to viscous losses in the shell and liquid the subsequent oscillations decay over time. The oscillation frequency increases as bubble size is decreased. In addition, the amplitude of the radial oscillations increases with increasing bubble diameter. These features will be studied in more detail below.

The resonant frequency, which was measured by performing a Fourier transform on the time-domain response, is plotted in Figure 2(c). In addition, the eigenfrequency (undamped natural frequency) is plotted and is related to the resonant frequency by the following expression:

$$\omega_0 = \frac{\omega_r}{\sqrt{1-\varsigma^2}}. \tag{45}$$

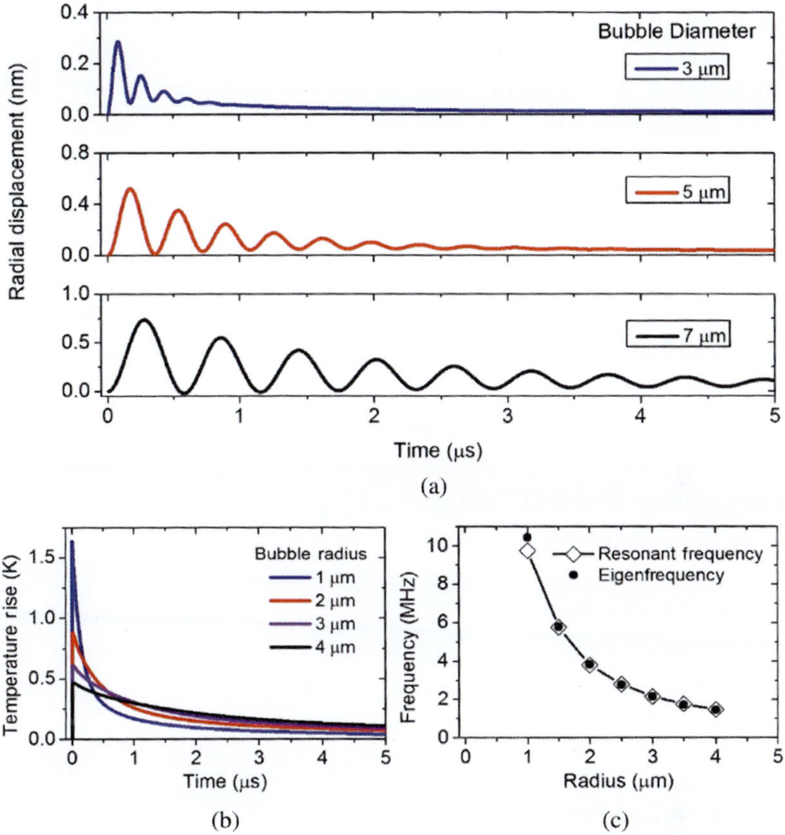

Fig. 2: (a) The transient response of a bubble (diameter of 3, 5, and 7 μm) to pulsed laser illumination. (b) The transient temperature rise in the gas core for bubbles with different radii (c) The resonant frequency, open diamonds, of the bubble oscillations and eigenfrequency, black circles, are plotted as a function of bubble radius.

The eigenfrequency can be found by linearizing Eq. (42) for small amplitude fluctuations, $x(t)$, about the resting radius R_0 ($R = x(t)+R_0$), such that the dynamic motion of the bubble wall can be expressed as a second-order system. The eigenfrequency from the linearized model can be expressed as:

$$f_0 = \frac{1}{2\pi}\sqrt{\frac{1}{\rho_L R_0^2}\left(3P_0 + \frac{4(\sigma + \chi)}{R_0}\right)}. \tag{46}$$

Comparing the predicted eigenfrequencies (Eq. (46)) from the linearized model to the resonant frequency of the time-domain response, the differences are close to those predicted by Eq. (45).

The result that the resonant frequencies fall into the low megahertz regime is important. The acoustic attenuation of tissue is frequency dependent, with high frequencies receiving more attenuation. An optically driven bubble produces a strong response in the low megahertz regime, where acoustic attenuation is minimal. This is a promising result for deep tissue imaging. In addition, the importance of a monomodal size distribution is evident. The signal-to-noise ratio may be improved by minimizing destructive interference effects from bubbles with different radii by utilizing a population of bubbles with similar sizes. Here, the photoacoustic emission from similar sized bubbles (spaced less than half a wavelength away $c_s/2f_0$, where c_s is the speed of sound in water) will sum coherently leading to an improved photoacoustic response from the population of bubbles.

As the bubble diameter is increased, the amplitude of the oscillations increases as shown in Figure 2(a). This is in contrast to the maximum temperature the gas core reaches, which decreases as bubble size increases as shown in Figure 2(b).

3.3.3. *Influence of the heating function*

The temporal profile of the heating function influences the response of a bubble. To understand the impact of the heating function on bubble response two limiting cases, an impulse heating function and a step rise in temperature, are studied.

In the case of the step increase in temperature, the maximum radial displacement increases with bubble radius. Following the ideal gas law ($V/V_0 = T/T_0$), it is apparent that given a constant increase in temperature, the larger the bubble, the larger the change in radius. For an impulse heating function, the maximum radial displacement decreases with increasing radius. Here, the bubble response follows a similar trend to the maximum temperature rise in the gas core (i.e., the amplitude of the forcing function). In this regime, all the heating occurs before bubbles complete one oscillation.

3.3.4. *Influence of shell properties on bubble dynamics*

The dynamic response of the bubble wall radius depends on the properties of the encapsulating shell. From Eq. (42), the shell viscosity, κ_s, influences the damping of the bubble oscillations. As the shell viscosity increases, e.g., from 0 to 1×10^{-8} kg/s, the settling time for the bubble response decreases. The resonance peak does not shift in frequency but broadens as shell viscosity is increased. The quality factor ($Q = f_0/\Delta f$), which is related to the damping ratio, $Q = 1/2\zeta$, is a measure of the stored energy over the dissipated energy. A resonator with a high Q factor will undergo more oscillations than a resonator with a lower Q factor. As shell viscosity is increased, the Q factor of the bubble is lowered. Considering an optically driven bubble as a photoacoustic contrast agent, the higher the Q factor the more acoustic power is radiated from bubble. Hence, an encapsulating shell that minimizes viscous losses would be ideal.

The shell elasticity, χ, adds an additional restoring force causing the eigenfrequency to shift to higher values. As a result of the changing elasticity, the resonance frequency shifts. The resonance peak shifts from 1.08 MHz to 2.76 MHz as the shell elasticity is increased from 0 N/m to 1.0 N/m, respectively. This is an important result, as populations of bubbles that all have exactly a 2.5 μm radius but exhibit variations in shell elasticity will produce a photoacoustic response over a wide frequency band. It would be beneficial to minimize the variations in shell elasticity such that photoacoustic emission is over a narrow bandwidth, and destructive interference effects are minimized.

4. Experimental Observations of Optically Induced Resonance

We have recently developed a convenient method to measure the dynamic response of individual nanoparticle-templated microbubbles.[26] The experimental setup, shown in Figure 3(a), consists of a modified dark-field optical microscope with three optical ports housing a pulsed excitation laser, a continuous wave probe laser, and a CCD camera. The microbubbles were held between a microscope slide

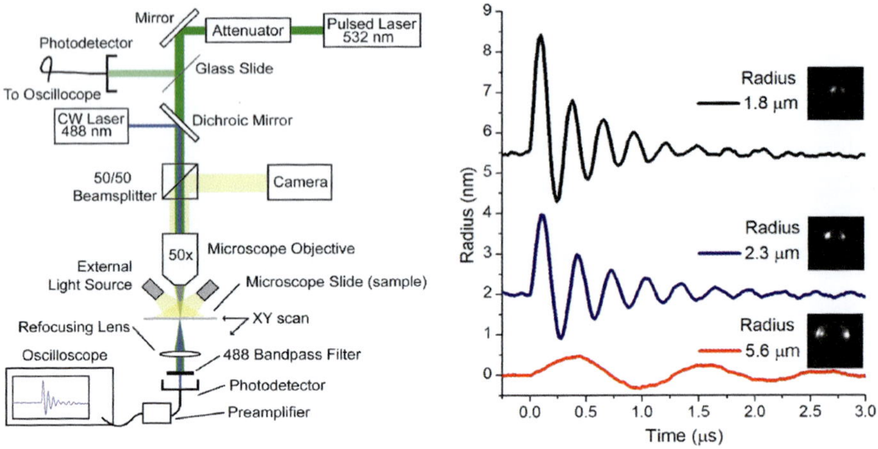

(a) (b)

Fig. 3: (a) The experimental setup used to measure the dynamic response of individual microbubbles and (b) the time domain responses of gold-coated microbubbles to pulsed laser excitation for different microbubble sizes. The dark field images of the microbubbles are shown above the measured responses. Taken from Dove *et al.*[26]

and cover slip and placed in the focal plane of a 50× long working distance objective. A pulsed microchip laser with a wavelength of 532 nm was used to excite microbubbles into resonant oscillations. The laser had a pulse width of 1.5 ns and a repetition rate of 3.0 kHz. The spot size of the excitation beam at the focal plane of the objective was 30 μm and a variable attenuator was used to adjust the laser fluence to approximately 4.5 mJ/cm^2.

The dynamic microbubble response was found using forward light scattering using a continuous wave laser operating at a wavelength of 488 nm. The beam is sent through the same 50× objective to the microbubble surface. The optical power was 2.4 mW and the spot size was approximately 20 μm. The transmitted and forward scattered light is collected using a lens, and directed through a 488 nm band-pass filter to a photodiode. The photodiode output is sent through an amplifier to an oscilloscope where the signal is digitized. The third optical port on the microscope houses a CCD camera. The camera is used to locate, position, and size microbubbles within the field of view of the microscope.

The basic principle used in the detection of microbubble oscillations is straightforward. The light at the detector decreases due to optical scattering when a microbubble is positioned at the center of the detection probe, and this decrease in detected light depends on the microbubble size. In order to calibrate our system, we measured the change in optical power at the photodetector as a function of microbubble radius in the static case. The slope of this curve gives the sensitivity of the measurement system (in units of mW/μm) as a function of microbubble resting radius R_0. The absolute sensitivity is found to increase with microbubble size. We assume that the detection system is linear for small amplitude oscillations about the resting radius. For a given microbubble size, the dynamic power changes measured at the photodetector when a microbubble is stimulated using the pulsed laser source can thus be converted to microbubble displacement by simply dividing by the sensitivity.

For the experimental measurements, a microbubble was first located within the field of view of the darkfield microscope. The position and size of the microbubble were determined through analysis of the dark-field image, and a computer controlled positioning stage was then used to move the microbubble to the center of the probe beam. The microbubble was excited by the pulsed laser and the optical response at the photodetector was recorded and converted to displacement. The results of these experiments for three microbubbles of radius R = 1.8, 2.3 and 5.6 μm are shown in Figure 3(b), where the optical images used to determine the microbubble radii are also provided. Note that the signals are artificially offset for ease of viewing. The signals were averaged 130,000 times (at a repetition rate of 200 Hz, limited by the oscilloscope) reducing the *RMS* noise-equivalent displacement level to 35 pm and 14 pm for 1.8 μm and 5.6 μm microbubbles, respectively. The uncertainty in the measurement of oscillation amplitude is a function of bubble radius and ranged from 5% to 9% of the measured value for bubble radii in the 1–6 μm range. The primary error sources are those associated with the calibration procedure, error in bubble radius determination and random noise in the measurement.

The stimulation of microbubble oscillation using a pulsed laser source is clearly demonstrated, and the oscillation frequency increases with decreasing bubble size as expected (Figure 2). The mechanism through which the pulsed laser drives microbubbles into oscillation is believed to be photothermal, as predicted by the theory presented above. Note that oscillations were not observed on bubbles without nanoparticle loading, nor were they observed when the microbubbles were excited at an optical wavelength of 1064 nm (where gold nanospheres have weak absorption).

The all-optical platform is very attractive for the study of microbubble physics and lipid mechanics, so long as an optically absorbing species is incorporated onto the microbubble shell. The approach combines displacement sensitivity (with signal averaging) in the tens of picometer range with micron scale spatial resolution. We have found that the microbubbles are exceptionally stable under laser irradiation at low laser fluence (<5 mJ/cm^2), with the bubble size and dynamic response remaining constant over hundreds of thousands of laser shots. At higher laser fluence ($\sim$10–20 mJ/cm^2), other effects were observed including changes in the microbubble size or complete dissolution. One limitation in the current experimental approach is that the measured bubbles are in contact with the bottom surface of the glass cover slip, and the presence of this surface may affect the dynamic response. One may be able to circumvent this limitation by using, for example, optical tweezers to translate the bubbles a sufficient distance from the boundary for the measurement.[40]

5. Dual Modality Imaging

The measurements on individual nanoparticle-loaded microbubbles demonstrate that the plasmonic microbubbles can be excited using a pulsed laser source. In addition, strong oscillations were observed at the microbubble resonance frequency. In this section, we explore the optical and acoustic responses of nanoparticle template microbubble populations with an aim towards using them as dual modality (ultrasound + photoacoustic) contrast agents.

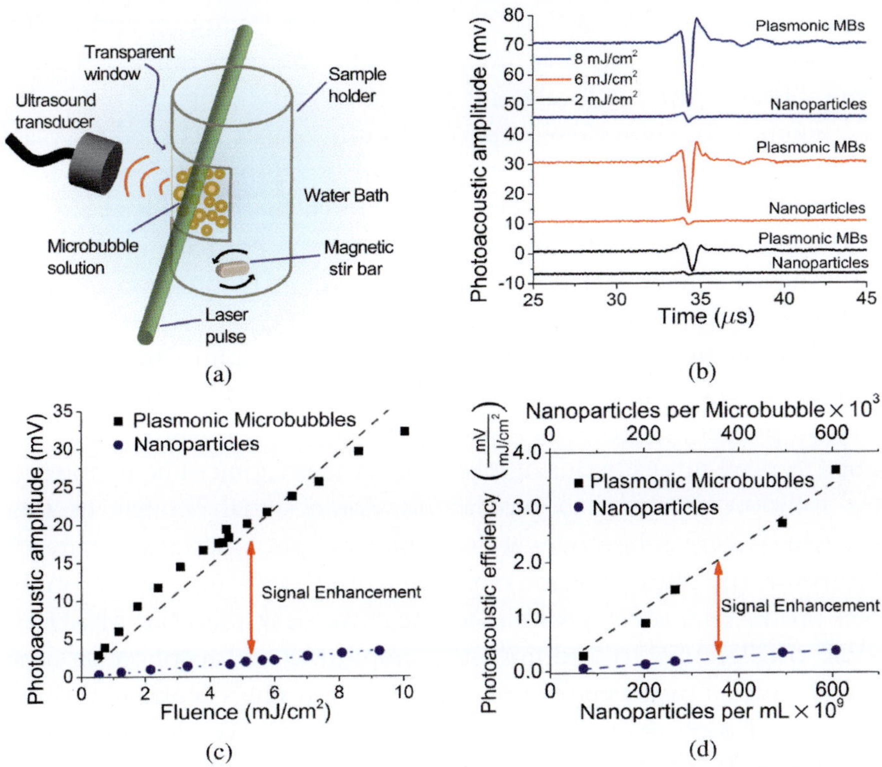

Fig. 4: (a) A schematic outlining the experimental approach to measure the photoacoustic response. (b) Signal averaged (100 times) photoacoustic waveforms from Plasmonic microbubbles at a 0.75% biotin mole fraction, and nanoparticles at the same concentration illuminated with laser fluences of 2, 6 and 8 mJ/cm^2. (c) Peak-to-peak amplitude of the photoacoustic waveforms recorded at varying fluences for the same Plasmonic microbubbles and nanoparticles. (d) Photoacoustic efficiency for varying the number of nanoparticles per microbubble and nanoparticles at the same concentration for all five biotin mole fractions. Taken from Dove *et al.*[25]

The experimental apparatus for measuring the photoacoustic response from the plasmonic microbubbles is shown in Figure 4(a). To characterize the response at varying laser fluences, 25 mL of the plasmonic microbubbles (at a concentration of 10^6 mL^{-1}) were held in a plastic vial with acoustically and optically transparent windows. The solution was continually mixed while subjected to pulsed laser illumination. The laser source had a wavelength of 532 nm and a pulse width of 5 ns. The photoacoustic signals were detected with an ultrasound transducer with a 2.25 MHz center frequency and a 50.8 mm focal length. The transducer was aligned perpendicular to the optical beam, with the focal point positioned at the center of the beam.

Figure 4(b) shows typical photoacoustic signals recorded for plasmonic microbubbles with a biotin mole fraction of 0.75% at laser fluences of 2, 6 and 8 mJ/cm^2. Also shown in Figure 4(b) are the photoacoustic signals measured from free nanoparticles in solution, with the same nanoparticle concentration as for the plasmonic microbubbles. The photoacoustic signals were delayed with respect to laser illumination by approximately 33.8 μs, corresponding to the ultrasound propagation time from the focal position to the transducer. The amplitude, given in mV and proportional to pressure, is analogous to pixel intensity during photoacoustic imaging. The nanoparticle solution produced a bipolar ultrasonic signal, similar to that expected from a homogeneous cylindrical photoacoustic source.[41] However, the photoacoustic emission from the plasmonic microbubbles produced a more pronounced negative peak followed by several weak oscillations. In addition, the amplitude of the photoacoustic signal emitted by plasmonic microbubbles was consistently higher, by a factor of 8–9, than that of free nanoparticles. We also noted that photoacoustic experiments on microbubbles alone yielded a response below the noise level due to the lack of optical absorption, while experiments on mixtures of unconjugated microbubbles and free nanoparticles produced a photoacoustic response similar to that of free nanoparticles alone.

Figure 4(c) shows the peak-to-peak amplitudes of the photoacoustic signals as a function of fluence over the 0.5–10 mJ/cm^2 range, with the dotted line showing a linear fit to the data. The free nanoparticles showed a linear increase in signal amplitude with fluence. The plasmonic microbubbles showed some deviations from linearity, with a larger increase in photoacoustic amplitude at lower fluences. The slope of the linear fits in Figure 4(c) provided a measure of the photoacoustic efficiency, giving the photoacoustic signal amplitude achievable for a given laser fluence. Figure 4(d) shows the photoacoustic efficiency for all five biotin mole fractions of plasmonic microbubbles and the corresponding free nanoparticle solutions at the same gold content. In both cases, the efficiency was found to be proportional to the overall nanoparticle concentration. However, the efficiency was 8.9-fold higher for plasmonic microbubbles than free nanoparticles.

The increase in signal amplitude and efficiency is explained by a coupling between the gold nanoparticles and the compressible microbubble gas core, as described above. With a spatially confined photoacoustic source (small with respect to the acoustic wavelength) the photoacoustic response is expected to be dictated by the total nanoparticle concentration, leading to similar responses for the plasmonic microbubbles and nanoparticles. However, the fact that the nanoparticles are arrayed around a compressible gas core may provide enhancement through photoacoustic or photothermal coupling to the microbubble itself (i.e., that microbubble oscillation is driven by optical illumination). As the microbubble resonance (1.5–3 MHz for microbubble diameters of 4–6 μm)[42] falls within the frequency band of the detection transducer (2.25 MHz center frequency), optically driven microbubbles would act to focus the broadband excitation frequencies to those within the detection band, providing an enhancement.[43] Further evidence of coupling is provided from the fact that the shape of the photoacoustic signal of the plasmonic microbubbles differs from that of the free nanoparticles.

Our results indicate that plasmonic microbubbles may have the potential to be a powerful multi-modal contrast agent, producing signal enhancement in both ultrasound and photoacoustic imaging.[25] To demonstrate this, we performed *in vitro* multimodal imaging in an agarose tissue phantom. The phantom was fabricated with a 2.3 mm diameter cylindrical channel to accommodate the flow of microbubbles and nanoparticles. We first compared the photoacoustic response of nanoparticles, microbubbles and plasmonic microbubbles under a laser fluence of 10 mJ/cm^2. Here the concentration of nanoparticles was 1.33×10^{13} mL^{-1}, approximately 15 times the nanoparticle concentration in the plasmonic microbubbles. The concentration of microbubbles was 10^6 mL^{-1}, identical to the concentration of plasmonic microbubbles. The photoacoustic image was formed by aligning the detection transducer to the center of the channel and scanning the sample about the transducer focal plane, creating an image of the axial cross section of the channel. At each spatial position, the maximum intensity of the photoacoustic signal was captured and plotted to produce an image. All signals were digitally filtered to suppress frequencies below 2 MHz and above 8 MHz.

The results of this experiment are shown in Figures 5(a)–5(c). The nanoparticle solution alone produced a weak photoacoustic response localized to the region of the tube, as shown in the image (Figure 5(a)). Microbubbles alone did not produce a detectable photoacoustic response, as expected, due to the lack of optical absorption (Figure 5(b)). The plasmonic microbubbles produced the largest photoacoustic response, and the border of the channel is clearly observed (Figure 5(c)). The mean pixel intensity for the plasmonic microbubbles was a factor of 4.7 greater than that observed from the free nanoparticle solution. Considering the fact that the nanoparticle concentration was greater in the free nanoparticle solution than the plasmonic microbubble solution, the signal enhancement normalized to nanoparticle concentration was approximately 70.5 for the maximum intensity projection, or 8.4-fold enhancement of the photoacoustic amplitude.

Similar experiments were performed to determine the ultrasound response of nanoparticles, control microbubbles and plasmonic microbubbles in the same flow-through phantom. Here the ultrasound probe was aligned perpendicular to the flow channel to image the circular cross section. The results for B-mode ultrasound imaging for nanoparticles, microbubbles and plasmonic microbubbles are shown in Figures 5(d)–5(f), respectively. The free nanoparticle solution was not seen in the ultrasound image due to the lack of echogenicity of the nanoparticles. The microbubble and plasmonic microbubble images were similar, with the overall pixel intensity varying by less than 13% between the two images. The gold loading on the microbubbles was found to have little effect on the echogenicity of the microbubbles, indicating that they can be used effectively as ultrasound contrast agents. We also looked at the non-linear ultrasound response of the different solutions using CPS. The results are nearly identical to those observed for B-mode ultrasound imaging

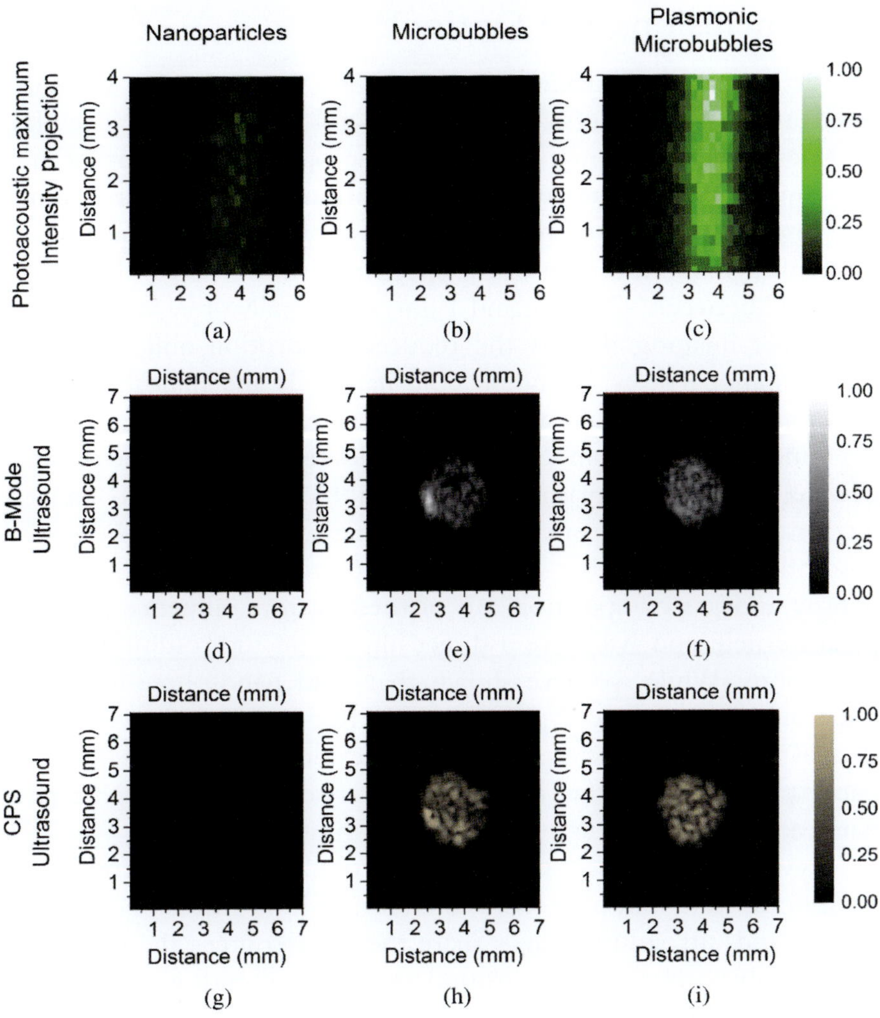

Fig. 5: (a)–(c) Photoacoustic maximum intensity projection image, from a custom photoacoustic imaging setup (d)–(f) B-mode ultrasound and (g)–(i) CPS ultrasound images acquired from a Siemens Sequoia Imaging System. Images of gold nanoparticles, microbubbles and plasmonic microbubbles were recorded for all modalities.

(Figure 5(g)–5(i)). Here the difference in pixel intensity between the images for microbubbles and plasmonic microbubbles was less than 10%, indicating a minimal effect of nanoparticle loading on the microbubble non-linear ultrasound response.

6. Conclusions and Outlook

This article has focused almost exclusively on the fabrication and characterization of microbubbles coated with gold nanospheres. The plasmon resonance wavelength, where strong optical absorption occurs, is around 530 nm. Unfortunately, absorption in blood severely limits the penetration of light into biological tissue at this wavelength. Light in the near infrared region of the spectrum (the so-called "biological window" between ~700 nm and 1 μm) is generally preferred for photoacoustic imaging due to the reduced absorption and scattering. Several nanoparticles, including gold nanorods and nanoshells, have plasmon resonance peaks within this wavelength range and are attractive candidates for plasmonic microbubbles. Futhermore, the photoacoustic efficiency of plasmonic microbubbles, or ability to convert incident light into acoustic waves, is a function of not only the optical absorption efficiency but also the nanoparticle size, shape, loading density and gas composition. All of these factors influence the temperature field and will have a direct impact on the resulting bubble oscillations. While we have shown that gold nanosphere-templated microbubbles produce a photoacoustic response that is well above that of free nanoparticles, we have not explored loading with other nanoparticles, and further improvements are expected through careful nanoparticle selection and surface structuring.

As we have discussed, plasmonic microbubbles provide contrast in both ultrasound and photoacoustic imaging modalities. The photoacoustic and ultrasound signals share the same source (the plasmonic microbubbles) but the background signals from endogeneous ultrasound scattering and optical absorption are unique to the two modalities. Combining the information from both images may allow for the signals from the plasmonic microbubbles to be better distinguished from the background, leading to improved specificity and contrast. Plasmonic microbubbles may also find application in therapeutic applications. Although the microbubbles are confined to the vasculature, the nanoparticles are small enough to transport outside of the vasculature and interrogate tumors through the enhanced permeability and retention effect. One could track the plasmonic microbubbles, through ultrasound or photoacoustic imaging, and release the nanoparticles at a particular location through microbubble destruction using an external ultrasound field. The nanoparticles could be tracked in the extravascular space allowing for tumor imaging or therapy. In the latter case, therapeutic effects could be induced by photothermal heating,[44] photothermolysis,[45] photoacoustic cavitation,[46] or the co-delivery of a particular drug.

In addition to plasmonic microbubbles, plasmonic droplets are promising candidates for a wide variety of imaging and therapeutic applications. Phase change droplets comprised of low boiling point perfluorocarbons (PFCs) have received widespread interest from the ultrasound imaging community for diagnostic and molecular imaging applications, and for potential use as therapeutic agents.[47,48] They can be made small enough to extravasate and have long circulation times. The liquid core is converted to a gas and expands in order to provide ultrasound contrast or create a therapeutic effect. Droplet vaporization can be achieved through ultrasound by applying a peak negative pressure sufficiently large to induce the phase transformation. Recently, phase change agents have been proposed as photoacoustic contrast agents.[49–55] Here, plasmonic nanoparticles are incorporated within the droplet or on the periphery. Optical absorption of a pulsed laser creates a local temperature rise within the droplet through the photothermal effect that leads to vaporization. This vaporization event produces an exceptionally strong photoacoustic response. After vaporization, a plasmonic microbubble can be produced. In fact, we have shown that droplets fabricated by condensation of plasmonic microbubbles (of the form described in this chapter) retain nanoparticle loading upon vaporization and hence are optically active.[56] We believe that interest in plasmonic droplets will continue to build in the coming years; as photoacoustic contrast agents, dual modality contrast agents, and theranostic agents.

In conclusion, we have provided an overview of the fabrication and characterization of plasmonic microbubbles. In addition, the physical mechanisms governing the response of plasmonic microbubbles to pulsed laser excitation have been elucidated, and we have presented a simple model describing this behavior. Plasmonic microbubbles offer excellent contrast in both photoacoustic and ultrasound imaging modalities, and provide a new tool for visualizing and affecting biological processes for theranostic applications.

Acknowledgments

This work was supported by NSF Grant CBET-1133687 to M.A.B.

References

1. Link, El-Sayed, *Annu. Rev. Phys. Chem.*, 331 (2003).
2. Everts, Saini, Leddon, Kok, Stoff-Khalili, Preuss, Millican, Perkins, Brown, Bagaria, Nikles, Johnson, Zharov, Curiel, *Nano Lett.*, 587 (2006).
3. El-Sayed, Huang, El-Sayed, *Nano Lett.*, 829 (2005).
4. Pitsillides, Joe, Wei, Anderson, Lin, *Biophys. J.*, 4023 (2003).
5. Yang, Skrabalak, Li, Xia, Wang, *Nano Lett.*, 3798 (2007).
6. Loo, Lowery, Halas, West, Drezek, *Nano Lett.*, 709 (2005).
7. Wang, Xie, Wang, Ku, Gill, O'Neal, Stoica, Wang, *Nano Lett.*, 1689 (2004).
8. Eghtedari, Oraevsky, Copland, Kotov, Conjusteau, Motamedi, *Nano Lett.*, 1914 (2007).
9. Huang, El-Sayed, Qian, El-Sayed, *J. Am. Chem. Soc.*, 2115 (2006).
10. Kam, O'Connell, Wisdom, Dai, *Proc. Natl. Acad. Sci. USA.*, 11600 (2005).
11. Beard, *Interface Focus*, 602 (2011).
12. Wang, Hu, *Science*, 1458 (2012).
13. Esenaliev, Larina, Larin, Deyo, Motamedi, Prough, *Appl. Opt.*, 4722 (2002).
14. Luke, Yeager, Emelianov, *Ann. Biomed. Eng.*, 422 (2012).
15. Goldberg, Raichlen, Forsberg, *Ultrasound Contrast Agents: Basic Principles and Clinical Applications*, CRC Press, 2001.
16. Qin, Caskey, Ferrara, *Phys. Med. Biol.*, R27 (2009).
17. Sirsi, Borden, *Bubble Sci. Eng. Technol.*, 3 (2009).
18. Unger, Porter, Culp, Labell, Matsunaga, Zutshi, *Adv. Drug Deliv. Rev.*, 1291 (2004).
19. Ferrara, Pollard, Borden, *Annu. Rev. Biomed. Eng.*, 415 (2007).
20. Sirsi, Borden, *Adv. Drug Deliv. Rev.*, 3 (2014).
21. Feshitan, Vlachos, Sirsi, Konofagou, Borden, *Biomater.,* 247 (2012).
22. Yang, Li, Chen, Zhang, Wu, Gu, *Biomater.s*, 3882 (2009).

23. Yuan, Uchiyama, Liu, Nguyen, Alexandrakis, *Appl. Phys. Lett.*, 33703 (2012).
24. Jeon, Song, Huynh, Kim, Kim, Helfield, Leung, Goertz, Zheng, Oh, Lovell, Kim, *J. Biomed. Opt.*, 16005 (2014).
25. Dove, Murray, Borden, *Soft Matter*, 7743 (2013).
26. Dove, Borden, Murray, *Opt. Lett.*, 3732 (2014).
27. Feshitan, Chen, Kwan, Borden, *J. Colloid Interface Sci.*, 316 (2009).
28. Kim, Costello, Duncan, Needham, *Langmuir*, 8455 (2003).
29. Satinover, Dove, Borden, *Ultrasound Med. Biol.*, 138 (2014).
30. Klibanov, *Bioconjug. Chem.*, 9 (2005).
31. Leckband, Schmitt, Israelachvili, Knoll, *Biochem.* (*Mosc.*), 4611 (1994).
32. Kerker, *The Scattering of Light, and Other Electromagnetic Radiation*, Academic Press, 1969.
33. C. F., Bohren, E. Clothiaux, D. R., Huffman, *Absorption and Scattering of Light by Small Particles*, Wiley-VCH, 2010.
34. Jain, Lee, El-Sayed, El-Sayed, *J. Phys. Chem. B*, 7238 (2006).
35. Richardson, Carlson, Tandler, Hernandez, Govorov, *Nano Lett.*, 1139 (2009).
36. U. Schleichert, K. J. Langenberg, W. Arnold, S. Fabbender, in *Rev. Prog. Quant. Nondestruct. Eval.*, 489 (1989).
37. Marmottant, Meer, Emmer, Versluis, Jong, Hilgenfeldt, Lohse, *J. Acoust. Soc. Am.*, 3499 (2005).
38. Rayleigh, *Philos. Mag. Ser.*, 94 (1917).
39. Plesset, Prosperetti, *Annu. Rev. Fluid Mech.* 145 (1977).
40. Garbin, Cojoc, Ferrari, Fabrizio, Overvelde, Meer, Jong, Lohse, Versluis, *Appl. Phys. Lett.*, 114103 (2007).
41. Tam, *Rev. Mod. Phys.*, 381 (1986).
42. Van der Meer, Dollet, Voormolen, Chin, Bouakaz, de Jong, Versluis, Lohse, *J. Acoust. Soc. Am*, 648 (2007).
43. Sassaroli, Li, O'Neill, *J. Acoust. Soc. Am.*, 2802 (2009).
44. Huff, Tong, Zhao, Hansen, Cheng, Wei, *Nanomed.*, 125 (2007).
45. Lapotko, Lukianova & Oraevsky, *Lasers Surg. Med.*, 631 (2006).
46. Ju, Roy, Murray, *Biomed. Opt. Express*, 66 (2013).
47. Matsunaga, Sheeran, Luois, Streeter, Mullin, Banerjee, Dayton, *Theranostics*, 1185 (2012).

48. Rapoport, *Wiley Interdiscip. Rev. Nanomed. Nanobiotechnol.*, 492 (2012).
49. Hannah, Luke, Wilson, Homan, Emelianov, *ACS Nano*, 250 (2014).
50. Hannah, VanderLaan, Chen, Emelianov, *Biomed. Opt. Express*, 3042 (2014).
51. Wilson, Homan, Emelianov, *Nat Commun*, 618 (2012).
52. Wei, Xia, Lombardo, Perez, Arnal, Larson-Smith, Pelivanov, Matula, Pozzo, O'Donnell, *Opt. Lett.*, 2599 (2014).
53. Wei, Lombardo, Larson-Smith, Pelivanov, Perez, Xia, Matula, Pozzo, O'Donnell, *Appl. Phys. Lett.*, 033701 (2014).
54. Jian, Liu, Gong, Su, Zhang, Wang, wang, Zhou, Xu, Li, Zheng, Song, Zhou, *Theranostics*, 1026 (2014).
55. Strohm, Rui, Gorelikov, Matsuura, Kolios, *Biomed. Opt. Exp.*, 1432 (2011).
56. Dove, Mountford, Murray, Borden, *Biomed. Opt. Exp.*, 4417 (2014).

CHAPTER 7

CONTRIBUTION OF NUCLEAR MEDICINE TO CANCER NANOTHERANOSTICS

Thomas Lars Andresen*,‡, Anncatrine L. Petersen*, Anders E. Hansen* and Jonas R. Henriksen†

**Department of Micro- and Nanotechnology, Center for Nanomedicine and Theranostics, Technical University of Denmark, 2800 Lyngby, Denmark*

†Deptartment of Chemistry, Center for Nanomedicine and Theranostics, Technical University of Denmark, 2800 Lyngby, Denmark

‡Thomas.andresen@nanotech.dtu.dk

The importance of molecular and diagnostic imaging has increased dramatically over the last decade. Today molecular imaging is used routinely in treatment planning and for evaluation of treatment response within a range of disease indications, and in particular in cancer therapy. Nuclear medicine plays a central role in this development and further offers unique possibilities for treating cancer through new tumor targeted innovations. Within nanomedicine there are particularly interesting possibilities for combining imaging and therapy. Engineered nanocarriers that target tumor tissue can transport both therapeutic radionuclides and imaging agents, which allows for theranostic approaches with interesting potential in personalized medicine. Advanced imaging systems now provide new possibilities for non-invasive monitoring of nanocarrier biodistribution in animals and humans and it is clear that future nanomedicines will be co-developed with companion diagnostics. Thus, advances in imaging and developments in nanocarrier radiolabeling techniques allows us to enter a new arena where we start to consider how to use imaging for patient selection and treatment monitoring in connection to nanocarrier-based medicines. Nanocarrier imaging agents could furthermore have interesting properties for disease diagnostics and staging of cancer.

1. Introduction

Theranostic nanocarriers provide a range of new treatment prospects for cancer patients. Particularly, the development of companion diagnostics and disease monitoring systems in conjugation with nano-therapeutics is highly interesting. Over the last few years, there has been an increasing interest in developing and testing theranostic nanoparticles in small animal models where cancer imaging and therapy is combined.[1] As an example of the high focus on new nano-particle imaging probes, the Food and Drug Administration (FDA) has approved more than 35 imaging or therapeutic nanoparticles for clinical trials in recent years.[2] Currently, there are no approved thera-nostic nanoparticles combining imaging and therapy capabilities in one formulation on the market. However, we can expect this to occur within the next three years. A main reason for why such imaging agents are important is that it is not certain that all cancer patients will benefit from nanotherapeutics as there may be large heterogeneity in nanoparticle accumulation between patients. In current clinical trials with nanotherapeutics, it is not determined if the used drug reaches the target site of action in a relevant therapeutic dose.[3] Data from preclinical imaging studies suggest that poor therapeutic response may be coursed by lack of effective accumulation of drugs in tumors.[4,5]

Thus, with the increasing amount of therapeutic nanoparticles in clinical development, there is a high demand of developing theranostic nanoparticles that are useful for predicting the therapeutic potential of the nano-delivered drugs on a general basis as well as on a personalized level. The most obvious theranostic nanomedicines at the moment are based on liposomes and polymer nanoparticles but other examples of suggested nanoparticles have been hard shell systems based on quantum dots, gold nanostructures and iron oxides that all can be conjugated with targeted therapies and diagnostic imaging agents. Furthermore, nanoparticle imaging probes for magnetic resonance or X-ray-based computed tomography (CT) imaging can be envisaged to have potential in evaluating individual patient benefit of nanotherapeutics.

In vivo imaging using radiolabeled pharmaceuticals has a central position in disease diagnostics, drug development and cancer treatment planning. During the last decade radiolabeled molecular and functional imaging agents have been developed to characterize the tumor microenvironment, guide therapies and evaluate therapeutic interactions.[6–9] Single photon emission computed tomography (SPECT) imaging, which is based on gamma-rays, remains the most widely used radioisotope-based imaging technique due to the high number of scanners in hospitals throughout the world. The advantage of this technique in comparison to positron emission tomography (PET) imaging is that the radioisotopes are generally longer lived and image resolution can be higher than for PET. However, PET has become the fastest growing clinical imaging technique due to its quantitative nature and high sensitivity, and PET is today a modern tool in cancer diagnostics and in planning of cancer treatments.[10,11] Compared to SPECT, PET has a higher detection sensitivity, which makes it possible to visualize radiotracer concentrations as low as 10^{-12} M.[10–12] Developments of new radiolabeling methods for PET imaging that can be utilized in nanoparticle technology as diagnostic and theranostic agents are therefore of great importance.

Today, the most widely used PET radiotracer is radioactive ^{18}F labeled deoxyglucose (^{18}FDG) for imaging of tumors. Even though ^{18}FDG has been, and still is, highly successful in diagnosing cancer and shows high imaging quality in many tumor types, there are several cancer forms where ^{18}FDG is not successful, including highly differentiated neuroendocrine (NE) tumors[13,14] and prostatic tumors.[15] In addition, there is a strong demand for improving molecular imaging tools for staging disease and evaluating treatment efficacy as early as possible. Development of new PET imaging agents and other radiotracers is therefore currently attracting enormous interest in research and industry. The main advantage of nuclear imaging techniques, and in particular PET imaging, is the ability to monitor radiolabeled agents at tracer quantities, where the used doses are not associated with pharmacological effects. The use of nuclear imaging has also become an essential tool in drug discovery and drug development, in screening and for identifying new drug candidates.[16] It is also without doubt that currently available molecular imaging probes can benefit the development of nanotherapeutics and should be considered for early integration into clinical development programs of nanotherapeutics.

Radiolabeled theranostic nanoparticles hold the potential to determine the biodistribution of a nanoparticle delivered drug, which in addition could be important for other treatments strategies, including radiation therapy and anti-angiogenic agents in cancer patients.[17] Nanotheranostic technologies could provide unique features and new methodologies to monitor, evaluate and individualize treatment in real-time.[18]

Future directions in development of diagnostic protocols does not only include imaging agents for new molecular targets, but may also focus on improving the understanding of how imaging agent combinations can give a more precise phenotypic characterization, including information on intra-tumor heterogeneities. The aim is not only to localize and stage the cancer, but also to aid the selection of the optimal treatment protocols. In this regard, radiolabeled tumor-targeted nanoparticles could potentially have interesting imaging properties and supplement existing imaging agents as they have different mechanisms of accumulation than the existing systems. Given the focus on personalized medicine and tumor-targeting agents new targets for nanoparticle delivery of therapeutic agents will surely emerge, making radiolabeled nanoparticles an increasingly important tool for the evaluation of drug delivery capabilities. Theranostic nanoparticles will additionally provide biodistribution data on concurrent accumulation in non-targeted tissues to assess the potential toxicity profile and pharmacological effect, which is highly important in early clinical development.

2. Nuclear Imaging Techniques

Radiolabeled nanoparticles can be traced *in vivo* by two imaging techniques, SPECT and PET. In Table 1 radionuclides used in SPECT and PET imaging applications are listed with their half-life, photon energy and method of production.

Table 1. Common used radionuclides in SPECT and PET imaging.

Radionuclide/ Imaging method	**Half-life**[a]	**γ: Photon energy β^+: Maximum positron energy (E_{max}) [keV (% fraction)]**[a]
^{67}Ga/SPECT	3.26 d	γ: 93 (39%), 184 (21%), 300 (17%)
^{111}In/ SPECT	2.81 d	γ: 171 (91%), 245 (94%)
^{123}I/SPECT	13.22 h	γ: 159 (83%)
^{186}Re/SPECT	3.72 d	γ: 137 (10%)
^{99m}Tc/SPECT	6.01 h	γ: 140 (89%)
^{201}Tl/SPECT	3.04 d	γ: 71 (37%)
^{11}C/PET	20.33 min	β^+: 960 (100%)
^{61}Cu/PET	3.3 h	β^+: 1215 (51%)
^{62}Cu/PET	9.67 min	β^+: 2926 (97%)
^{64}Cu/PET	12.7 h	β^+: 653 (17%)
^{18}F/PET	109.77 min	β^+: 634 (97%)
^{68}Ga/PET	67.71 min	γ: 1900 (88%)
^{124}I/PET	4.18 d	β^+: 1535 (12%), 2137 (11%)
^{13}N/PET	9.97 min	β^+: 1199 (100%)
^{15}O/PET	2.07 min	β^+: 1732 (100%)
^{82}Rb/PET	1.26 min	β^+: 3378 (82%), 2601 (13%)
^{89}Zr/PET	78 h	β^+: 902 (23%)

[a] Data derived from Refs. 19 and 20.

2.1. *SPECT imaging*

Nanoparticles can be labeled with various single photon emitters allowing SPECT imaging of the nanoparticles. SPECT isotopes are generally cheaper, more readily available and are longer lived than most PET isotopes. In order to determine the position of the emitted photon within a subject after administration of a radiolabeled nanoparticle, a gamma camera and collimators integrated in the SPECT scanner are needed. In SPECT, physical collimators filter the photons emitted from single photon emitting radionuclides and only photons perpendicular to the scanner is thereby are registered (Figure 1). As a consequence, the collimators only direct a fraction of the high-energy photons allowing their interaction with the NaI crystal and photo multiplier tubes (PMT) in the gamma camera (Figure 1).

The photons registered by the NaI crystal is converted into an emitted light and registered by the PMT resulting in an electrical pulse. Through data reconstruction, images are then constructed showing the distribution of the radiolabeled nanoparticle within the subject. Because the emitted light is proportional to the type of radiation energy that hits the NaI crystal, simultaneous dual-tracer imaging is possibly in SPECT imaging.[20,21] This enables detection of nanoparticles labeled with two different single photon emitters or two different nanoparticles that are labeled differently within the same experiment. Dual-imaging cannot be performed for PET imaging since the registered photons from the annihilation all have the same energy.

The photon filtration by the collimators results in lower detection sensitivity of SPECT compared to PET scanners. Even though SPECT has lower detection sensitivity, the longer half-lives of single photon emitters offers the possibility to observe biodistribution of radiolabeled nanoparticles several days or weeks after administration. However, 3D images are more difficult to obtain, and 2D projections are needed in many angles by rotating the gamma camera around the subject, where each scan can take from seconds to minutes to perform. The nanoparticle biodistribution is therefore assumed to be constant throughout the duration of the scan, and this makes dynamic image acquisition difficult in SPECT imaging.[20]

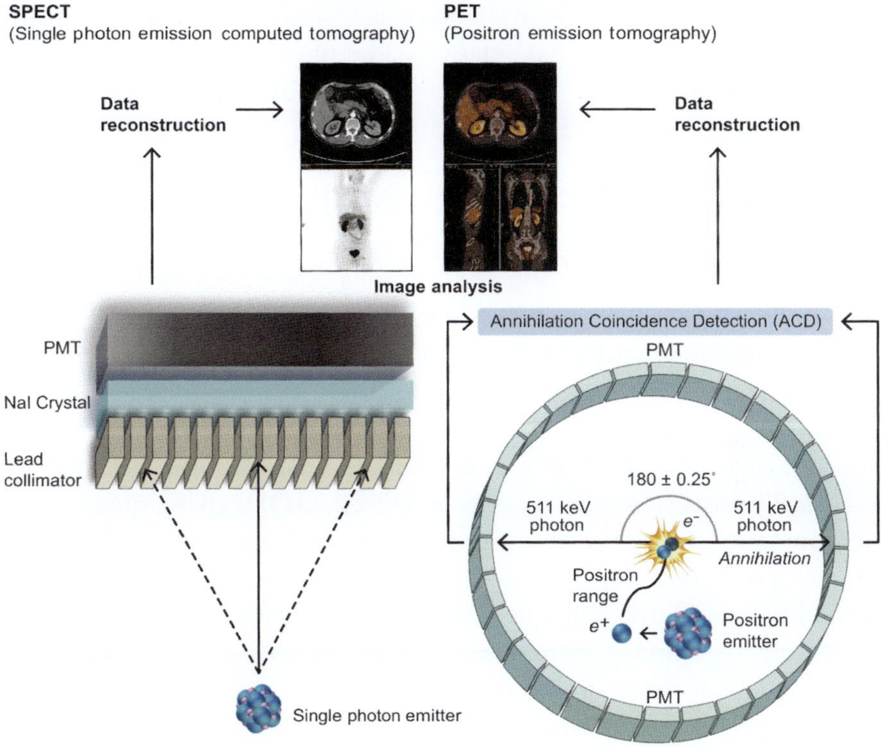

Fig. 1: Schematic diagram of the typical components required in SPECT imaging (*left panel*) and PET imaging (*right panel*). In SPECT imaging the photons emitted from the single photon emitters are filtered by physical lead collimators, and only a fraction of the photons enter and interact with the NaI crystal and PMT in the gamma camera. In PET imaging the positron (e^+) emitted from the positron emitter travels a short distance (positron range) depending on its positron energy, and annihilate with an electron (e^-) producing two 511 keV photons moving in opposite directions. Opposite PMTs in the PET scanner must register the two photons at the same time in annihilation coincidence detection (ACD) in order to accept the signal. When the two photons are detected by the two detectors, the decay can be localized to the line connecting the two detectors. After each scanning procedure, data from the scanners are reconstructed using scanner specific algorithms followed by data analysis and image interpretations.

Examples of single photon emitting radionuclides are ^{99m}Tc ($T_{1/2}$ = 6.01 h), ^{123}I ($T_{1/2}$ = 13.22 h), ^{111}In ($T_{1/2}$ = 2.81 d), ^{201}Tl ($T_{1/2}$ = 3.04 d) and ^{67}Ga ($T_{1/2}$ = 3.26 d). ^{99m}Tc is the most widely used radionuclide in nuclear medicine due to its favorable half-life, photon energy and readily availability as a generator produced radionuclide (Table 1). ^{99m}Tc has relatively low photon energy (140 keV), and is therefore highly suitable for SPECT imaging as the patient thereby receives relatively low radiation doses.

2.2. *PET imaging*

PET is based on the detection of γ-photons that are emitted after annihilation between a positron emitted from a radionuclide and an electron in close proximity in the surroundings. In contrast to single photon emitters, most positron emitters have relatively short half-lives (Table 1), which makes the radiolabeling of the imaging agent challenging. In contrast to SPECT, PET allows direct image analysis of the radioactivity specifically sequestered in a region of interest (ROI), giving quantitative determination of biodistribution based on differences in pixel intensities. This difference is particular important for clinical translation, which should be considered when developing nanotheranostics.

Positrons emitted from the decaying positron emitting radionuclide travels a short distance (depending on the positron energy) before it undergoes annihilation with an electron producing a pair of 511 keV photons emitted at an angle of 180° in opposite directions (Figure 1). A typical PET scanner consists of scintillators placed in a ring around the subject. Opposite detectors must register both photons at the same time in a so-called annihilation coincidence detection (ACD) in order to accept the signal as one that originates from an annihilation event[11] (Figure 1). When the two photons are detected by two detectors in annihilation coincidence, the decay can be localized on the line connecting the two detectors in the so called line of response (LOR), and the PET image quantitatively reflects the localization and concentration of the radiolabeled agent within the subject. The ability to register the pair of 511 keV photons in ACD allows detection of the photons without using collimators as in SPECT imaging. The PET scanner thereby registers more photons per radioactive dose administered to a patient. In addition, due to the ring structure of the PET scanner, detection of multiple LOR at different angles from the same decaying nuclide permits direct 3D imaging as well as dynamic imaging.[22] A drawback of PET is that the short physical half-life of positron emitters (Table 1) requires fast and efficient radiolabeling. Thus, for successful imaging, the half-life of the radionuclide must be long enough to carry out the desired labeling procedure and long enough to allow accumulation in the target site e.g., tumor tissue.

Examples of short-lived positron emitters are ^{15}O ($T_{½}$ = 2.07 min), ^{13}N ($T_{½}$ = 9.97 min), ^{11}C ($T_{½}$ = 20.33 min), ^{68}Ga ($T_{½}$ = 67.71 min) and ^{18}F ($T_{½}$ = 110.77 min). Longer lived positron emitters have attractive attributes for use in nanoparticle PET imaging since there is sufficient time for radiolabeling and for the nanoparticles to be distributed *in vivo* and monitored hours or days after administration. Examples of longer-lived positron emitters are ^{64}Cu ($T_{½}$ = 12.7 h), ^{89}Zr ($T_{½}$ = 78 h) and ^{124}I ($T_{½}$ = 4.18 d). An advantage of radio-metals such as ^{68}Ga, ^{89}Zr and ^{64}Cu compared to non-metal radionuclides is the relatively simple chelation chemistry that can be utilized in the labeling procedure.

In the last few years significant research effort has been devoted to the radio-metal ^{64}Cu, because of its relatively long half-life compared to other positron emitters, making imaging 48 h after administration easily achievable,[23] and because of its relatively straightforward chelation chemistry and low positron range. Similar to ^{18}F, ^{64}Cu has a fairly low positron range (Table 1: E_{max} = 653 keV) resulting in PET images of high quality.[24]

3. Radiolabeling Techniques of Nanoparticles

A large variety of techniques have been developed to label nanoparticles with radionuclides, but for nanoparticles to serve as carriers of radionuclides for imaging and diagnostic application several features of the labelling technique are important: (1) high incorporation efficiency, (2) simple and fast preparation, preferably at room temperature, (3) readily available isotopes with good imaging characteristics, (4) high radionuclide labelling stability *in vitro* and *in vivo* and (5) generic applicability to same type of nanoparticles.[25,26] Several techniques have been developed for incorporating radionuclides into nanoparticles for *in vivo* imaging using SPECT and PET, and examples are outlined in Tables 2 and 3.

Table 2. Examples of radiolabeling methods of nanoparticles for SPECT imaging.

Radionuclide/ Nanoparticle	Labeling method	Refs.
^{67}Ga/Liposome	Remote loading by lipophilic chelator oxine into preformed liposomes.	63, 64, 67
^{67}Ga/Liposome	Surface chelation by labeling DTPA-lipid in preformed liposome.	29
^{111}In/Liposome	Encapsulation of ^{111}In-DTPA added to lipid film followed by liposome manufacture.	50, 51
^{111}In/Liposome	Remote loading of ^{111}In by chelation to lipophilic oxine into preformed liposomes.	58, 61, 62, 64
^{111}In/Liposome	Remote loading of ^{111}In by chelation to ionophore A23187 into preformed liposomes.	66, 70
^{111}In/Iron oxide	Surface chelation on iron oxide nanoparticles (SPIONs).	37
^{111}In/Micelle	Surface ^{111}In-labeled annexin A5 on core cross-linked polymeric micelles.	38
^{111}In/AuNP	Surface ^{111}In-labeled DTPA on PEG-coated AuNPs.	71
^{123}I/Liposome	Encapsulating ^{123}I attached to lipid molecule followed by liposome manufacture.	49
^{123}I/Liposome	Remote loading using Bolton–Hunter reagent.	65
^{99m}Tc/Liposome	Passive encapsulation by adding $^{99m}TcO_4^-$ to lipid film.	72
^{99m}Tc/Liposome	Membrane labeling of preformed liposomes using stannous chloride.	55, 56
^{99m}Tc/Liposome	Surface chelation of chelator-lipid in preformed liposomes.	27–30, 36
^{99m}Tc/Liposome	Remote loading of ^{99m}Tc into preformed liposomes by chelation to a lipophilic chelator.	59, 60, 73
^{99m}Tc/AuNP	Surface chelation by labeling HYNIC or DTPA.	39–41, 71
^{67}Ga/Cobalt-ferrite	Surface chelation of chelating agent *p*-SCN-bn-NOTA by ^{67}Ga-citrate.	42

Table 3. Examples of radiolabeling methods of nanoparticles for PET imaging.

Radionuclide/ Nanoparticle	Labeling method	Refs.
^{18}F/Liposome	Membrane labeling of ^{18}F attached to lipid molecule followed by liposome manufacture.	52
^{18}F/Liposome	FDG encapsulation during manufacture.	53
^{18}F/Liposome	Surface chelation by labeling of chelator-lipid in preformed liposomes.	31, 32
^{18}F/Quantum dots	Surface incorporation via a nucleophilic *hetero*aromatic substitution using a [^{18}F] FPyME reagent.	74
^{18}F/AuNP	Covalently surface labeling using [^{18}F]-fluorobenzoate.	75
^{64}Cu/Liposome	Surface chelation by labeling chelator-lipid in preformed liposomes.	33–35
^{64}Cu/Liposome	Remote loading of ^{64}Cu into preformed liposomes by chelation to 2-hydroxyquinoline.	69
^{64}Cu/Liposome	Gradient remote loading of ^{64}Cu into preformed liposomes by chelation to 4-DEAP-ATSC.	3
^{64}Cu/Iron oxide	Surface chelation by radiolabeling a chelator.	44–46
^{64}Cu/Quantum dots	Surface chelation by radiolabeling a chelator.	43
^{64}Cu/Ferritin	Direct loading of ^{64}Cu into the cavity of the ferritin nanostructure.	76
^{64}Cu/Micelle	Surface chelation by radiolabeling a chelator.	48
^{124}I/Liposome	Remote loading using Bolton–Hunter reagent with arginine-containing liposomes.	65
^{124}I/Iron oxide	Surface labeling by Iodo-beads iodination.	47
^{89}Zr/Liposome	Membrane labeling using chelator-free liposomes.	57

The radiolabeling methods can be divided into four general approaches depending on the type of nanoparticle (Figure 2). In general, surface chelation[27–48] can be used to label all nanoparticles as outlined in Figure 2, whereas passive encapsulation[49–53], membrane labeling[54–57] and remote loading[3,58–69] are methods used in liposome

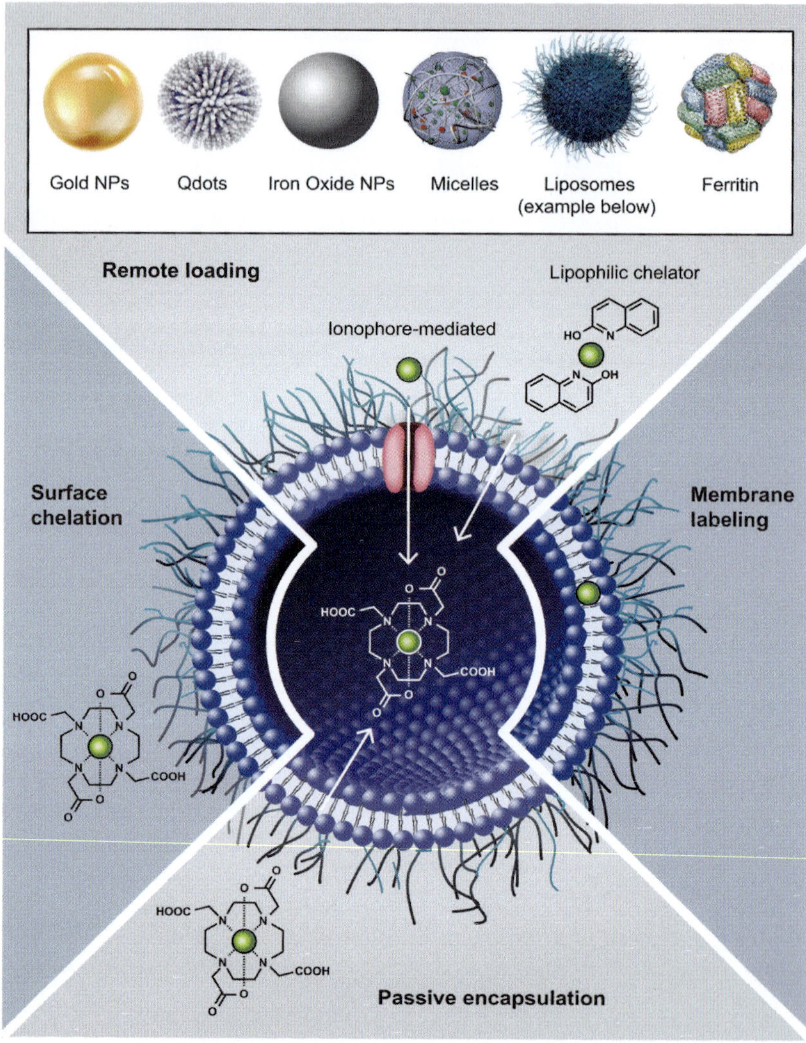

Fig. 2: Schematic diagram of labeling methods for preparing radioactive nanoparticles. Remote loading, membrane labeling and passive encapsulation are labeling approaches used on liposomes, and surface chelation is a labeling method utilized on all nanoparticles. The green circle symbolizes a radionuclide.

and polymersome radiolabeling. Surface chelation of nanoparticles can be achieved by incorporating chelator conjugates that bind the radionuclides onto the surface of the nanoparticle during preparation (Figure 2).

In surface chelation the radionuclides are attached to the surface of the nanoparticles, and the radionuclides are therefore exposed to proteins and macromolecules in the blood stream during circulation, which potentially can result in release of the radionuclides from the nanoparticle surface. The *in vivo* stability of surface labeled nanoparticles e.g., liposomes, gold and iron oxide particles are therefore very dependent on the radionuclide-chelator binding constant. Possible trans-chelation or trans-metalation of nanoparticles associated radionuclides can be investigated by incubating nanoparticles with competing chelating agents[30] or metal entities. A surface chelation approach was developed in order to label SPIONs with an ^{111}In-mAbMB antibody. The SPIONs have a magnetic core and are coated with carboxylic acid groups for antibody conjugation through a carbodiimide coupling reaction.[37] Labeling using surface chelation on preformed liposomes often gives labeling efficiencies as high as 90%. An example is the ^{64}Cu labeling approach by Seo *et al.* where two bifunctional ^{64}Cu chelators (TETA–PDP and CB–TE2A–PDEA) were synthesized and conjugated to long-circulating liposomes.[34]

In general, it should be expected that the *in vivo* stability of surface labeled nanoparticles is not as high as when the radionuclide is encapsulated inside the nanoparticles, e.g., in liposomes. Remote loading of radionuclides into the aqueous phase of preformed (premanufactured) liposomes, can utilize ionophores or lipophilic chelators to transport the radionuclide over the membrane of the liposomes, and the radionuclide is then traped inside by chelation to a pre-encapsulated chelator (Figure 2). Remote loading can also include a gradient-based loading of the radionuclide such as a pH-gradient[60] or a chelator gradient-based remote loading.[3] In general, the remote loading approaches concentrate radionuclides in the internal aqueous compartment of the liposomes providing high loading efficiencies (>90%), and seems to provide the greatest *in vivo* stability compared to other labeling approaches, due to the protected location which prevents exchange of the radionuclide with the biological environment.[77]

Methods for remote loading of radionuclides into the interior aqueous phase of preformed liposomes can be divided into two categories.

Firstly, the radionuclide can be carried by a lipophilic chelator through the lipid bilayer of the preformed liposomes into the aqueous phase, where the radionuclide is bound to a chelator and becomes entrapped. Such a remote loading approach was developed in order to load ^{67}Ga and ^{111}In into preformed liposomes containing nitrilotri-acetic acid (NTA)[61,64] or deferoxamine (DF)[63] as chelator. In this approach 8-hydroxyquinoline (oxine) was used as lipophilic chelator to carry ^{67}Ga (or ^{111}In) through the lipid bilayer in a radionuclide-lipophilic chelator form, from where ^{67}Ga (or ^{111}In) is trapped with encapsulated NTA or DF. Alternatively, the lipophilic chelator can also be converted from a membrane permeable form to a membrane impermeable form after interaction with an encapsulated molecule. One example of this is the use of hexamethyl propylene amine oxime (HMPAO) to load ^{99m}Tc into preformed liposomes encapsulating glutathione (GSH).[68] HMPAO chelates ^{99m}Tc into a membrane permeable ^{99m}Tc-HMPAO complex, and HMPAO then carries ^{99m}Tc into the preformed liposomes, where it interacts with GSH resulting in its conversion to a membrane impermeable ^{99m}Tc-HMPAO complex. The exact mechanism for this is not clear but is hypothesized to be a reduction of the complex by GSH.[68] Liposomes loaded with this method have been tested clinically for detection of infection and inflammation.[78] Other lipophilic chelators, *N*-*N*-bis(2-mercaptoethyl)-*N'*,*N'*-diethylethylenediamine (BMEDA) and diisopropyl iminodi-acetic acid (DISIDA), have similar features as HMPAO, and have been used to load ^{99m}Tc into preformed liposomes encapsulating GSH.[59,73] A pH gradient can also be utilized in chelator-radionuclide transport and entrapment within liposomes. In a study, the lipophilic chelator BMEDA has been reported to label liposomes with ^{99m}Tc radionuclides using a pH gradient method.[60] The liposomes are prepared containing ammonium sulphate in the interior phase (pH 5.5) and phosphate-buffered saline (PBS) in the exterior phase (pH 7.4). At pH 7.4 BMEDA is lipophilic and chelates ^{99m}Tc and the complex becomes neutral. The neutral lipophilic complex will permeate the lipid membrane. BMEDA contains three amine groups that inside the vesicles at pH 5.5 are protonated by proton exchange with NH_4^+ ions, and becomes trapped inside the liposomes, whereas free resulting

NH_3 crosses the lipid bilayer and thereby escapes the liposome.[60] Lee *et al.* reported a gradient-based method using a liposome-loadable Cu chelator, 4-DEAP-ATSC. During the ^{64}Cu loading process, the tertiary amine groups of the ^{64}Cu:4-DEAP-ATSC complex become protonated after crossing the liposomal membrane and remain stably entrapped within the liposome.[3] This approach is currently being utilized as part of an ongoing clinical study.[79]

Secondly, an ionophore can be included in the liposome bilayer introducing a hydrophilic pore in the membrane allowing radionuclides to cross the lipid bilayer. The ionophore A23187 has been reported for use in liposome membranes to transport externally added $^{111}InCl_3$ across the membrane, where the radionuclide becomes trapped when it interacts with encapsulated chelators such as NTA.[70] This method was the basis for the Vescan™ product tested as a liposomal cancer-imaging agent in patients.[80–85]

In passive encapsulation the radionuclide labeling is performed during manufacture of the liposomes. The radionuclide is included in the buffer solution (most often associated with a chelator) from where the liposomes are formed, and since passive entrapment strongly depends on the entrapped aqueous volume of the liposomes, the particle size is important for loading efficiencies. The loading efficiency is normally <10% for 100 nm liposomes, why this method is rarely used.

In membrane labeling the radionuclides are conjugated to the surface or embedded within the bilayer of liposomes. The radionuclides can either be conjugated to preformed liposomes or be conjugated to a lipid that is formulated into the liposomes. Alternatively a radionuclide containing hydrophobic molecule can be added to preformed liposomes that has high affinity to a hydrophobic membrane environment. Typical radionuclides for the conjugation are iodide and fluoride isotopes; however, the chemistry involved will often require purification processes. In the membrane labeling approach, there is often a risk of unstable liposome radiolabeling. A loss of radioactivity from the liposomes *in vivo* can result in an incorrect estimation of the biodistribution of the liposomes and it can also reduce the quality of the diagnostic images. Abou *et al.* reported a membrane labeling of the PET isotope, ^{89}Zr, by an interaction of the radio-metal with the lipids' phosphate head groups, a chelator-free strategy.[57] Here the radiolabeled liposomes were challenged with EDTA resulting in only 40% of the total radioactivity associated to the liposomes, and also incubation in serum demonstrated the moderate stability of the liposomes when using a membrane labeling approach.[57]

Radioactive nanoparticles often have to be produced within strict time limits due to the radioactive decay of the radionuclides used and it is therefore best to incorporate the radionuclides into nanoparticles through surface chelation or into preformed liposomes via remote loading immediately prior to use.

3.1. *In vivo studies on nanoparticles labeled by remote loading and surface chelation*

Even though no diagnostic nanoparticle radiotracer has reached the market, radiolabeling methods have been developed for studying nanoparticles in mammals and humans to provide detailed information on the pharmacokinetics and biodistribution of potential nanotherapeutics.[17]

Several radiolabeled liposomes with various radionuclides have been investigated in cancer patients. The single photon emitting radionuclides, ^{99m}Tc and ^{111}In, have been used in clinical studies in diagnostic SPECT imaging for inflammation and infection[78,86–90] as well as cancer[54,80–85,91–95] (Table 4).

The first clinical study using ^{64}Cu radiolabeled liposomes for PET imaging was initiated in 2014 by Merrimack Pharmaceuticals (Table 4).[79] This study aims at providing new insights into the biodistribution and tumor deposition kinetics of liposomes in human tumors including variability across patients and/or tumor types. Assessment of these parameters may aid in identifying cancer patients that are well-suited for treatment with liposomal therapies. Extending this concept, Merrimack Pharmaceuticals are developing a drug-free ^{64}Cu-liposomal diagnostic agent with the intent of prospectively selecting patients for liposomal therapies and potentially other nanomedicines.[3,79]

Table 4. Clinical studies of radiolabeled liposomes for diagnostic/theranostic imaging of cancer using SPECT and PET.

Radionuclide/ Nanoparticle	Labeling method	Study	Refs.
^{111}In/Liposome	Remote loading by oxine into preformed liposomes.	Clinical	91, 92
^{111}In/Liposome	Remote loading by ionophore A23187 into preformed liposomes.	Clinical	80–85
^{99m}Tc/Liposome	Membrane labeling of preformed liposomes using stannous chloride.	Clinical	54, 93–95
^{64}Cu/Liposome	Gradient-based method using a liposome-loadable Cu chelator (4-DEAP-ATSC).	Clinical	79

Among the current methods tested in humans, remote loading[3,78,80–85,91,92] and surface chelation[86,87] appears to be the most successful. Several clinical studies of membrane labeled liposomes were performed in the 1980's for diagnostic SPECT imaging of cancer[54,93–95]; however, several of the utilized methods were considered problematic for further clinical studies due to low *in vivo* radionuclide retention.

Studies in mice and rats have been reported with positron emitting radionuclides, ^{18}F and ^{64}Cu, for evaluating the biodistribution and tumor accumulation of different nanoparticles using PET imaging[3,32–35,43,47,52,53,57,69,76] (Table 3). In a study by Marik *et al.*, quantitative biodistribution data of [^{18}F]FDP-radiolabeled liposomes were obtained from PET images (Figure 3), where the biodistribution of radiolabeled liposomes was compared to radiolabeled diglyceride, 3-[^{18}F]fluoro-1,2-dipalmitoylglycerol [[^{18}F]fluorodipalmitin ([^{18}F] FDP)] in healthy rats.[52]

In another study, a labeling method was developed for remote loading of ^{64}Cu into preformed PEGylated liposomes using DOTA as the encapsulated copper chelator and the lipophilic chelator 2-hydroxyquinoloine to transport ^{64}Cu across the membrane. This resulted in high loading efficiencies (>95%) and the loading method could be

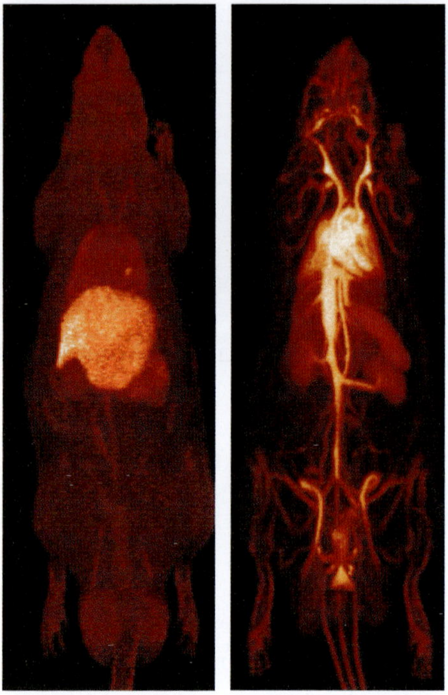

Fig. 3: Full-body maximum intensity projections (MIPs) for [^{18}F]FDP and [^{18}F] FDP liposomes in a rat model. A MIP of free [^{18}F]FDP is shown in the left image with uptake in the liver, spleen and lungs. The right image shows a MIP of liposomal [^{18}F]FDP, which remains circulating in the blood for the duration of the 90-min scan (reprinted with permission).[52]

used in a broad temperature range. The ^{64}Cu PEGylated liposomes were studied in healthy mice and tumor-bearing mice using a HT29 colon adenocarcinoma xenograft model (Figure 4), and the accumulation of the liposomes in the different organs was determined.[69] This method has further been developed as a non-assisted loading method (without use of ionophore) and used for evaluating liposome biodistribution in dogs with various cancer types and is planned for a study in cancer patients as a companion diagnostic.

Lee and coworkers developed another ^{64}Cu remote loading approach where a gradient-loadable chelator, 4-DEAP–ATSC, was used for incorporating ^{64}Cu into liposomal therapeutics for PET imaging.[3] ^{64}Cu chelated to 4-DEAP–ATSC (>94%) was loaded into

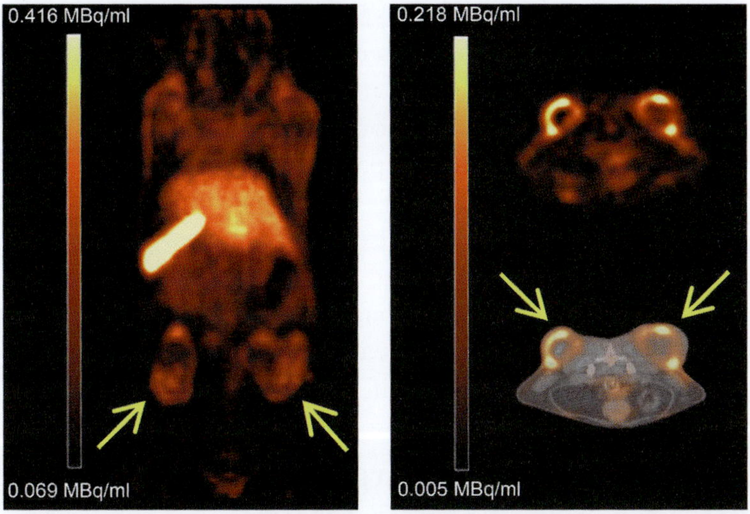

Fig. 4: PET/CT-images of ^{64}Cu-liposomes distribution in tumor-bearing mice. *Left*: Coronal PET image 24 h post-injection of ^{64}Cu-liposomes into a mouse bearing colon adenocarcinoma (HT29; marked with arrows) on right and left flank. *Right*: Axial PET image (top) and axial PET/CT-fusion (bottom) images 24 h post-injection of ^{64}Cu-liposomes into a mouse bearing colon adenocarcinoma (HT29; marked with arrows) on right and left flank (reprinted with permission).[69]

PEGylated liposomal doxorubicin (PLD) and HER2-targeted PLD (MM-302) with efficiencies >90%, and PET/CT imaging of xenograft mice injected with ^{64}Cu-MM-302 revealed ^{64}Cu positively correlated with liposomal drug deposition.[3]

To label liposomes with ^{99m}Tc,[30] a surface chelation method was developed using *N*-hydroxysuccinimidyl hydrazine nicotinate hydrochloride (HYNIC) conjugated to the amino group of distearoyl phosphatidylethanolamine (DSPE) and subsequently incorporated into the liposome during hydration. A mixture of tricine and stannous chloride was added to $^{99m}TcO_4^-$ and subsequently added to HYNIC-liposomes yielding high labeling efficiency (>95%). Liposomes labeled with this method have been tested clinically for detection of infection and inflammation.[86,87]

Pharmacokinetic and imaging studies have been reported in patients receiving liposomal adriamycin. Liposomes were remote loaded with ^{111}In by use of the lipophilic chelator oxine and with

DF as the encapsulated chelator.[91] Similarly, diethylene triamine pentaacetic acid (DTPA) has been used as the encapsulated chelator for ligand exchange with ^{111}In-oxine in PEGylated liposomes.[96] A study using these PEGylated ^{111}In-liposomes has been reported with effective targeting of solid tumors in patients with locally advanced cancers.[92] Simultaneous loading of ^{99m}Tc and ^{111}In into liposomes encapsulating DF and GSH has also been reported.[58] This dual labeling method can be used to image the distribution of liposomes out to 10 days. ^{99m}Tc gives good images <24 h scan times due to its short half-life ($T_{½}$ = 6 h), whereas ^{111}In is suitable for prolonged imaging because of its long half-life ($T_{½}$ = 68 h).

4. Passive and Active Targeting in Radio-Nanoparticle Design

Several important features concerning the design of passively and active targeted nanoparticles need to be taken into consideration to control biodistribution and for obtaining a high degree of tumor accumulation. These include physical and chemical characteristics where surface chemistry, particle size as well as nanoparticle shape and softness influence their biological behavior. In addition, the administered nanoparticle dose is a factor that influences to which degree the nanoparticle properties affect biodistribution, opsonization and clearance by immune cells. After intravenous injection, nanoparticles interact with blood components such as lipoproteins and macromolecules. The interaction with lipoproteins may involve lipid exchange or enzymatic hydrolysis, which eventually could lead to breakdown of the nanoparticles and especially liposomes composed of phospholipids and protein-based nanoparticles.[97–100] Protein opsonization, or adsorption of marker macromolecules such as immunoglobulins, is part of the body's defense mechanism. The spleen and liver are the dominating organs responsible for nanoparticle blood clearance[101–103] due to the high concentration of macrophages that migrates to these organs as monocytes from the bone marrow, as well as hepatocytes (in the liver).

PEGylation and surface conjugation of other hydrophilic polymers reduces nanoparticle interaction with lipoproteins and RES and thereby increases the blood half-life.[104,105] The circulation time can more or less be modulated by tuning the surface coating by varying the degree of PEGylation. The optimal level of PEGylation on for example liposomes for long circulation half-life has been extensively studied.[104–107] From a drug delivery point of view, the generally accepted hypothesis is that a longer blood circulation half-life results in repeated liposome (or nanoparticle) passages through the vasculature at the tumor site, and thereby results in greater extravasation into the tumor tissue.[91,108] While the higher degree of PEGylation result in longer circulation time and higher tumor accumulation, which is beneficial for drug delivery purposes, it may not prove to be optimal, if the aim is to use radiolabeled nanoparticles as imaging agents. In this case background clearance of the radiolabeled nanoparticles from blood will generally improve imaging quality. Therefore, from an imaging point of view, a compromise between tumor accumulation and blood circulation time is preferred in order to obtain optimal images by lowering the background signal from the blood.

The *particle size* is another important parameter when designing nanoparticles for *in vivo* applications to prevent opsonization and clearance. Several studies have investigated the optimal size of non-PEGylated liposomes,[62,109,110] and liposomes that are 50–100 nm in diameter have been shown to have longer circulation and higher tumor accumulation compared to larger liposomes.[111] In general, studies in mice show that larger nanoparticles are eliminated from the blood circulation more rapidly than smaller nanoparticles of similar compositions[103,112,113] due to higher RES recognition. PEGylation of liposomes results in clearance rates that are relatively insensitive to the size in the range of 50 to 250 nm.[111,114–116] However, no clinical studies are available to determine the effect of particle size on tumor accumulation.

An important factor in nanoparticle design is determination of the dose needed to obtain optimal accumulation characteristics of nanoparticles at the target site relative to background activity (activity in normal tissues) for imaging purposes. In a study by Laverman *et al.* very low lipid doses were shown to alter the biodistribution of ^{99m}Tc-PEG liposomes dramatically in rats, rabbits as well as in humans.[87]

The main differences in the clearance profiles were observed in the initial clearance phase ($T_{½\alpha}$), whereas the clearance during the terminal phase or elimination phase ($T_{½\beta}$) was less affected by the lipid dose levels.[87] In humans injected with a lipid dose (0.1 μmol/kg) an increased activity within the liver, spleen and bone marrow within the first 4 h was observed compared to humans injected with higher lipid doses (0.5 μmol/kg).[87]

4.1. *Passive in vivo targeting*

Cancerous tissue is characterized by leaky blood vessels with gaps between the endothelial cell layers that are up to 700 nm, allowing nanoparticles to extravasate into the extracellular space in the diseased tissue.[117,118] This leakiness is caused by the fast and uncontrolled tumor growth, with a contributing effect from the inflamed condition in the tissue. Furthermore, nanoparticles become trapped in the extracellular space due to the ineffective lymphatic drainage within tumor tissue and the difference in the pressure between the interstitial space and the blood stream. The combined effects are referred to as the enhanced permeability and retention effect (EPR-effect), and the utilization of the EPR effect is generally referred to as passive tumor targeting (Figure 5).

The ability of various nanoparticles labeled with ^{99m}Tc, ^{111}In, ^{67}Ga, ^{18}F and ^{64}Cu, to localize in tumor tissues due to the EPR-effect has been reported in several preclinical studies in rats and mice using SPECT imaging[56,63,67,70,71,119] as well as PET imaging[32,53,69,120] (Table 5).

The relatively long half-life of ^{64}Cu makes it one of few PET isotopes that are suitable for *in vivo* imaging of nanoparticles as it allows sufficient time to reach maximum nanoparticles accumulation in the tumor tissue before imaging. In a study the ability of ^{64}Cu loaded PEGylated liposomes to accumulate in tumor tissue due to the EPR-effect was investigated in tumor bearing mice using PET imaging, where the tumors were clearly visualized from coronal and axial view (Figure 4).[69] In another study, passively targeted ^{64}Cu labeled micelles also showed high accumulation in tumors due to the EPR-effect (Figure 6).[48] Here the micelles were coated with a PEG corona reducing RES recognition and were only 30 nm in size.

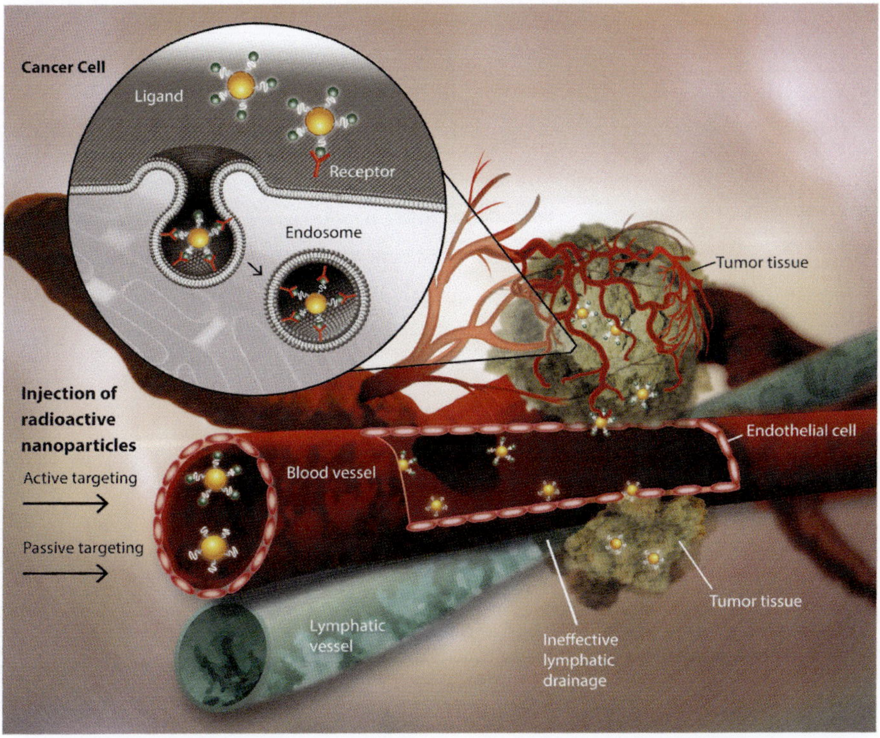

Fig. 5: Passive and active targeting of nanoparticles in tumor tissue.

Clinical studies using passively targeted radiolabeled liposomes and SPECT imaging, have showed positive tumor identification, which in many cases can be attributed to tumor accumulation by the EPR effect and in some cases it could be that it is only nanoparticles in the blood pool that gives rise to signal (Table 4). Figure 7 shows a patient with stage $T_1I_1S_1$ AIDS related Kaposis sarcoma that was injected with passively targeted ^{111}In-labeled DTPA liposomes where several tumors in the left foot and leg, right arm and face are visualized.[92] They also demonstrated that liposome deposition was very variable across tumor types and among patients with the same tumor type.[92] This indicates the potential variability in therapeutic outcome of variable liposome deposition in tumors.

Thus, to successfully design radiolabeled nanoparticles for clinical use, a balance must be achieved between preserving a

Table 5. Examples of passively targeted radiolabeled nanoparticles in preclinical cancer studies.

Radionuclide/imaging technique/nanoparticle	Tumor model	Refs.
^{67}Ga/SPECT/Liposome	SL2 lymphoma in mice	63
^{67}Ga/SPECT/Liposome	Yoshida sarcoma in rats	67
^{111}In/SPECT/AuNP	Human squamous carcinoma A431 in mice	71
^{111}In/SPECT/Liposome	EMT6 tumors in mice	70
^{99m}Tc/SPECT/Liposome	Walker 256 carcinoma in rats	56
^{99m}Tc/SPECT/Iron oxide	Sentinel lymph node in Wister male rats	121
^{67}Ga/SPECT/Liposome	Ehrlich solid tumors in mice	119
^{18}F/PET/Micelle	Walker 256 carcinoma in rats	122
^{64}Cu/PET/Liposome	Human colon adenocarcinoma (HT29) in mice	69
^{64}Cu/PET/Micelle	U87MG glioblastoma in mice	48
^{64}Cu/PET/Liposome	Met-1 tumors in mice	120
^{64}Cu/PET/Liposome	Meth A sarcoma in mice	53

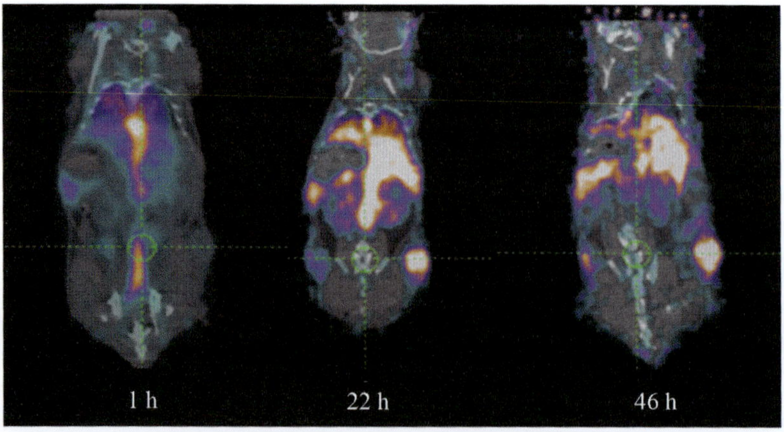

Fig. 6: PET/CT-images of ^{64}Cu labeled DOTA conjugated micelles in mice with U87MG tumor xenograft (tumor in right flank on displayed slices). The images reveal the biodistribution at 1, 22 and 46 h post-injection with good tumor accumulation and modest uptake in liver and spleen (reprinted with permission).[48]

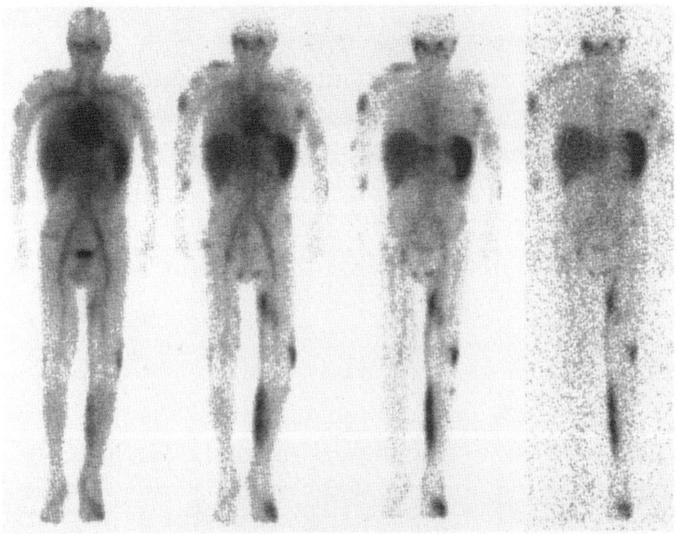

Fig. 7: Serial whole body gamma camera images over 7 days of a patient with stage $T_1I_1S_1$ AIDS–KS. Multiple areas of uptake of radiolabeled liposomes are seen in the left foot and leg, right arm, and face. Each of these areas corresponded with a typical Kaposis sarcoma lesion. Prolonged retention of the radiolabel is seen despite significant clearance of circulating liposomes, as demonstrated by disappearance of radiolabel from the cardiac blood pool (reprinted with permission).[92]

favorable circulation half-life, i.e., maximum tumor accumulation and blood clearance to reduce background signal. The retention of radioisotope payload is naturally an important factor to ensure high quality images. Regulatory approval of a radiolabeled nanoparticles requires toxicity testing and approval of all the individual components in the drug formulations. It is therefore, a great advantage to investigate a radiolabeled nanoparticle that is based on an already approved drug delivery system. The loading approach developed by Lee *et al.*[3] using a gradient-loadable chelator, 4-DEAP–ATSC, for liposomal ^{64}Cu labeling is suitable for labeling existing liposomal therapeutics, and can potentially transform these into theranostics to evaluate the potential as a prognostic tool for predicting treatment outcome.[3]

4.2. *Active in vivo targeting*

While nanoparticles passively accumulate in tumor sites due to the EPR-effect, the attachment of targeting ligands has been proposed to enhance tumor accumulation and cellular uptake (Figure 5). Targeting strategies using ligands that are directed towards over-expressed receptors on tumor cells or highly expressed markers on the endothelium of tumor vasculature can potentially improve the disease specific targeting of nanoparticles[18,123] and work additively with the EPR-effect to increase tumor accumulation. The targeting ligands can include antibodies, antibody fragments, peptides, aptamers and small molecules such as folic acid or carbohydrates that target the cancer cells/tissue.[18] The aim of using targeting ligands in diagnostic applications is to increase the imaging agent concentration in diseased tissue relatively to healthy organs and tissue, preferably at an early time-point after injection. However, it is not clear how much the use of targeting ligands improve liposome tumor accumulation. While some studies have shown that active targeting of nanoparticles increase accumulation in tumors.[124,125] Other studies report nanoparticles with targeting ligands that improve the intracellular delivery of their cargo to the target cells, but with a biodistribution and tumor accumulation similar to the non-targeted systems.[126–129] Targeting strategies of cancer cells and tumor tissue have so far included targeting ligands for a number of receptors, e.g., transferrin[130,131], folate[128,129,132,133], integrin[39,43,44,46,76,134–136], epidermal growth factor (EGFR)[3,127,137–141], vasoactive intestinal peptide receptors (VIP-R)[142–144], somatostatin[145,146], membrane matrix metalloprotease[147,148], annexin A5[38] and nucleosome specific monoclonal antibody 2C5[124,125] have been reported. Despite the significant efforts that have been made in targeting strategies, only passive targeting delivery systems have been tested in clinical studies with radiolabeling liposomes using SPECT imaging. The first clinical study using ^{64}Cu-radiolabeled liposomes for PET imaging are testing ^{64}Cu radiolabeled HER2-targeted liposomal doxorubicin (MM-302) in breast cancer patients.[79]

Among the preclinical studies on targeted nanoparticles both SPECT[38,39,42,124,125,142,143,147–149] and PET[3,32,43,44,46,76,146–148,150] imaging studies have been reported (Table 6). Targeted ^{3}H- and ^{10}B labeled

Table 6. Examples of active targeted radiolabeled nanoparticles in preclinical cancer studies.

Imaging technique/Nanoparticle	Targeting agent/Cell surface target	Tumor model	Refs.
^{99m}Tc/SPECT/Liposome	Vasoactive intestinal peptide (VIP)/VIP receptors	MNU-induced mammary cancer in rats	143
^{99m}Tc/SPECT/Liposome	Cyclic peptide inhibitor CTTHWG-FTLC (CTT)/Matrix metalloproteinases and gelatinases (MMP-2 and MMP-9)	KS1767 Kaposi's sarcoma in mice	148
^{99m}Tc/SPECT/AuNP	RGD-peptide/Integrin	C6 glioma in mice	39
^{111}In/SPECT/Liposome	Monoclonal antibody (mAb 2C5) and polychelating amphiphilic polymer (PEP)/Nucleosomes	Lewis lung carcinoma and breast adenocarcinoma (HT29) in mice	124, 125
^{111}In/SPECT/Liposome	Mesothelioma-targeting human single chain antibody (scFv), M1/Melanoma cell adhesion molecule (MCAM)	Epithelioid (M28) and sarcomatoid (VAMT-1) in mice	149
^{111}In/SPECT/Iron oxide	Annexin A5/Phosphatidylserine	EL4 lymphoma and MDA-MB-468 breast tumor in mice	38
^{67}Ga/SPECT/Cobalt-ferrite	DNA aptamer (AS1411)/Nucleolin	C6 glioma in mice	42
^{18}F/PET/Liposome	Angiogenic homing peptide, APRPG/Integrins	C6 glioma in mice	32,150
^{64}Cu/PET/Liposome	Somatostatin peptide analog, Ocreotate (TATE)/Somatostatin receptors	Human neuroendocrine tumors (NCI-H727) in mice	146
^{64}Cu/PET/Liposome	HER2 antibody (scFv)/HER2 receptors	Human HER2-overexpressing breast carcinoma (BT474-M3) in mice	3
^{64}Cu/PET/Quantum dots, Iron ioxide, Ferritin	RGD-peptide/Integrin	U87MG glioblastoma tumor model in mice	43,44,46,76

liposomes have also been exploited in several *in vivo* preclinical studies tracking the biodistribution and tumor targeting effect of liposomes with ligands as folate[128,129,132,133], transferrin[131], anti-vascular cell adhesion molecule-1 (anti-VCAM-1)[151] and cyclic NGR peptide for aminopeptidase N receptor targeting[152] (Table 6).

An example of enhancing tumor accumulation by active targeting of long-circulating was reported for ^{111}In-labeled liposomes modified with the nucleosome-specific monoclonal antibody 2C5. Tumor-bearing mice were tail vain injected with the targeted liposomes and biodistribution was visualized through gamma-imaging studies.[124,125] The data clearly demonstrated enhanced tumor accumulation of 2C5-modified ^{111}In-labeled liposomes compared with non-targeted controls.

In an animal imaging study performed by Lee *et al.*[3] HER2 over-expressing tumors were targeted in a xenograft mice model with theranostic liposomes (PEGylated HER2-targeted liposomes encapsulating doxorubicin (MM-302)) visualized using PET/CT imaging.[3] Here the ^{64}Cu-MM-302 targeted the over-expressed receptors on the tumors and showed tumor-to-muscle (T/M) ratios of 6.3 ± 2 and 7.1 ± 3 at 5 h and 20 h post-injection.[3]

Another theranostic agent was prepared by Yang *et al.*[46], a cRGD-functionalized, doxorubicin-conjugated and ^{64}Cu-labelled superparamagnetic iron oxide nanoparticle (SPION) for targeted anticancer drug delivery and PET/magnetic resonance imaging (MRI) of tumors with integrin expression.[46]

In another imaging study NE tumors were targeted in a xenograft mice model with diagnostic PEGylated ^{64}Cu-liposomes visualized using PET imaging.[146] Here the PEGylated ^{64}Cu-liposomes modified with a somatostatin analog (octreotate, TATE) targeted the over-expressed receptors on NE tumors and showed higher T/M ratio (12.7 ± 1.0) than the control-liposomes without TATE (8.9 ± 0.9). The targeted liposomes showed same tumor accumulation as the controls but had a slightly shorter blood circulation half-life.[146]

Active targeting has been investigated in multiple studies, however, the increase in solid tumor accumulation relative to levels obtained with passive targeting based on the EPR-effect is not clear and it is not obvious how relevant optimization of targeting in mouse xenograft models is to human cancers. However, the active targeting may prove more effective in humans than in xenograft models where the EPR-effect results in a very high accumulation by itself. In order to test this, more clinical studies using active targeted radiolabeled nanoparticles are warranted to provide new knowledge on how active targeted nanoparticle technology can be used in medical diagnostic as well as in therapeutic clinical applications. Targeted nanoparticles are likely to have great potential in personalized medicine where therapy can be tailored to the individual patient based on tumor expression of specific biomarkers.

5. Dosimetric Safety Assessment of Liposomal Radiopharmaceuticals

Radiation dosimetric data and safety assessment are required by the FDA during review of applications for approval of new radiopharmaceuticals. The amount of radiation that is absorbed within different organs and the body as whole from radiotracer administration should be calculated by standardized methods described by the International Committee on Radiation Protection (ICRP) and Medical Internal Radiation Dose (MIRD) committee. One of the standardized methods is the computer software for internal dose assessment called OLINDA/EXM (Organ Level Internal Dose Assessment/Exponential Modeling).[154] In order to estimate absorbed doses, whole human body phantom libraries as well as decay data of more than 800 radionuclides are integrated in the code of OLINDA/EXM.[154] Relatively accurate dosimetric safety assessments can be obtained from biodistribution and kinetic data from animal or human studies, especially from quantitative PET imaging data, allowing estimation of radiation exposures to a patient during a diagnostic scanning procedure.

5.1. *Calculating radiation doses according to OLINDA/EXM*

Several factors determine the amount of radiation absorbed within an organ (referred to as target organ) including the physical characteristics of the radionuclide as $T_{½}$, emission type, penetration ability and the biological characteristics of the radiotracer such as kinetics and retention in organs (referred to as source organs) over time.[154,155] The absorbed dose to a target organ is the sum of all radiation from inside the target organ (self-irradiation) plus radiation from all neighboring source organs. A source organ is defined as an organ having radiotracer uptake significantly above background on medical images. Typically source organs from an administration of a nanoparticle radiotracer are the kidneys, liver, spleen, lung, bone marrow and heart. Another source organ is the blood stream due to the long circulating properties of many types of PEGylated nanoparticles. In order to estimate the absorbed doses, the residence time (T_R) is calculated for each source organ corresponding to the total cumulated activity (A_c) in a source organ divided by the total activity dose (D) administered to the subject. The residence time (T_R) is defined in Eq. (2). The cumulated activity is the total number of disintegrations within the source organs, and is calculated by integrating the time-activity curve from VOIs. The cumulated activity (A_c) is calculated using Eq. (1):

$$A_c = V_{\text{organ}} \cdot \int_0^{\infty} \hat{A}\, dt; [\text{Bq} \cdot \text{h}], \tag{1}$$

where $\hat{A}$ is the activity concentration [Bq/ml] in the source organ as function of time, uncorrected for radioactive decay and V_{organ} is the volume of the organ [ml]. The volume of the organ can be determined from a CT scan.

The residence time (T_R) is calculated by dividing the cumulated activity (A_c) for the particular source organ by the total activity dose administered (D):

$$T_R = \frac{A_c}{D}; [h]. \tag{2}$$

The calculated T_R values are the principal input in the OLINDA/EXM software. The output allows a number of different important dosimetric assessments, such as identifying the most critical organs and estimating the total effective dose (ED_T). The different contributions from alpha particles, beta particles and ***photons*** as well as the total dose (D_T) to the target organs can also be obtained. The effective dose (*ED*) for each target organ is calculated by multiplying D_T delivered to each target organ by its tissue weighting factor (w_T) defined in Eq. (3). The tissue weighting factor represents relative sensitivity of organs to biological damage[156]:

$$ED = w_T \cdot D_T; \quad [mSv]. \tag{3}$$

The aim of calculating each single *ED* for all organs is to identify the most critical organs. The most critical organs are thereby the organs, which are most susceptible to biological damage and for developing cancer, which in the end may limit the administrative dose of a radiopharmaceutical to a patient. Organs containing cells that are reproducing fast in the body are the most vulnerable to radiation damage, and it is therefore important to keep the dose delivery to these organs or tissues to a minimum.[154,155] The organs obtaining the highest *ED*, so called critical organs, from radiolabeled nanoparticle administration are typically the spleen, liver, stomach and intestine walls, red marrow and lungs. By summing the *ED* for all the organs, the ED_T can be achieved. For most diagnostic radiopharmaceuticals, the ED_T values are in the range of 2–10 milli Sievert (mSv).[157] Different dose limit ranges expressed as ED_T have been defined by ICRP, and can be used as guidelines when designing clinical imaging studies.

While an evaluation of the absorbed radiation dose to a patient based on preclinical studies provides a reasonable guideline, especially for identifying the most critical organs, caution must be exercised in interpreting the approximated absorbed radiation doses. A clinical biodistribution study with absorbed dose calculations is required of a particular radiopharmaceutical in order to make safe dosimetric assessing of the diagnostic potential prior to clinical diagnostic use. While a few preclinical dosimetry studies on liposomes for radiotherapeutic applications have been reported,[158–161] an evaluation of the absorbed doses from diagnostic liposomal radiopharmaceuticals have not yet been published.

6. Cancer Imaging and Personalized Therapy using Nanoparticle Radiopharmaceuticals

Several clinical trials on radiolabeled liposomal formulations have in the past been carried out using SPECT imaging; however, most of these studies were done in the 1990's and the quality of the generated images was not high. Scanner technology and imaging quality have evolved in recent years and this provides many new possibilities for theranostic approaches and nanoparticle radiotracers are highly interesting in this regard. The first clinical study using the very promising theranostic ^{64}Cu radiolabeled liposomes for PET imaging was initiated in 2014 by Merrimack Pharmaceuticals.[79] With the improved radiolabeling methodologies developed in the last decade additional clinical studies are warranted to further increase the knowledge of nanoparticle *in vivo* behavior and tumor specificity, where clinical PET imaging studies will be of great importance due to the higher detection sensitivity compared to SPECT imaging. Radiolabeled nanoparticle technology may not only provide information on biodistribution and pharmacokinetics of nanoparticle drugs, but may also be a significant addition to the currently available arsenal of imaging agents for cancer diagnostics. A number of malignancies are not optimally visualized with currently available radiotracers, including prostate and ovarian cancers.[162] The biodistribution and circulation properties of radiolabeled nanoparticles compared to other imaging agents, such as ^{18}FDG and radiolabeled peptides, potentially makes radiolabeled nanoparticles interesting as diagnostic agents, besides the obvious importance of their use as companion diagnostics in nanomedicine.

The evaluation of radiolabeled nanoparticles in various preclinical models has generally provided promising results from a diagnostic as well as a drug delivery perspective, both for passive and active targeting systems (Tables 5 and 6). However, the discrepancy between spontaneous syngenic human cancer and xenograft models, in regards to tumor microenvironment, angiogenesis and tumor growth and invasion, makes the direct translation of preclinical results difficult. There is a strong need to quantify differences in nanoparticle accumulation in tumors based on passive targeting (EPR-effect), in large animals with spontaneous cancers and in humans. Investigations of active targeting in large animals with spontaneous tumors would also be highly valuable as we currently have very little information on targeting from studies other than mouse xenograft models. Currently, no publications exists on differences in targeting ligand benefit for accumulation of nanoparticles in tumors in large animals or humans that have developed cancer spontaneously, in comparison to non-targeted systems, which is highly warranted to understand differences in comparison to mouse models. Imaging studies using spontaneous cancer-bearing dogs may provide the opportunity to improve on current knowledge on biodistribution of nanoparticle drugs by serving as spontaneous clinical cancer models. Dogs develop several cancer types that are directly comparable to cancers in humans, which make dogs attractive as direct large animal models.[163–165]

6.1. *Molecular and functional imaging strategies used in drug development and targeted therapies*

During the last decade radiolabeled molecular and functional imaging agents have been developed to characterize the tumor microenvironment, guide therapies and evaluate therapeutic interactions.[6–9]

Identification of tumor characteristics and targets, including gene-expression profiles, mutational status and phenotypical characteristics, is often based on multiple tumor biopsies. This approach was recently identified as being insufficient in many cases to fully describe the whole tumor due to large intra-tumor heterogeneities in the parameters being evaluated.[166] Novel cancer imaging agents target cancer tissue by being sensitive to tumor specific micro-environmental conditions or phenotypical characteristics. Future directions in development of diagnostic protocols does not only include imaging agents for new molecular targets but may also focus on improving the understanding of how imaging agent combinations can give a more precise phenotypic characterization, including information on intra-tumor heterogeneities.

6.2. *Nanoparticle imaging for monitoring therapy and personalized treatment*

The unique possibility to predict the biodistribution of drug delivery systems by radiolabeled nanoparticles may serve as a method to individualize and optimize cancer therapy during the treatment period. Ideally, patients that are planned to receive nanoparticle-based chemotherapeutics, should be evaluated individually for tumor accumulation and be selected for treatment on the basis of this. It would be a very important step forward in nanomedicine to conduct a clinical study of a nanoparticle chemotherapeutic agent and image the nanoparticle biodistribution as part of the first injection. The patient should follow then current standardized treatment and the accumulated patient data can then be part of a comparison study where treatment benefit, including toxicity parameters, is correlated with degree of accumulation and biodistribution of the nanoparticle formulation. In addition it would be important to evaluate how nanoparticle tumor accumulation changes over a treatment period, i.e., will the nanoparticle accumulate less in tumors after a few treatment cycles? Such studies would identify which and when cancer patients may benefit from delivery of chemotherapeutics by nanoparticle systems. During the course of therapy, changes in the tumor microenvironment, including vascularization, may change the optimal delivery method for chemotherapy. Therapy using nanoparticle drugs may be affected by concurrent therapies targeting the tumor blood vessels or tumor angiogenesis,[167] as well as by numerous pharmacologic agents affecting blood pressure and vascular permeability. Furthermore, several of the most commonly used therapeutic modalities may influence bloods vessels and endothelial cells within solid tumors. Knowledge on vascular condition and its influence on nanoparticle drug accumulation are therefore highly important to optimally plan drug delivery approaches and radiolabeled nanoparticle could serve to monitor treatment in real-time allowing adjustment of the delivery type and dosing during therapy.

7. Conclusions and Outlook

The developments in nanomedicine over the last decade has resulted in a dramatic increase in the number of clinical trials that have been initiated with nanotherapeutics for treating cancer and new nanodrugs are reaching market. There are now indications that nanoparticle imaging systems for companion diagnostics is going to occur in clinical trials and eventually reach market as co-developed systems in conjugation to nanotherapeutics. The benefit of this is likely to be large, both for patients, society and companies that decide to utilize the benefits that imaging systems can provide in patient selection and monitoring of therapy. Nanoparticle systems provide an optimal platform within the theranostic area due to the functionality that can be engineered relatively easily into nanoparticles allowing the same carrier to function both as drug delivery systems and as imaging probes. In research articles many aim to add both drugs and imaging probes into the same particle, but it is more likely in a clinical and commercial setting that a few nanoparticle imaging probes will be developed and commercialized that can function to evaluate treatment benefit and used in patient selection in combination with a range of nanoparticle drug delivery systems. It is going to be interesting to follow this development in the coming years due to the obvious impact nanoparticle imaging probes can have on cancer treatment with nanotherapeutics, in particular for patient selection and thereby individualized therapy.

References

1. F. Chen, E. B. Ehlerding, W. Cai, *J. Nucl. Med.*, 1919 (2014).
2. A. S. Thakor, S. S. Gambhir, *Ca. Cancer J. Clin.*, 395 (2013).
3. H. Lee, J. Zheng, D. Gaddy, K. D. Orcutt, S. Leonard, E. Geretti, J. Hesterman, C. Harwell, J. Hoppin, D. A. Jaffray, T. Wickham, B. S. Hendriks, D. Kirpotin, *Nanomedicine: NBM*, 155 (2015).
4. A. L. Kesner, W. Hsueh, N. L. Htet, B. S. Pio, J. Czernin, M. D. Pegram, M. E. Phelps, D. H. S. Silverman, *J. Nucl. Med.*, 2021 (2007).

5. W. A. Hsueh, A. L. Kesner, A. Gangloff, M. D. Pegram, M. Beryt, J. Czernin, M. E. Phelps, D. H. S. Silverman, *J. Nucl. Med.*, 1995 (2006).
6. J. K. Willmann, N. van Bruggen, L. M. Dinkelborg, S. S. Gambhir, *Nat. Rev. Drug Discov.*, 591 (2008).
7. B. Turkbey, H. Kobayashi, M. Ogawa, M. Bernardo, P. L. Choyke, *Am. J. Roentgenol.*, 304 (2009).
8. L. Fass, *Mol. Oncol.*, 115 (2008).
9. G. Lappin, R. Garner, *Nat. Rev. Drug Discov.*, 233 (2003).
10. S. Gambhir, *Nat. Rev. Cancer*, 683 (2002).
11. M. E. Phelps, E. J. Hoffman, N. A. Mullani, M. M. Terpogossian, *J. Nucl. Med.*, 210 (1975).
12. S. Gambhir, H. Herschman, S. Cherry, J. Barrio, N. Satyamurthy, T. Toyokuni, M. Phelps, S. Larson, J. Balatoni, R. Finn, M. Sadelain, J. Tjuvajev, R. Blasberg, *Neoplasia*, 118 (2002).
13. T. Binderup, U. Knigge, A. Loft, B. Federspiel, A. Kjaer, *Clin. Cancer Res.*, 978 (2010).
14. E. Miele, G. P. Spinelli, F. Tomao, A. Zullo, F. De Marinis, G. Pasciuti, L. Rossi, F. Zoratto, S. Tomao, *J. Exp. Clin. Canc. Res.*, 52 (2008).
15. H. Schoder, S. M. Larson, *Semin. Nucl. Med.*, 274 (2004).
16. S. V. Smith, *J. Inorg. Biochem.*, 1874 (2004).
17. B. Goins, *Expert Opin. Med. Diagn.*, 853 (2008).
18. F. M. Kievit, M. Zhang, *Adv. Mater*, H217 (2011).
19. A. Sonzogni, *NuDat 2.6, National Nuclear Data Center*, Brookhaven National Laboratory, 2012.
20. S. Vallabhajosula, in Molecular Imaging: *Radiopharmaceuticals for PET and SPECT*, Springer, 2009.
21. A. Rahmim, H. Zaidi, *Nucl. Med. Commun.*, 193 (2008).
22. M. E. Phelps, *in PET: Physics, Instrumentation, and Scanners*, Springer, 2006.
23. M. Shokeen, C. J. Anderson, *Acc. Chem. Res.*, 832 (2009).
24. J. S. Lewis, R. Laforest, F. Dehdashti, P. W. Grigsby, M. J. Welch, B. A. Siegel, *J. Nucl. Med.*, 1177 (2008).
25. W. T. Phillips, *Adv. Drug Deliv. Rev.*, 13 (1999).
26. V. P. Torchilin, *Nat. Rev. Drug Discov.*, 145 (2005).
27. Q. Ahkong, C. Tilcock, *Nucl. Med. Biol.*, 831 (1992).

28. R. Goto, H. Kubo, S. Okada, *Chem. Pharm. Bull.*, 1351 (1989).
29. D. Hnatowich, B. Friedman, B. Clancy, M. Novak, *J. Nucl. Med.*, 810 (1981).
30. P. Laverman, E. Dams, W. Oyen, G. Storm, E. Koenders, R. Prevost, J. van der Meer, F. Corstens, O. Boerman, *J. Nucl. Med.*, 192 (1999).
31. T. Urakami, S. Akai, Y. Katayama, N. Harada, H. Tsukada, N. Oku, *J. Med. Chem.*, 6454 (2007).
32. N. Oku, M. Yamashita, Y. Katayama, T. Urakami, K. Hatanaka, K. Shimizu, T. Asai, H. Tsukada, S. Akai, H. Kanazawa, *Int. J. Pharm.*, 170 (2011).
33. J. W. Seo, S. Qin, L. M. Mahakian, K. D. Watson, A. Kheirolomoom, K. W. Ferrara, *J. Control. Release*, 28 (2011).
34. J. W. Seo, L. M. Mahakian, A. Kheirolomoom, H. Zhang, C. F. Meares, R. Ferdani, C. J. Anderson, K. W. Ferrara, *Bioconjug. Chem.*, 1206 (2010).
35. J. W. Seo, H. Zhang, D. L. Kukis, C. F. Meares, K. W. Ferrara, *Bioconjug. Chem.*, 2577 (2008).
36. C. Tilcock, Q. Ahkong, D. Fisher, *Nucl. Med. Biol.*, 89 (1994).
37. R. Misri, D. Meier, A. C. Yung, P. Kozlowski, U. O. Haefeli, *Nanomedicine: NBM*, 1007 (2012).
38. R. Zhang, W. Lu, X. Wen, M. Huang, M. Zhou, D. Liang, C. Li, *J. Nucl. Med.*, 958 (2011).
39. E. Morales-Avila, G. Ferro-Flores, B. E. Ocampo-García, L. M. De León-Rodríguez, C. Santos-Cuevas, R. García-Becerra, L. A. Medina, L. Gómez-Oliván, *Bioconjug. Chem.*, 913 (2011).
40. B. Ocampo-García, G. Ferro-Flores, E. Morales-Avila, F. Ramírez De Mar, *Nucl. Med. Commun.*, 1095 (2011).
41. B. E. Ocampo-García, F. d. Ramírez M., G. Ferro-Flores, L. M. De León-Rodrí¬guez, C. Santos-Cuevas, E. Morales-Avila, C. A. de Murphy, M. Pedraza-López, L. A. Medina, M. A. Camacho-López, *Nucl. Med. Biol.*, 1 (2011).
42. D. W. Hwang, H. Y. Ko, J. H. Lee, H. Kang, S. H. Ryu, I. C. Song, D. S. Lee, S. Kim, *J. Nucl. Med.*, 98 (2010).
43. W. Cai, K. Chen, Z. Li, S. S. Gambhir, X. Chen, *J. Nucl. Med.*, 1862 (2007).

44. H. Lee, Z. Li, K. Chen, A. R. Hsu, C. Xu, J. Xie, S. Sun, X. Chen, *J. Nucl. Med.*, 1371 (2008).
45. J. Xie, K. Chen, J. Huang, S. Lee, J. Wang, J. Gao, X. Li, X. Chen, *Biomater.*, 3016 (2010).
46. X. Yang, H. Hong, J. J. Grailer, I. J. Rowland, A. Javadi, S. A. Hurley, Y. Xiao, Y. Yang, Y. Zhang, R. J. Nickles, W. Cai, D. A. Steeber, S. Gong, *Biomater.*, 4151 (2011).
47. J. C. Park, M. K. Yu, G. I. An, S. I. Park, J. Oh, H. J. Kim, J. H. Kim, E. K. Wang, I. H. Hong, Y. S. Ha, T. H. Choi, K. S. Jeong, Y. Chang, M. J. Welch, S. Jon, J. Yoo, *Small*, 2863 (2010).
48. A. I. Jensen, T. Binderup, P. E. K. Kumar, A. Kjaer, P. H. Rasmussen, T. L. Andresen, *Biomacromol.*, 1625 (2014).
49. J. Hardy, I. Kellaway, J. Rogers, C. Wilson, *J. Pharm. Pharmacol.*, 309 (1980).
50. E. Holmberg, K. Maruyama, D. Litzinger, S. Wright, M. Davis, G. Kabalka, S. Kennel, L. Huang, *Biochem. Biophys. Res. Commun.*, 1272 (1989).
51. A. Klibanow, K. Maruyama, V. Torchilin, L. Huang, *FEBS Lett.*, 235 (1990).
52. J. Marik, M. S. Tartis, H. Zhang, J. Y. Fung, A. Kheirolomoom, J. L. Sutcliffe, K. W. Ferrara, *Nucl. Med. Biol.*, 165 (2007).
53. N. Oku, Y. Tokudome, H. Tsukada, T. Kosugi, Y. Namba, S. Okada, *Biopharm. Drug Dispos.*, 435 (1996).
54. G. Lopezberestein, L. Kasi, M. G. Rosenblum, T. Haynie, M. Jahns, H. Glenn, R. Mehta, G. M. Mavligit, E. M. Hersh, *Cancer Res.*, 375 (1984).
55. J. R. Morgan, K. E. Williams, R. L. Davies, K. Leach, M. Thomson, L. A. P. Williams, *J. Med. Microbiol.*, 213 (1981).
56. V. Richardson, K. Jeyasingh, R. Jewkes, B. Ryman, M. Tattersall, *Biochem. Soc. Trans.*, 290 (1977).
57. D. S. Abou, D. L. J. Thorek, N. N. Ramos, M. W. H. Pinkse, H. T. Wolterbeek, S. D. Carlin, B. J. Beattie, J. S. Lewis, *Pharm. Res.*, 878 (2013).
58. V. Awasthi, B. Goins, R. Klipper, W. Phillips, *Nucl. Med. Biol.*, 155 (1998).
59. A. Bao, B. Goins, R. Klipper, G. Negrete, M. Mahindaratne, W. Phillips, *J. Pharm. Sci.*, 1893 (2003).
60. A. Bao, B. Goins, R. Klipper, G. Negrete, W. Phillips, *J. Pharmacol. Exp. Ther.*, 419 (2004).

61. P. Beaumier, K. Hwang, *J. Nucl. Med.*, 810 (1982).
62. O. Boerman, G. Storm, W. Oyen, L. Vanbloois, J. Vandermeer, R. Claessens, D. Crommelin, F. Corstens, *J. Nucl. Med.*, 1639 (1995).
63. A. Gabizon, J. Huberty, R. M. Straubinger, D. C. Price, D. Papahadjopoulus, *J. Liposome Res.*, 123 (1988).
64. K. Hwang, J. Merriam, P. Beaumier, K. Luk, *Biochim. Biophys. Acta*, 101 (1982).
65. M. Mougin-Degraef, E. Jestin, D. Bruel, P. Remaud-Le Saec, L. Morandeau, A. Faivre-Chauvet, J. Barbet, *J. Liposome Res.*, 91 (2006).
66. M. R. Mauk, R. C. Gamble, *Anal. Biochem.*, 302 (1979).
67. I. Ogihara, S. Kojima, M. Jay, *J. Nucl. Med.*, 1300 (1986).
68. W. T. Phillips, A. S. Rudolph, B. Goins, J. H. Timmons, R. Klipper, R. Blumhardt, *Nucl. Med. Biol.*, 539 (1992).
69. A. L. Petersen, T. Binderup, P. Rasmussen, J. R. Henriksen, D. R. Elema, A. Kjaer, T. L. Andresen, *Biomater.*, 2334 (2011).
70. R. T. Proffitt, L. E. Williams, C. A. Presant, G. W. Tin, J. A. Uliana, R. C. Gamble, J. D. Baldeschwieler, *J. Nucl. Med.*, 45 (1983).
71. G. Zhang, Z. Yang, W. Lu, R. Zhang, Q. Huang, M. Tian, L. Li, D. Liang, C. Li, *Biomater.*, 1928 (2009).
72. I. McDougal, J. Dunnick, M. McNamee, J. Kriss, *Proc. Natl. Acad. Sci. U. S. A.*, 3487 (1974).
73. M. Suresh, Y. Cao, J. *Pharm. Pharm. Sci.*, 31 (1998).
74. F. Duconge, T. Pons, C. Pestourie, L. Herin, B. Theze, K. Gombert, B. Mahler, F. Hinnen, B. Kuhnast, F. Dolle, B. Dubertret, B. Tavitian, *Bioconjug. Chem.*, 1921 (2008).
75. S. Guerrero, J. Raul Herance, S. Rojas, J. F. Mena, J. Domingo Gispert, G. A. Acosta, F. Albericio, M. J. Kogan, *Bioconjug. Chem.*, 399 (2012).
76. X. Lin, J. Xie, G. Niu, F. Zhang, H. Gao, M. Yang, Q. Quan, M. A. Aronova, G. Zhang, S. Lee, R. Leapman, X. Chen, *Nano Lett.*, 814 (2011).
77. B. Goins, W. Phillips, *Prog. Lipid Res.*, 95 (2001).
78. E. Dams, W. Oyen, O. Boerman, G. Storm, P. Laverman, P. Kok, W. Buijs, H. Bakker, J. van der Meer, F. Corstens, *J. Nucl. Med.*, 622 (2000).

79. National Institute of Health, U.S., (https://clinicaltrials.gov), Study ID: NCT01304797 (2014).
80. C. A. Presant, R. T. Proffitt, A. F. Turner, L. E. Williams, D. Winsor, J. L. Werner, P. Kennedy, C. Wiseman, K. Gala, R. J. Mckenna, J. D. Smith, S. A. Bouzaglou, R. A. Callahan, J. Baldeschwieler, R. J. Crossley, *Cancer*, 905 (1988).
81. C. A. Presant, D. Blayney, R. Proffitt, A. Turner, L. Williams, H. Nadel, P. Kennedy, C. Wiseman, K. Gala, R. Crossley, S. Preiss, G. Ksionski, S. Presant, *Lancet*, 1307 (1990).
82. C. A. Presant, A. F. Turner, R. T. Proffitt, *J. Liposome Res.*, 985 (1994).
83. A. Turner, C. Presant, R. Proffitt, L. Williams, D. Winsor, J. Werner, *Radiology*, 761 (1988).
84. A. Kubo, K. Nakamura, T. Sammiya, M. Katayama, T. Hashimoto, S. Hashimoto, H. Kobayashi, T. Teramoto, *Eur. J. Nucl. Med.*, 107 (1993).
85. A. Khalifa, D. Dodds, R. Rampling, J. Paterson, T. Murray, *Nucl. Med. Commun.*, 17 (1997).
86. A. Brouwers, D. De Jong, E. Dams, W. Oyen, O. Boerman, P. Laverman, T. Naber, G. Storm, F. Corstens, *J. Drug Target.*, 225 (2000).
87. P. Laverman, A. H. Brouwers, E. T. M. Dams, W. J. G. Oyen, G. Storm, N. Van Rooijen, F. H. M. Corstens, O. C. Boerman, *J. Pharmacol. Exp. Ther.*, 996 (2000).
88. J. Morgan, L. Williams, C. Howard, *Br. J. Radiol.*, 35 (1985).
89. M. Osullivan, N. Powell, A. French, K. Williams, J. Morgan, B. Williams, *Ann. Rheum. Dis.*, 485 (1988).
90. B. Williams, M. Osullivan, G. Saggu, K. Williams, L. Williams, J. Morgan, *Ann. Rheum. Dis.*, 314 (1987).
91. A. Gabizon, R. Chisin, S. Amselem, S. Druckmann, R. Cohen, D. Goren, I. Fromer, T. Peretz, A. Sulkes, Y. Barenholz, *Br. J. Cancer*, 1125 (1991).
92. K. Harrington, S. Mohammadtaghi, P. Uster, D. Glass, A. Peters, R. Vile, J. Stewart, *Clin. Cancer Res.*, 243 (2001).
93. J. Murray, E. Kleinerman, J. Cunningham, J. Tatom, K. Andrejcio, J. Lepezuniga, L. Lamki, M. Rosenblum, H. Frost, J. Gutterman, I. Fidler, I. Krakoff, *J. Clin. Oncol.*, 1915 (1989).

94. R. Perezsoler, G. Lopezberestein, L. P. Kasi, F. Cabanillas, M. Jahns, H. Glenn, E. M. Hersh, T. Haynie, *J. Nucl. Med.*, 743 (1985).
95. V. J. Richardson, B. E. Ryman, R. F. Jewkes, K. Jeyasingh, M. N. H. Tattersall, E. S. Newlands, S. B. Kaye, *Br. J. Cancer*, 35 (1979).
96. K. Harrington, G. Rowlinson-Busza, K. Syrigos, R. Abra, P. Uster, A. Peters, J. Stewart, *Br. J. Cancer*, 684 (2000).
97. D. Fugman, K. Shirak, R. Jackson, J. Johnson, *Biochim. Biophys. Acta*, 191 (1984).
98. M. Jones, A. Nicholas, *Biochem. Biophys. Acta*, 145 (1991).
99. P. C. Noordam, A. Killian, R. F. M. O. Elferink, J. Degier, *Chem. Phys. Lipids*, 191 (1982).
100. T. L. Andresen, D. H. Thompson, T. Kaasgaard, *Mol. Membr. Biol.*, 353 (2010).
101. G. Gregoriadis, *N. Engl. J. Med.*, 765 (1976).
102. J. N. Weinstein, *Cancer Treat. Rep.*, 127 (1984).
103. J. H. Senior, *CRC Crit. Rev. Ther. Drug Carrier Syst.*, 123 (1987).
104. T. Allen, C. Hansen, F. Martin, C. Redemann, A. Yauyoung, *Biochim. Biophys. Acta*, 29 (1991).
105. D. Papahadjopoulos, T. M. Allen, A. Gabizon, E. Mayhew, K. Matthay, S. K. Huang, K. D. Lee, M. C. Woodle, D. D. Lasic, C. Redemann, F. J. Martin, *Proc. Natl. Acad. Sci. U. S. A.*, 11460 (1991).
106. T. Chow, Y. Lin, J. Hwang, H. Wang, Y. Tseng, V. F. Pang, R. Liu, W. Lin, C. Yang, G. Ting, *J. Nucl. Med.*, 2073 (2009).
107. C. M. Lee, Y. D. Choi, E. J. Huh, K. Y. Lee, H. C. Song, M. J. Sun, H. J. Jeong, C. S. Cho, H. S. Bom, *Cancer Biother. Radio.*, 620 (2005).
108. A. Gabizon, *Clin.Cancer Res.*, 223 (2001).
109. T. Allen, C. Hansen, J. Rutledge, *Biochim. Biophys. Acta*, 27 (1989).
110. T. Allen, C. Hansen, *Biochim. Biophys. Acta*, 133 (1991).
111. D. Drummond, O. Meyer, K. Hong, D. Kirpotin, D. Papahadjopoulos, *Pharmacol. Rev.*, 691 (1999).
112. R. Abra, C. Hunt, *Biochim. Biophys. Acta*, 493 (1981).
113. K. Hwang, in *Liposomes: From Biophysics to Therapeutics*, Marcel Dekker Inc., 109, 1987.
114. D. Liu, A. Mori, L. Huang, *Biochim. Biophys. Acta*, 95 (1992).

115. M. C. Woodle, D. D. Lasic, *Biochim. Biophys. Acta*, 171 (1992).
116. T. Allen, D. Stuart, in *Liposomes: Rational design*, Marcel Dekker Inc., 63, 1998.
117. T. Andresen, S. Jensen, K. Jorgensen, *Prog. Lipid Res.*, 68 (2005).
118. T. Kaasgaard, T. L. Andresen, *Exp. Opinion on Drug Delivery*, 225 (2010).
119. I. Ogiharaumeda, S. Kojima, *J. Nucl. Med.*, 516 (1988).
120. A. Wong, E. Ormsby, H. Zhang, J. W. Seo, *J. Invest. Med.*, 234 (2012).
121. R. Madru, P. Kjellman, F. Olsson, K. Wingardh, C. Ingvar, F. Stahlberg, J. Olsrud, J. Latt, S. Fredriksson, L. Knutsson, S. Strand, *J Nucl. Med.*, 459 (2012).
122. M. Allmeroth, D. Moderegger, D. Guendel, H. Buchholz, N. Mohr, K. Koynov, F. Roesch, O. Thews, R. Zentel, *J. Control. Release*, 77 (2013).
123. F. Danhier, O. Feron, V. Preat, *J. Control. Release*, 135 (2010).
124. T. A. Elbayoumi, V. P. Torchilin, *Eur. J. Nucl. Med. Mol. I.*, 1196 (2006).
125. S. Erdogan, A. Roby, V. P. Torchilin, *Mol. Pharmaceut.*, 525 (2006).
126. D. W. Bartlett, H. Su, I. J. Hildebrandt, W. A. Weber, M. E. Davis, *Proc. Natl. Acad. Sci. U. S. A.*, 15549 (2007).
127. D. B. Kirpotin, D. C. Drummond, Y. Shao, M. R. Shalaby, K. Hong, U. B. Nielsen, J. D. Marks, C. C. Benz, J. W. Park, *Cancer Res.*, 6732 (2006).
128. M. O. Oyewumi, R. A. Yokel, M. Jay, T. Coakley, R. J. Mumper, *J. Control. Release*, 613 (2004).
129. X. Wang, J. Li, Y. Wang, K. J. Cho, G. Kim, A. Gjyrezi, L. Koenig, P. Giannakakou, H. J. C. Shin, M. Tighiouart, S. Nie, Z. Chen, D. M. Shin, *ACS Nano*, 3165 (2009).
130. M. Freedman, E. H. Chang, Q. Zhou, K. F. Pirollo, *Acad. Radiol.*, 627 (2009).
131. S. Miyata, S. Kawabata, R. Hiramatsu, A. Doi, N. Ikeda, T. Yamashita, T. Kuroiwa, S. Kasaoka, K. Maruyama, S. Miyatake, *Neurosurg.*, 1380 (2011).
132. A. Gabizon, A. Horowitz, D. Goren, D. Tzemach, H. Shmeeda, S. Zalipsky, *Clin. Cancer Res.*, 6551 (2003).
133. G. Henriksen, B. Schoultz, T. Michaelsen, O. Bruland, R. Larsen, *Nucl. Med. Biol.*, 441 (2004).

134. S. Du, H. Pan, W. Lu, J. Wang, J. Wu, J. Wang, *J. Pharmacol. Exp. Ther.*, 560 (2007).
135. G. Huang, Z. Zhou, R. Srinivasan, M. S. Penn, K. Kottke-Marchant, R. E. Marchant, A. S. Gupta, *Biomater.*, 1676 (2008).
136. R. Schiffelers, G. Koning, T. ten Hagen, M. Fens, A. Schraa, A. Janssen, R. Kok, G. Molema, G. Storm, *J. Control. Release*, 115 (2003).
137. J. Beuttler, M. Rothdiener, D. Mueller, F. Y. Frejd, R. E. Kontermann, *Bioconjug. Chem.*, 1201 (2009).
138. A. Fondell, K. Edwards, L. M. Ickenstein, S. Sjoberg, J. Carlsson, L. Gedda, *Eur. J. Nucl. Med. Mol. I.*, 114 (2010).
139. J. Gao, W. Liu, Y. Xia, W. Li, J. Sun, H. Chen, B. Li, D. Zhang, W. Qian, Y. Meng, L. Deng, H. Wang, J. Chen, Y. Guo, *Biomater.*, 3459 (2011).
140. C. Mamot, D. Drummond, C. Noble, V. Kallab, Z. Guo, K. Hong, D. Kirpotin, J. Park, *Cancer Res.*, 11631 (2005).
141. E. Portnoy, S. Lecht, P. Lazarovici, D. Danino, S. Magdassi, *Nanomed.-Nanotechnol.*, 480 (2011).
142. S. Dagar, M. Sekosan, B. Lee, I. Rubinstein, H. Onyuksel, *J. Control. Release*, 129 (2001).
143. S. Dagar, A. Krishnadas, I. Rubinstein, M. Blend, H. Onyuksel, *J. Control. Release*, 123 (2003).
144. E. Refai, C. Jonsson, M. Andersson, H. Jacobsson, S. Larsson, P. Kogner, M. Hassan, *Nucl. Med. Biol.*, 931 (1999).
145. J. Zhang, W. Jin, X. Wang, J. Wang, X. Zhang, Q. Zhang, *Mol. Pharm.*, 1159 (2007).
146. A. L. Petersen, T. Binderup, R. Jølck, P. Rasmussen, J. Henriksen, A. Pfeifer, A. Kjær, T. Andresen, *J. Control. Release*, 254 (2012).
147. M. Kondo, T. Asai, Y. Katanasaka, Y. Sadzuka, H. Tsukada, K. Ogino, T. Taki, K. Baba, N. Oku, *Int. J. Cancer*, 301 (2004).
148. O. Medina, K. Kairemo, H. Valtanen, A. Kangasniemi, S. Kaukinen, I. Ahonen, P. Permi, A. Annila, M. Sneck, J. Holopainen, S. Karonen, P. Kinnunen, E. Koivunen, *Anticancer Res.*, 33 (2005).
149. A. K. Iyer, Y. Su, J. Feng, X. Lan, X. Zhu, Y. Liu, D. Gao, Y. Seo, H. F. VanBrocklin, V. C. Broaddus, B. Liu, J. He, *Biomater.*, 2605 (2011).
150. N. Maeda, S. Miyazawa, K. Shimizu, T. Asai, S. Yonezawa, S. Kitazawa, Y. Namba, H. Tsukada, N. Oku, *Biol. Pharm. Bull.*, 1936 (2006).

151. S. Gosk, T. Moos, C. Gottstein, G. Bendas, *Biochim. Biophys. Acta*, 854 (2008).
152. F. Pastorino, C. Brignole, D. Marimpietri, M. Cilli, C. Gambini, D. Ribatti, R. Longhi, T. Allen, A. Corti, M. Ponzoni, *Cancer Res.*, 7400 (2003).
153. V. P. Torchilin, *AAPS Journal*, E128 (2007).
154. M. G. Stabin, R. B. Sparks, E. Crowe, *J. Nucl. Med.*, 1023 (2005).
155. D. Fisher, *Semin. Radiat. Oncol.*, 123 (2000).
156. International commission on radiation protection, in *Annual ICRP* 37:2–4, 103, (2007).
157. International commission on radiation protection, in *Annual ICRP* 22:3, 62, (1992).
158. D. Emfietzoglou, K. Kostarelos, G. Sgouros, *J. Nucl. Med.*, 499 (2001).
159. K. Kostarelos, D. Emfietzoglou, *Anticancer Res.*, 3339 (2000).
160. L. Chen, Y. Wu, I. Liu, C. Ho, W. Lee, C. Chang, K. Lan, G. Ting, T. Lee, J. Shien, *Nucl. Med. Biol.*, 35 (2012).
161. H. Wang, H. Yu, Y. Lu, N. Heish, Y. Tseng, K. Huang, K. Chuang, C. Chen, J. Hwang, W. Lin, S. Wang, G. Ting, J. Whang-Peng, W. Deng, *Nucl. Instrum. Meth. A.*, 533 (2006).
162. P. De Iaco, A. Musto, L. Orazi, C. Zamagni, M. Rosati, V. Allegri, N. Cacciari, A. Al-Nahhas, D. Rubello, S. Venturoli, S. Fanti, *Eur. J. Radiol.*, E98 (2011).
163. C. Khanna, C. London, D. Vail, C. Mazcko, S. Hirschfeld, *Clin. Cancer Res.*, 5671 (2009).
164. M. Paoloni, C. Khanna, *Nat. Rev. Cancer*, 147 (2008).
165. B. E. LeRoy, N. Northrup, *Vet. J.*, 149 (2009).
166. M. Gerlinger, A. J. Rowan, S. Horswell, J. Larkin, D. Endesfelder, E. Gronroos, P. Martinez, N. Matthews, A. Stewart, P. Tarpey, I. Varela, B. Phillimore, S. Begum, N. Q. McDonald, A. Butler, D. Jones, K. Raine, C. Latimer, C. R. Santos, M. Nohadani, A. C. Eklund, B. Spencer-Dene, G. Clark, L. Pickering, G. Stamp, M. Gore, Z. Szallasi, J. Downward, P. A. Futreal, C. Swanton, *N. Engl. J. Med.*, 883 (2012).
167. S. M. Weis, D. A. Cheresh, *Nat. Med.*, 1359 (2011).

CHAPTER 8

NANOTHERANOSTICS IN GENE THERAPY

Madhura Deshpande*, Shravan Kumar Sriraman*
and Vladimir Torchilin*,†,‡

*Center for Pharmaceutical Biotechnology and Nanomedicine, Northeastern University, Boston, MA 02115, USA
†Department of Biochemistry, Faculty of Science, King Abdulaziz University, Jeddah 21589, Saudi Arabia
‡v.torchilin@neu.edu

Over the last few years, the efficiency of nanoparticles has been widely demonstrated with a number of nanoparticle-based drugs being approved for clinical use. They have proved most useful in the delivery of labile drugs such as genes which when delivered specifically to the target site can elicit potent therapeutic effects. However, there still exist a number of barriers for the delivery of these agents to effect patient outcomes. These nanoparticles have also been widely used as diagnostic imaging agents. Therefore with patient compliance in mind the ability to combine both functions of diagnosis and therapy into a single platform would prove extremely useful. This emerging field of 'nanotheranostics' has gained a lot of interest in recent years with the overall aim of being able to provide personalized treatments to patients. This chapter thus aims to facilitate a better understanding of the various components of such a complex multifunctional platform and to subsequently equip the reader with all the latest developments in the emerging field of nanotheranostics specifically employing gene therapy to overcome and treat the various disease states.

1. Introduction

Nanomedicine represents an emerging field which combines nanotechnology, biomedicine and molecular engineering to attain improved strategies for drug delivery and diagnosis of disease states, such as cancer, which pose enormous challenges in terms of their treatment and management. Nanomedicines possess favorable properties such as increased drug stability, biocompatibility, weak immunogenicity, improved biodistribution and pharmacokinetics, ability to effectively carry the desired payload as well as specifically targeting it to the disease site.[1–4] They help to overcome problems associated with free drugs and conventional delivery systems such as non-selectivity, dose-limiting toxicity and off-site side effects, limited solubility of therapeutic molecules as well as multi-drug resistance.[5–7] Research in nanotechnology is aimed at developing methods to detect disease conditions in the human body non-invasively, monitor the condition and selectively deliver agents to effectively treat it. Nanoscale agents can help to image or detect abnormal physiological conditions at an early stage. Once detected, nanocarriers can carry the drug payloads, target it to the desired site and deliver it for maximum therapeutic effect. Multifunctional nanocarriers are being successfully developed that can simultaneously achieve all of this. Traditionally, diagnostic and therapeutic agents have been studied and developed independently. However, more recently nanocarriers that can combine both diagnosis and delivery of a therapy have been developed giving rise to the term 'nanotheranostics'.[8] Nanotheranostics have the capability of using nanoscale carriers for (1) concomitant early detection of disease states, (2) targeting a therapy to the disease site based on the diagnosis, (3) successful delivery of the payload at the disease site and

(4) monitoring of the response to treatment and disease progression by imaging or other diagnostic modalities. Thus, imaging can be done to obtain monitoring before, during and after treatment to follow the delivery and biodistribution of therapeutics and their elicited response. Research in this promising field of nanotheranostics focuses on integration of nanosensors and nanomedicines and efforts are aimed towards developing effective diagnostic biomarkers and imaging probes, targeting moieties and techniques, and molecular imaging-guided nanocarriers for delivery of various therapies to build a complete nanotheranostic platform system.[9]

The ultimate goal of nanotheranostics is to provide personalized medicine to patients so that an optimal treatment tailored to an individual patient's needs can be provided thus circumventing problems due to individual variability. Since a single therapeutic agent does not exert similar effect on different patients with the same diagnosis, the aim of personalized medicine is to draw out a treatment best suited for a particular patient based on the patients' genes, proteins and metabolites.[10] Nanotheranostics can help provide maximum personalized therapeutic benefit and safety by making possible the screening of patients who have the potential to favorably respond to a therapy based on early diagnosis and treatment leading to the possibility of improved results.[10–14] Additionally, sequencing of the human genome and recent advances in cancer genomics have opened up numerous attractive opportunities of utilizing nanotheranostics delivering genetic material for personalized medicine.[14] Development of a disease, such as cancer, in a patient due to his/her susceptibility to that disease, based on the patient's genetic make-up, can trigger the delivery of a nanotheranostic for diagnosis and targeting of a gene therapy that could potentially repair the genetic abnormality in the patient that was responsible for the development of the disease. Recent progress in cancer biology has identified that the large degree of molecular heterogeneity in tumors of the same type, among the cells of the same tumors and even between the primary and metastatic tumors, along with the development of multi-drug resistance by cancer cells, are responsible for the increased cancer malignancies and limited effects of conventional monotherapies.[15,16] Diagnosis of these tumor-related genetic mutations while simultaneously treating them with effective modalities such as gene therapy can be achieved by employing nanotheranostics. The amalgamation of biomolecular imaging and gene-based therapeutics has the promise of overcoming the challenges of cancer heterogeneity and adaptation.[17] The therapeutic prospects of nanotheranostics making use of gene therapy are thus substantial because of their considerable potential in the treatment of numerous diseases, either inherited or acquired, caused by genetic deficiencies and mutations, such as cancer, cardiovascular diseases, acquired immune deficiency syndrome (AIDS), or some autoimmune disorders.

This book chapter provides a review focusing on the recent development of nanotheranostic systems employing gene therapy as a means to effect personalized medicinal treatment.

2. Composition of a Nanotheranostic

Various nanocarriers containing either diagnostic or therapeutic properties have evolved to combine both these functionalities into one nanotheranostic particle.

A large variety of nanotheranostics have been developed which differ greatly in their size, shape, functionality, targeting moiety, mechanism of action and imaging modality. Even with such a broad variety of nanotheranostics being available, a typical nanotheranostic has certain characteristic components: a therapeutic agent, a nanocarrier made of polymers, lipids, etc. which provides a matrix for encapsulation of the therapeutic agent and attachment of various ligands or functional groups, a targeting ligand and finally a detection agent as a non-invasive imaging modality (Figure 1). These have been reviewed in more detail below.

2.1. *Therapeutic agent*

Recent knowledge about cancer diagnostics, tumor pathology, genes expressed in tumors and availability of high throughput methods can allow us to determine which genes need to be silenced or expressed in individual patients, thus enabling us to control the expression of

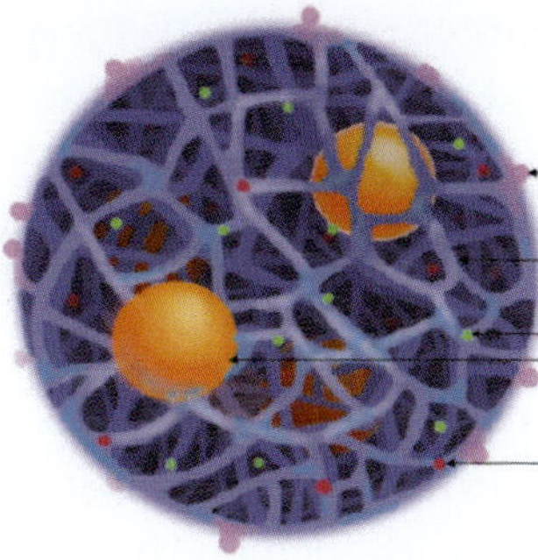

Fig. 1: Schematic representation of the structure of a typical nanotheranostic. (Reprinted with permission from reference.[25] Copyright 2015 American Chemical Society.)

specific genes.[13,18] Gene therapy involves the use of genetic material to modify cells *in vitro* or *in vivo* to obtain a favorable therapeutic outcome and is a promising alternative therapy to the use of conventional drugs. In gene therapy, genes are introduced in a person's cells to complement certain genes or modify certain abnormal genes so as to control or treat a disease condition thereby restoring biological functions.[19] For this, nucleotide drugs such as plasmid DNA (pDNA),[20] complementary DNA (cDNA),[21] messenger RNA (mRNA),[22] antisense oligonucleotides (AS-ODN),[23] as well as small interfering RNA (siRNA)[24] can be delivered in order to restore normalcy to the disease site or quell further progression of the disease. Physical encapsulation or entrapment in a nanocarrier matrix, electrostatic interactions with components of the nanotheranostic, chemical modifications of gene of interest or covalent conjugation to an imaging agent or nanocarrier are routinely used methods to load genes in a nanotheranostic.[25]

2.2. *Nanocarrier*

One of the most important challenges in gene therapy is the generation of an optimal delivery vehicle for the specific, effective and safe targeting of the gene to the desired site. Such an ideal nanodelivery system should possess several characteristics such as biocompatibility, biodegradability, no toxicity or immunogenicity, desired size range

(20–200 nm) to accumulate at the target site, ability to specifically bind and target the gene to the desired site and then release it effectively intracellularly in the cytosol by endosomal escape, stability against enzymatic degradation and rapid clearance by liver and kidneys.[26,27] To achieve this, physicochemical properties of nanocarriers such as size and surface charge can be optimized. Surface modification with polyethylene glycol (PEG) helps reduce opsonization and uptake by the cells of the mononuclear-phagocytic system.[28] Positive surface charge of nanocarriers aids interaction with negatively charged cell surface thereby assisting endocytosis.[29] Genes can be delivered by viral vectors such as retrovirus, adenovirus, lentivirus, etc. or non-viral vectors.[30,31] Various non-viral vectors include polymeric and lipid-based nanocarriers such as liposomes, gold nanoparticles, magnetic nanoparticles, dendrimers, etc. Use of viral vectors for gene therapy poses challenges such as reversion of virus to virulent form leading to undesirable immune response and toxicity; hence research is advancing towards development of alternative carriers, especially non-viral nanoscale carriers for administering genes into target cells effectively.[32]

2.3. *Targeting ligand*

Most nanoparticles are expected to accumulate in tumors by passive targeting mediated by the enhanced permeability and retention (EPR) effect.[33] However passive targeting can have several limitations such as irregularities in targeting due to differences in tumor vasculature with tumor type, reduced interaction between nanoparticle and cell surfaces, lack of control leading to drug expulsion, reduced therapeutic effect and multidrug resistance.[34] To prevent this, several ligands with therapeutic, diagnostic, or barrier-avoiding properties can be conjugated to the surface of a nanoparticle system.[35] Nanoparticles that are functionalized with targeting bodies can attach to target cells through ligand-receptor binding that induce receptor-mediated endocytosis and drug release inside the cell.[36] Depending on the chemical nature of the nanocarrier coating, functional groups such as amines, sulfhydryls, or carboxyl groups can be present for bioconjugation to fluorescent labels or targeting ligands.[37] Examples of targeting ligands include proteins (antibodies and their fragments), peptides, small molecules, nucleic acids (aptamers), or others (vitamins or carbohydrates).[38–40]

2.4. *Imaging moiety*

Molecular imaging allows visualizing nanoparticles cellularly and subcellularly *in vivo* non-invasively to assess the mechanism of action, biodistribution as well as clearance of the nanoparticles in the body. This data can shed light upon specificity of nanoparticle uptake, the uptake rate, the distribution of the system within the heterogeneous tumor microenvironment, and the clearance rates and routes from the target site of action.[41] It could thus play a vital role in the selection of patients and therapies, especially in the case of nanoparticle-based treatment of cancer where the vascularization of the tumor is what determines if the nanoparticles will be able to effectively target the cancer by EPR.[42] Unlike small molecules, nanotheranostics can easily incorporate diagnostic and therapeutic moieties in a single system, thus permitting the use of nanotheranostics in personalized medicine to ensure effective delivery, effect and diagnostic monitoring at the target site of action.[43] Various imaging ligands (e.g., radiotracers, fluorophores/absorbers, T1/T2 magnetic resonance (MR) contrast agents etc.) have been included into nanoparticles to aid their *in vivo* visualization[43–50] based on imaging modalities such as MRI, computed tomography (CT), ultrasound (US), optical imaging (bioluminescence and fluorescence), single photon emission computed tomography (SPECT) and positron emission tomography (PET).[51,52]

3. Applications of Nanotheranostics in Gene Therapy

As discussed above, a nanotheranostic can be developed to provide non-invasive assessment of carrier biodistribution, quantification of localized accumulation and therapeutic agent release by incorporation of a gene of interest in a nanocarrier matrix functionalized with targeting ligand and imaging modality. Many nanotheranostics are composed of a combination of more than one type of component like the biomaterial used for nanocarrier matrix, the presence of more than one imaging moiety or the type of targeting ligand used to aid in therapeutic and diagnostic functions. Described below are the different applications of nanotheranostics in the field of gene therapy.

3.1. *Polymer-based nanotheranostics*

Polymeric nanomaterials have been used widely as the matrix material of nanotheranostics. Their physicochemical properties are dependent on the chain length of the polymer backbone and the structural morphology and mechanical properties of the polymer. Cationic polymers encapsulating genetic materials through electrostatic interactions can be additionally functionalized to form theranostic nanoparticles.[53–55]

A polymer-based nanocarrier for gene delivery typically possesses cationic sections, organelle-escape units and degradable segments. Examples of these cationic segments include polyamines such as polylysine, polyarginine, chitosan, polyethylenimine (PEI) and polyamidoamine dendrimers, etc.[56–61] The anionic charge of the nucleic acid helps them to easily complex with the positively charged cationic polymers to form condensed polymer-nucleic acid complexes. The cationic polymers thus protect the genetic material from degradation and aid in the endocytosis of the nanocarriers by endosomal vesicles. The transfection efficiency of the polymer-based nanocarriers can be regulated by modifying their effective size and charge by fine tuning the N/P ratio (ratio of nitrogen of polymer to phosphate of DNA).[55,62] The organelle-escape units improve the gene transfection efficiency of cationic complexes by conferring endosomal escape while the degradable segments are required for the release of the complexed DNA by the nanocarriers upon entry in the cytoplasm.[61]

However, some cationic polymers also show rapid clearance by the MPS upon binding with plasma proteins during circulation and dose-dependent cytotoxicity after intravenous administration.[63] This can be prevented by the PEGylation of nanocarriers as PEG forms a shielding layer on the nanocarrier surface, thus protecting it from immune recognition by steric hindrance thereby improving its pharmacokinetic profile.[64,65] Additionally, PEGylation improves the hydrophilicity and hydrodynamic radius of the nanocarriers thus increasing their solubility and decreasing their clearance respectively.[55]

Huh *et al.* prepared self-assembled nanoparticles using cationic polymers such as hydrophobically modified glycol chitosan (GC) and PEI.[66] The cationic polymer PEI helped in improved siRNA binding by providing the cationic charge to effect its effective complexation. GC helped to decrease the interaction of the nanocarrier with serum proteins and thus reduce possible formation of aggregates during blood circulation.[67] The diagnostic agent Cy5.5 was attached to the siRNA by chemical modification and helped to monitor the siRNA for its biodistribution and gene silencing both *in vitro* and *in vivo* in mouse models by means of optical imaging. Significant increase in accumulation of siRNA *in vivo* in mouse models bearing tumors was determined using NIR fluorescence of Cy5.5. Similarly, a tumor-targeted siRNA nanotheranostic was developed using red fluorescence protein (RFP)-expressing B16F10 tumor cells and a RFP-target siRNA sequence. This helped to track the targeted effect of gene silencing in tumor tissue by changes in the degree of red fluorescence.[66,68]

Polymer-based nanocarriers are effective in overcoming the several challenges associated with oligonucleotide delivery by facilitating entry into the cells and release in the cytosol along with protection of the encapsulated oligonucleotides from degradation and rapid clearance.[69] A novel example of this is polymers forming vesicles or 'polymerosomes' (Psomes) with controlled release properties as shown by Kim *et al.*[70] Block copolymers like PEG-polylactic acid (OLA) and inert PEG-polybutadiene were used to prepare nano-transforming Psomes to deliver fluorescently labeled siRNA. These nanocarriers were degradable and allowed passive entry into cultured cells. The vesicles then transformed into micelles which escaped endo-lysosomes and delivered siRNA into the cytosol. The 30% encapsulation efficiency of fluorescently labeled siRNA in OLA Psomes, as quantified by spectrofluorimetry, was similar to the encapsulation efficiency of oligonucleotides in nanocomplexes that use the commercially available cationic lipid transfection reagent Lipofectamine 2000. The OLA Psomes targeted the mRNA corresponding to the expression of lamin A/C proteins. The gene silencing by siRNA-Psomes was determined *in vitro* in human A549 lung cancer epithelial cells. The distribution of fluorescently labeled Psomes and the fluorescent siRNA was monitored by two-color epifluorescence microscopy imaging. siRNA and the copolymers were seen to co-localize in the endolysosomes. The siRNA Psomes led to a 40% gene knockdown of the lamin A/C proteins comparable to the effect by Lipofectamine 2000, while the naked siRNA did not show any gene silencing, as observed by both imaging and quantification, compared to the controls. The *in vitro* data thus indicated that gene silencing mediated by OLA Psomes was very effective, comparable to that by common cationic-lipid transfection.

Another example of a polymeric nanotheranostics are dendrimers.[71] Dendrimers are highly branched 3D structured macromolecules with properties such as water solubility, uniform size and molecular weight. They are multivalent and possess many openings internally making them highly surface-functional and adaptable for both diagnostic and gene delivery purposes.[72] Poly(amido amine) (PAMAM) dendrimer-conjugated magnetofluorescent nanoworms called 'dendriworms' are one such application of theranostic dendrimers.[73] The siRNA-dendriworms, in a wide range of siRNA loading doses, were found to readily enter the cells *in vitro* and *in vivo*, escape endosomes and silence target protein expression, whereas dendrimers or nanoworms by themselves were ineffective. The siRNA dendriworms with 100 nM siRNA targeted against epidermal growth factor receptor (EGFR) suppressed the protein levels of EGFR by 70–80% *in vitro* in human glioblastoma cells, which was 2.5-fold more efficient than common cationic lipids. For theranostic application of these siRNA-dendriworms, fluorescent dendriworms (0.5 mg/mL) containing 0.115 mg/mL siRNA were administered by an intracranial infusion for 3 days and 7 days with the help of an osmotic pump with 0.5 μL/h administration rate. Interestingly, it was found that their biodistribution in the CNS tissues of healthy CD-1 outbred mice was found out to be in the perinuclear region. Consistent with the *in vitro* results, the siRNA-dendriworms decreased the levels of EGFR expression significantly *in vivo* in a transgenic mouse model of glioblastoma.

3.2 *Lipid-based nanotheranostics*

Lipid-based nanocarriers such as micelles and liposomes have been known to be efficient systems for delivery of therapeutic agents *in vivo*.[74] Such vectors can encapsulate nucleic acids into lipoplex nanoparticles due to charge–charge interactions between the cationic lipids and anionic nucleic acids, thus protecting the nucleic acids from enzymatic degradation and non-specific blood uptake.[75] However, the lipid-based nanocarriers can have certain drawbacks such as recognition by the immune cells as well as colloidal instability leading to aggregation in biological fluids. In addition, they may not be target cell-specific and hence chemical modifications may be needed for their effective use *in vivo*.[76] As mentioned earlier, for lipid-based nanocarriers, their *in vivo* stability and circulation half-life can be improved and interactions with the MPS can be decreased by using a polymer coating such as PEG to cover the outer surface of these systems.[28] In addition these lipid-based nanotheranostics can be further functionalized with ligands for targeting and imaging.

Kenny *et al.* formulated PEGylated liposomes encapsulating siRNA called as liposome-entrapped siRNA (LEsiRNA).[77] In these liposomes, the lipids conjugated with Gadolinium (Gd) (III) and siRNA attached with AlexaFluor® were MR and fluorescence imaging contrast agents, respectively. The PEGylated liposomes were prepared from the combination of individual lipids Gd. 2-[4,7-bis-carboxymethyl-10-[(N,N-distearylamidomethyl-Nα-amido-methyl]-1,4,7,10-tetra azacyclododec-1-yl]-acetic acid (DOTA.DSA), *N1*-cholesteryloxycarbonyl-3,7-diazanonane-1,9-diamine (CDAN), 1,2-dioleoyl-sn-glycero-3-phosphocholine (DOPC), 1,2-distearoyl-sn-glycero-3-phosphoethanolamine-N-methoxy(PEG)-2000 ($DSPE\text{-}PEG^{2000}$) and 1,2-dioleoyl-sn-glycero-3-phosphoethanolamine-N-(lissamine rhodamine B sulfonyl) (DOPE-Rhodamine) in the following molar ratios 30:31:31:7.5:0.5 m/m/m/m/m (mol%). MR images of mice bearing OVCAR-3 human ovarian cancer xenografts showed accumulation of LEsiRNA 24 h after intravenous administration. Fluorescence microscopy also showed co-localization of liposomes and siRNA within tumors. The LEsiRNA-mediated uptake of the anti-cancer Survivin siRNA after 48 h and 72 h post injection correlated to a significant decrease in tumor growth compared to controls indicating effectiveness of this lipid-based nanotheranostic.

Another example of micellar nanotheranostics is nanomicelles developed by Kanazawa *et al.* for systemic siRNA delivery.[78] Amphiphilic diblock copolymers methoxy PEG (MPEG)/polycaprolactone (PCL) attached with a cell-penetrating peptide, TAT, through a disulfide bond were used to prepare micelles to deliver siRNA both *in vitro* and *in vivo*. siRNA was labeled with 6-carboxyfluorescein-aminohexyl (FAM) and incorporated in MPEG-PCL-SS-TAT micelles and these showed an uptake similar to that of commercially used LipoTrust at a nitrogen:phosphate (N/P) ratio of 30 and a significantly greater intracellular uptake of FAM-labeled siRNA than FAM-siRNA only. The MPEG-PCL-SS-TAT micelles that did not contain siRNA did not cause any significant cytotoxicity in S-180 sarcoma cells. Intravenous injection of MPEG-PCL-SS-TAT/anti vascular endothelial growth factor (VEGF) siRNA (siVEGF) micelles *in vivo* in mice bearing S-180 sarcoma tumors led to decrease in VEGF secretion from these tumors and significant suppression of tumor volumes compared to the effect of naked siVEGF or micelles containing control siRNA. The decreased VEGF secretion was determined to be due to increased siRNA release in the cytosol upon S–S bond cleavage by intracellular glutathione, which caused release of TAT peptide and dissociation of siRNA from the micelles.

Ko *et al.* reported a new gene carrier consisting of MNPs formed by the covalent conjugation between phospholipid and PEI (PLPEI) with PEG enveloping these complexes.[79] The low molecular weight PEI 1.8 kDa helped in nucleic acid condensation, aided endosomal escape and reduced cytotoxicity that is usually associated with larger molecular weight PEI. Similarly, our group has developed MNPs with PLPEI/1-Palmitoyl-2-oleoyl-sn-glycero-3-phosphocholine (POPC)/Cholesterol/DSPE–PEG^{2000} (4:3:3:0.3 mol/mol) encapsulating siRNA at N/P ratio of 10 (Figure 2).[80] siRNA was labeled with FAM and encapsulated in MNPs to study their cellular uptake. Fluorescence microscopy confirmed the internalization of FAM-siRNA mediated by MNPs (green dots in Figure 3). Once inside the cytosol, the

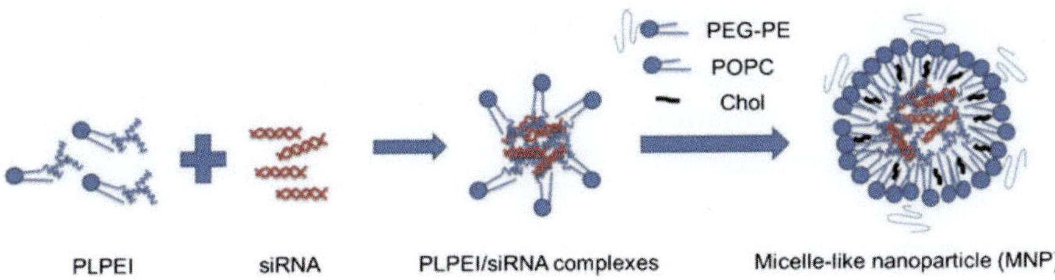

Fig. 2: Schematic representation of the self-assembly process of micelle-like nanoparticles (MNPs).

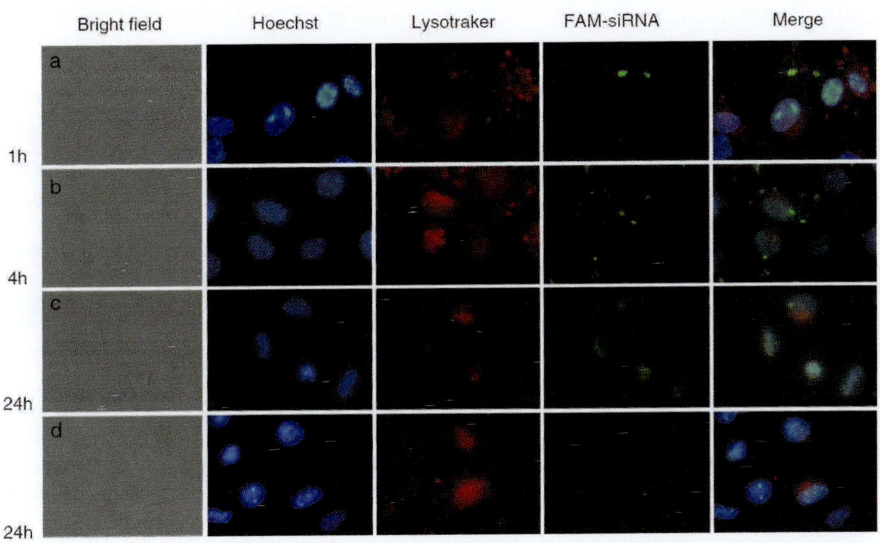

Fig. 3: Intracellular trafficking of a–c MNPs and d free FAM-siRNA after different incubation times with B16 cells. The nuclei (blue) were stained with Hoechst dye. The internalized FAM-siRNA appears green and the cytoplasmic boundaries (red) were marked with Lysotracker Red.

siRNA in the MNPs maintained their biological activity since MNPs downregulated GFP expression significantly compared with the control and with MNPs loaded with negative siRNA, respectively. These MNPs based on a dense PLPEI/siRNA core enveloped by a lipid/PEG layer were thus shown to be effective nanotheranostics as they exhibited properties of good complexation, preventing siRNA from serum degradation as that of PEI, but with better biocompatibility properties such a neutral surface charge and a lack of *in vitro* cytotoxicity. For more information on the use of lipid-based systems for gene delivery see references.[81–83]

3.3. *Antibody-based nanotheranostics*

Nanotheranostics utilizing antibodies as targeting ligands have been the focus of development over the last decade. An anti-EGFR deletion mutant antibody was used by Hadjipanayis *et al.* to develop iron oxide nanotheranostics for targeted imaging and therapeutic treatment of glioblastoma.[84] The EGFR variant III (EGFRvIII) deletion mutant protein shows expression selectively in malignant glioma cells but not in normal brain tissue. A polyclonal rabbit antibody toward the chemically synthesized 14-amino-acid fusion junction sequence (EGFRvIIIAb), which has specific binding to EGFRvIII protein, was covalently conjugated to the amphiphilic triblock copolymer-coated iron oxide nanoparticles (IONPs) to form a novel nanotheranostic (EGFRvIIIAb–IONPs) directed towards glioblastoma. The distribution of the EGFRvIIIAb–IONPs to the intratumoral and peritumoral regions in the brain was done using convection enhanced delivery (CED). CED utilizes a pressure gradient produced by the liquid containing the therapeutic agent to achieve a continuous injection and is used for delivery of therapeutic agents such as in the treatment of malignant gliomas because it is useful in bypassing the blood–brain barrier (BBB) and prevents the accumulation of nanoparticles in the RES organs of liver and spleen, or circulating macrophages after systemic delivery.[85,86] The T2-weighted MRI signal at the tumor site, in athymic nude mice bearing a human U87ΔEGFRvIII glioma model tumor, decreased after treatment with EGFRvIII–IONPs using CED indicating dispersion of the nanotheranostics. Animals treated with MRI-guided CED of EGFRvIIIAb–IONPs showed a significantly greater survival rate as compared with the CED of untreated control or IONPs as a result of the selective tumor targeting and inhibition of EGFR phosphorylation.

Another example is the use of a single-chain antibody as a targeting molecule by Chen *et al.* wherein a non-viral polymeric vector modified with a CD3 single chain antibody (scAbCD3) was used for gene delivery to T cells.[87] This polymeric vector had dual functional properties as it was first complexed with superparamagnetic iron oxide nanoparticles (SPIONs) and was used for T-lymphocyte targeted gene delivery by condensing a therapeutic gene plasmid. The scAbCD3-functionalized, PEG-grafted PEI (PEG-g-PEI)-coated SPIONs (scAbCD3–PEG–g–PEI–SPION) were synthesized by bioconjugation and ligand exchange methods. The targeting polyplexes (scAbCD3–PEG–g–PEI–SPION/DNA) were then prepared by including a diacylglycerol kinase (DGKα) gene that could impair T-cell receptor (TCR) signaling further leading to anergy of T-cells. In mature T-cells, involvement of the T-cell antigen receptor, such as the CD3 receptor, can result in anergy, and hence such receptors can be utilized for targeted gene delivery to T-cells.[87] The uptake of scAbCD3-conjugated polyplexes by the target T-cells (HB8521) was via CD3 receptor-mediated endocytosis as shown by the T2-weighted MRI and the gene transfection efficiency of scAbCD3-targeted polyplexes in T-cells was much higher compared to the non-targeted polyplexes as shown by quantitative flow cytometric analysis. Also, DGKα gene transfection into HB8521 cells led to lower levels of cell proliferation and IL-2 expression in response to immune stimulation in cells transfected with the scAbCD3-targeted polyplexes as compared to the cells that were not transfected previously during stimulation, indicating that MRI-visible targeted nanotheranostics can inhibit TCR-induced diacylglycerol signaling.

3.4. *Peptide-based nanotheranostics*

Nanotheranostics based on peptides and proteins are another example of targeted nanotheranostics for tumor-specific delivery of genetic material. EPPT synthetic peptides targeting under glycosylated mucin-1 (uMUC-1) antigen have been used since this antigen is overexpressed in more than 90% of breast cancers and in more than 50% of all cancers in humans.[88] Nanotheranostics employing these EPPT peptides (MN–EPPT–siBIRC5) were prepared which showed superparamagnetic and fluorescence properties. For this, amine-modified SPIONs with a cross-linked dextran coating (MN) were made first, followed by attachment of Cy5.5 dye to the surface of nanoparticles to prepare MN–Cy5.5 and then conjugation of thiol-modified, FITC-labeled EPPT peptides and siRNA to MN-Cy5.5 via a hetero-functional cross-linker, *N*-succinimidyl 3-(2-pyridyldithio) propionate (SPDP). The tumors in mice bearing BT-20 breast tumors could be monitored by T2 MRI and near-IR optical imaging upon systemic administration of the nanotheranostics to quantify tumor volume changes as well as optimize the treatment schedule for greater efficacy. Treatment with EPPT-peptide targeted nanotheranostics inhibited the anti-apoptotic proto-oncogene, survivin, by the action of siBIRC5, which developed significant necrosis and apoptosis in the tumors leading to a reduction in tumor growth rates. Similar approaches have been used to target other liposome-based and iron-oxide nanoparticles with peptides to allow for enhanced theranostic functionalities.[89–92]

3.5. *Small molecule-based nanotheranostics*

The diverse structural and functional properties of small molecules make them great targeting ligands for nanotheranostics. One of the most widely studied small molecules as a targeting ligand is folic acid (folate). Since folate receptors are overexpressed on tumor cells, folate-mediated targeting to tumors is characterized by a high binding affinity of folate for the folate receptor.[93] ^{111}In-DTPA-folate, ^{99m}Tc-folate conjugate (EC20), folate-linked fluorescent hepten (EC17), and diacetylvinylblastine hydrazide-folate conjugate (EC145) are currently being tested in clinical trials as cancer imaging and therapeutic moieties.[94,95] Folate has been combined with drug delivery vehicles or inorganic nanoparticles to produce targeted theranostic agents. An example of a folate-targeted nanotheranostic is the design of hollow gold nanospheres carrying siRNA directed towards NF-κB, a transcription factor involved in the expression of genes engaged in tumorigenesis, by Lu *et al.*[96] In this case, the photothermal effects of gold nanospheres were utilized to regulate drug release and as a therapeutic tool. The shells of the hollow gold nano-spheres (HAuNS, 40 nm) consisting of a thin gold wall with a hollow interior and exhibiting strong surface plasmon resonance (SPR) tunability in the NIR region[100–103] were prepared first. The surface of HAuNS was then functionalized with thiol-modified siRNA duplexes targeting the NF-κB p65 subunit and folates via a thioctic acid-terminated PEG linker to generate F–PEG–HAuNS–siRNA. A pulsed near-IR laser (800 nm) irradiation caused a photothermal effect and changed the absorption spectra of the HAuNS–siRNA solutions, pointing towards a structural loss and dissociation of siRNA from HAuNS, as shown by TEM and fluorescence microscopy. Significant down regulation of the NF-κB p65 subunit was shown only by the folate-targeted nanotheranostics with near-IR laser irradiation upon systemic administration in HeLa xenografts, indicating the specific targeting and endolysosomal escape of the nanotheranostics at the tumor site. The *in vivo* combination of gene therapy with a chemotherapeutic drug, irinotecan, which enhances the sensitivity to NF-κB inhibition, produced significantly higher apoptosis. *In vivo* micro-PET/CT imaging also suggested the effective folate-targeted nanotheranostic properties of the gold spheres at the tumor site.[97]

3.6. *Stimuli-based nanotheranostics*

Nanotheranostics can be actively targeted based on the presence of an environmental or chemical stimulus *in vivo* at a specific time to allow for site-specific release of the theranostic cargo. One example is pH-triggered nanotheranostic micelles formed with PEO–b–PCL block copolymers with modifications on both the blocks.[98] The PCL core of the micelles incorporated short polyamines, spermine (SP), to complex *mdr1* siRNA and attached doxorubicin (DOX) chemically via a pH-sensitive hydrazone (Hyd) linkage. The micelles could also attach fluorescent imaging agents to monitor micelles *in vitro* and *in vivo.* Two ligands were conjugated to the micellar shell, an active targeting ligand, RGD4C specific for integrin receptors ($\alpha v\beta 3$) and a cell penetrating peptide TAT for intracellular uptake. The micellar nanotheranostics were prepared by mixing plain or peptide-modified PEO–*b*–P(CL–g–SP)/siRNA and PEO-*b*- P(CLHyd–DOX) block copolymers. The cellular uptake of these micelles was by receptor-mediated endocytosis, and the siRNA was released in the cytoplasm because of endosomal rupture facilitated by spermine and TAT peptide. The nanotheranostic micelles were obtained by attaching a near-infrared fluorophore (Cy5.5) (NIRF) to the spermine side chain or by using fluorescently labeled (Dy677) siRNA, which facilitated the *in vivo* monitoring of the carrier as well as the encapsulated siRNA. The actively targeted nanotheranostic RGD/TAT-micelles containing MDR1-siRNA exhibited enhanced penetration, significant cellular uptake, and increased cytotoxicity of DOX in DOX-resistant cells. The efficacy was due to down- regulation of *P*-glycoprotein (*P*-gp) expression on cell and nuclear membranes caused by cytoplasmic delivery of siRNA and DOX through nanotheranostic micelles.[98] Similarly, Shim *et al.* developed a novel multi-functional theranostic comprising of siRNA-encapsulating polyplexes containing gold nanoparticles.[99] The gold nanoparticles were attached with acid-labile linkages to allow for release in the acidic tumor microenvironment causing efficient siRNA-polyplex entry into the cell as well as generating optical signal changes thereby allowing for the simultaneous diagnosis and treatment of the tumor. The various other stimuli-based systems such as magnetic-, ultrasound- and light-triggered theranostics have been discussed in greater detail in 3.7.

3.7. *Magnetic nanotheranostics*

Magnetic nanoparticles have been preferentially used in the field of theranostics as these can be manipulated by magnetic field gradients and can be applied in the field of biomedicine, for MRI as well as magnetic particle imaging.[55,100] MRI signal is based on the precession of water hydrogen nuclei within an applied magnetic field. After application of radiofrequency field, the relaxation process by which the nuclei return to the original aligned state is used to obtain an image.[51,101] Contrast agents used to shorten the relaxation parameters (T1 and T2) of water help to differentiate between tissues. Nanotheranostics attached with paramagnetic molecules such as Gd and manganese (Mn) or nanotheranostics that are inherently superparamagnetic such as those of iron oxide, are used to deliver the therapeutic agent.[51,102] An example of a targeted magnetic gene delivery nanotheranostic system is MnMEIO–siGFP–Cy5/PEG–RGD which includes 15 nm Mn-doped magnetism-engineered iron oxide (MnMEIO) particles to be tracked by MRI, bovine serum albumin coating for nanoparticle stability, siRNA, labeled with fluorescence dye Cy5, as the therapeutic gene to silence green fluorescent protein-expressing genes inside cells (siGFP), cancer cell-specific targeting ligand, RGD peptide, to target the integrin $\alpha v\beta 3$ overexpressed on certain metastatic tumor cells and tumor endothelial cells, and PEG (MW 3400) for increased *in vivo* time of plasma circulation.[103] Upon targeting the nanotheranostic particles to tumor cells by the RGD peptide, the nanotheranostic enters the cells by receptor-mediated endocytosis by RGD signaling and unloads siRNA in the endosome through the chemical hydrolysis of a bond between the siRNA and the nanoparticle. MRI could image the distribution of the siRNA because of the T2 contrast made available by the iron oxide particles and the fluorescent dye, Cy5, attached to the siRNA, making this a very efficient theranostic system.[10,103] For similar uses of magnetic nanotheranostics for delivery of genes see references.[104–107]

3.8. *Inorganic metal-based nanotheranostics*

Recent advances in synthesis and targeting have led to the development of nanoparticles based on inorganic metal materials for molecular imaging and therapeutic purposes. Inorganic metal-based nanoparticles have distinct optical and electronic properties, which are helpful in their use as nanoprobes for molecular diagnosis and biomedical analysis. Genetic material can be effectively incorporated onto these nanoparticle surfaces along with various other ligands such as targeting agents, fluorescent dyes, polymers, therapeutic drugs or nucleic acids to obtain an efficient nanotheranostic system. Nanotheranostics are being developed based on different inorganic metal-based nanoparticles such as gold nanoparticles, IONPs and quantum dots (QDs) which are reviewed below in detail.[108]

3.8.1. *Gold-based nanotheranostics*

Gold-based nanoparticles have been widely used for gene delivery because of their size, biocompatibility, efficient translocation and ease of surface functionalization using gold-thiol chemistry.[108,109] Thiolated nucleic acid strands can be efficiently attached to the gold nanoparticle surface. The unique surface of gold nanoparticles enables the efficient attachment of siRNA to it by chemisorptions and electrostatic interaction.[108] Surface-functionalized gold nanoparticles with cationic molecules also bind to nucleic acids enabling effective gene delivery.[55]

An example of gold-based nanotheranostics is the use of gold-nanobeacons (Au-nanobeacons) to silence a particular mRNA and monitor its efficacy by quantitative fluorescence signaling.[110] The antisense Au-nanobeacon was composed of a stem-looped oligonucleotide, double-labeled with 3′-Cy3 and 5′-Thiol-C6 linked to the surface of gold nanoparticles, which has a sequence blocking the enhanced green fluorescent protein (EGFP) expression. In these Au-nanobeacons, the fluorescently labeled hairpin DNA brings the fluorophore into close proximity with the AuNP, thus quenching its fluorescence. Hybridization of the Au-nanobeacon to the complementary target restores fluorescence with the fluorescence signal being proportional to the level of silencing. The Au-nanotheranostics thus blocked the EGFP expression efficiently in a colorectal cancer cell line and helped to evaluate the cellular toxicity.[110]

3.8.2. *Iron-oxide-based nanotheranostics*

IONPs are nanocrystals made from magnetite (Fe_3O_4) and its oxidized form maghemite (γ-Fe_2O_3).[111] IONPs are widely used in gene delivery as they have small and tunable size range, are biocompatible, biodegradable, possess good surface functionalization properties as well as MR imaging ability in response to external magnetic field providing increased spatial imaging modality with minimum invasion.[100,112] SPIONs (generally with diameter size smaller than 20 nm) can produce larger local inhomogeneities the applied magnetic field, thus making them better negative contrast agents for MRI.[112–114] Veiseh and coworkers constructed a nanovector made up of a SPION nanoparticle core coated with PEG-grafted chitosan, and PEI.[115] siRNA was covalently bound to the nanoparticles to avoid its enzymatic degradation and thus enhance its gene silencing efficiency. The tumor-targeting peptide chlorotoxin (CTX), which has high affinity for brain tumors, was covalently linked to the nanoparticles for tumor specificity and potency. The SPIONs were tested for their delivery of siRNA to the brain tumor cells via receptor-mediated endocytosis and for their knockdown of GFP transgene expression in C6/GFP+ glioma cells. The delivery of the nanotheranostic was tracked by MRI which produced specific contrast enhancement of brain tumor cells. Similarly, iron-oxide nanoparticles coated with cationic lipid-like materials have also been developed for the delivery of DNA and siRNA thus simultaneously providing MR imaging with gene delivery and magnetic hyperthermia thus allowing for an effective multifunctional theranostic.[116]

3.8.3. *QD-based theranostics*

QDs are light-emitting nanocrystals composed of a semiconductor core (e.g., CdSe, CdTe, InP, InAs and PbSe) with an outer layer of ZnS.[117] QDs have special properties such as increased signal brightness, improved photo- and chemical stability, broad adsorption, narrow emission spectrum and size-tunable light emission compared to organic dyes or fluorescent proteins thus making them ideal candidates for use as theranostic agents.[118,119] An example is the use of PEI-bound QDs by Lee *et al.* to study the intracellular localization and release of siRNA from the carrier using a FRET system.[120] These complexes were also functionalized with a protein transduction domain (Hph-1) peptide. The complexes without the peptide modification showed delayed dissociation and entered tumor cells via endocytosis and endosomal escape. On the other hand, the faster Cy5-siRNA release and dissociation of complexes possessing Hph-1 peptide indicated entry in the cells by transcytosis. QDs coated with polymeric materials for siRNA delivery were also recently developed.[121] These polymer coatings imparted a ‘proton sponge’ effect thus allowing for efficient endosomal escape while simultaneously allowing for the intracellular tracking of the nanotheranostic. Similarly, QDs were used in conjunction with a chitosan-based carrier to deliver and monitor siRNA for HER2 knockdown in SKBR3 breast cancer cells.[122] Thus QDs could be used as efficient nanotheranostics to deliver genes like DNA and siRNA as well as monitor their delivery non-invasively.[123–125] However, the assessment of toxicity associated with the use of QDs has been a major cause for concern as little was known about their pharmacokinetics, distribution and clearance *in vivo*. A number of studies have since attempted to assess these issues in detail.[126,127]

3.9. *Photothermal-based nanotheranostics*

Increased heat energy leads to cell death, making photothermal therapy and the resulting hyperthermia an effective strategy for clinical cancer therapy.[128–130] Some nanoparticles, with strong and tunable SPR absorption properties, can be stimulated by external near-infrared (NIR) light for imaging and therapeutic applications.[131] Activation by a NIR laser beam is needed for infiltration through the blood and tissues, identified as the 'biological optical window'. Gold- or carbon-based nanomaterials have the ability to transform optical energy into heat. If these nanoparticles are targeted to the tumor site, they can heat up the tissues and cause hyperthermia leading to targeted cell death. They can be additionally multifunctionalized simultaneously allowing therapeutic effects, diagnostic imaging and delivery of other therapeutics exerting synergistic effects in combination with photothermal therapy.[10]

Hyperthermia induced by gold nanorods is mainly localized, but a non-specific uptake of gold nanorods can also kill healthy cells. Hence, specific targeting of gold nanorods to the target site can help to prevent the photothermal ablation of normal cells while having a specific cytotoxic effect on the target cancer cells.[132] In the field of gene delivery, application of photothermal-based nanotheranostics is a relatively recent approach. Bonoiou and co-workers had developed gold-nanorods with DARPP-32 siRNA in order to target the dopaminergic signaling pathway in the brain.[133] Interestingly, the formulation was able to effect knockdown of the target proteins while not inducing non-specific cytotoxicity and trans-migrate across an *in vitro* model of the BBB. PEI-modified graphene oxide nanocomposites have also been developed for phothermally controlled gene delivery.[134] The nanocomposite was able to efficiently transfect the target cells with plasmid DNA with no observable cytotoxicity. It was also found that this gene transfection efficiency was further enhanced by NIR radiation thus allowing for endosomal escape mediated by the locally induced heat. Similarly, gold nanorods have also been developed to induce photo thermal ablation and gene delivery in prostate cancer cells while serving as an imaging modality as well.[135]

3.10. *Multimodal imaging-based nanotheranostics*

Recently, multimodal imaging has become a crucial non-invasive means of evaluating the efficiency of nanoparticle delivery. It involves the coupling of optical imaging with other imaging modalities such as PET/SPECT, CT, MRI and ultrasound.[43] Optical imaging is a non-ionizing, non-invasive method which utilizes photons emitted by bioluminescent and fluorescent probes and whose contrast mechanism is based on the optical properties of the tissue constituents such as absorption, scattering, fluorescence, transmission and reflectance. It is beneficial over other imaging techniques because its detection of low energy photons is relatively inexpensive and the visible to NIR light spectrum range allows good spatial resolution, without exposure to ionizing radiation. However, its main limitation is poor tissue penetration depth (0–2 cm) and high noise in fluorescent imaging due to the tissue scattering of photons in the visible light region (395–600 nm).[136] Using contrast agents in the NIR (700–900 nm) window helps overcome these limitations in *in vivo* imaging with reduced autofluorescence, reduced tissue scattering, and greater depth of penetration.[12,51] Further combination of optical imaging with other imaging modalities helps to improve its function. As an example, Medarova *et al.* used MRI and fluorescence imaging to track the local tumor accumulation and function of magnetic nanotheranostics covalently linked with siRNAs.[137] They developed magnetic nanoparticles (for MRI) labeled with Cy5.5 dye (for NIR optical imaging), modified with myristoylated polyarginine peptides (MPAP) acting as a membrane translocation unit and conjugated to a synthetic siRNA. By targeting model (GFP) and therapeutic (survivin) genes, they determined that the nanotheranostic delivery could be tracked *in vivo* by MRI and optical imaging, thus correlating distribution of therapeutic agents with their biological activity.[43,137]

3.11. *Ultrasound-based nanotheranostics*

Microbubbles and nanobubbles are <10 μM-sized spherical cavities filled with gas. These mirobubbles can be composed of different chemicals and can be caused to expand and contract in the presence of ultrasound allowing for triggered-release.[138] The commercial contrast agents may employ gases including perfluorocarbons (PF), such as octofluoropropane (C3F8), decafluorobutane (C4F10) and sulfur hexafluoride (SF6). The microbubble shell can be made up of denatured albumin, phospholipids, or various polymers and can be further conjugated with targeting ligands and therapeutic agents.[139] Nanotheranostics based on microbubbles and nanobubbles employ them as contrast agents and gene carriers in the presence of ultrasound.[139] Non-viral vectors such as lipid- and polymer-based nanocarriers help to prolong the plasma circulation of nucleic acids and facilitate intracellular delivery and thus improve gene transfection *in vivo* with the help of ultrasound.[140,141] A number of groups have utilized ultrasound for the effective site-specific delivery of nanotheranostics.[142,143] Sirsi *et al.* have used focused ultrasound to achieve tumor-specific delivery of *p*DNA complexed in a PEI- and PEG-based microbubble to solid tumors in a murine model.[20] Several strategies have been used to incorporate non-viral vectors with the microbubble shell to enhance gene loading capacity and *in vivo* gene transfection efficiency. Recently, microbubbles encapsulating VEGF-165 DNA were developed by Leong-Poi *et al.*[144] They had demonstrated that in a chronic ischemia rat model, contrast-enhanced ultrasound resulted in a significantly increased microvascular blood flow, with DNA transfection being localized to vascular endothelium at the target site. Polyelectrolyte-layered lipid microbubbles have also been used for the *in vivo* targeting of *p*DNA to the liver.[145] The *p*DNA, expressing a herpes simplex virus thymus kinase (HSV-TK), was added on polylysine-coated lipid microbubbles and then delivered intravenously into mice. A 2.2-fold increase in apoptotic effect was shown by the cell suicide inducing HSV-TK plasmids in tumors where ultrasound was applied to plasmid-loaded microbubbles compared to the plasmid alone. Tumor growth was significantly slower when ultrasound-mediated plasmid loaded-microbubbles were administered compared to controls as well. Similarly, 'bubble liposomes' encapsulating DNA and siRNA have also been developed for the simultaneous ultrasound-mediated imaging as well as the triggered release of its genetic cargo allowing for enhanced transfection.[146]

In order to further improve effectiveness, some groups have also combined the use of ultrasound as well as photothermal therapies as was elegantly shown by Ke *et al.*[147]

4. Conclusions

Nanotheranostics have great potential as multifunctional agents that can move towards achieving tailored treatment for individual patients. Along with gene therapy, the targeting and imaging properties of these nanotheranostics can help to effectively trigger the localized and targeted delivery of genetic material, according to an individual's unique molecular profile, and monitor the effects before, during, or after the therapy. However, all the components of a nanotheranostic need to be analyzed thoroughly in terms of their stability, toxicity and complex interaction with each other and the genetic payload over longer periods. Factors such as cost and regulatory issues also need to be considered.[148] Overall, nanotheranostics and gene therapy together could serve as a successful integration of therapy and diagnosis, which is important for the future development of personalized medicine.

References

1. V. P. Torchilin, *Adv. Drug Deliv. Rev.*, 302 (2012).
2. D. Peer *et al.*, *Nat. Nanotechnol.*, 751 (2007).
3. R. Duncan, R. Gaspar, *Mol. Pharm.*, 2101 (2011).
4. A. Schroeder *et al.*, *Nat. Rev. Cancer*, 39 (2012).
5. T. M. Allen, P. R. Cullis, *Science*, 1818 (2004).
6. L. S. Jabr-Milane, L. E. van Vlerken, S. Yadav, M. M. Amiji, *Cancer Treat. Rev.*, 592 (2008).
7. R. R. Sawant, A. M. Jhaveri, V. P. Torchilin, *Adv. Drug Deliv. Rev.*, 1436 (2012).
8. T. Lammers, S. Aime, W. E. Hennink, G. Storm, F. Kiessling, *Acc. Chem. Res.*, 1029 (2011).
9. M. Swierczewska, G. Liu, S. Lee, X. Chen, *Chem. Soc. Rev.*, 2641 (2012).
10. T. H. Kim, S. Lee, X. Chen, *Expert Rev. Mol. Diagn.*, 257 (2013).
11. J. Falk, Epigenetics & Sequencing — Gene Expression Systems' Second International Meeting. Chromatin methylation to disease biology & theranostics, Vol. 11, 650 (2008).
12. P. Rai *et al.*, *Adv. Drug Deliv. Rev.*, 1094 (2010).
13. R. R. Sawant, A. M. Jhaveri, V. P. Torchilin, *Adv. Drug Deliv. Rev.*, 1436 (2012).
14. S. Mura, P. Couvreur, *Adv. Drug Deliv. Rev.*, 1394 (2012).
15. K. H. Allison, G. Sledge Jr., *Oncology*, Williston Park, NY, 28 (2014).
16. S. Bhatia, J. V. Frangioni, R. M. Hoffman, A. J. Iafrate, K. Polyak, *Nat. Biotechnol.*, 604 (2012).
17. K. Shah, A. Jacobs, X. Breakefield, R. Weissleder, *Gene Ther.*, 1175 (2004).
18. D. T. Ross *et al.*, *Nat Genet.*, 227 (2000).
19. M. G. Toscano *et al.*, *Gene Ther.*, 117 (2011).
20. S. R. Sirsi *et al.*, *J. Control Release*, 224 (2012).
21. Z. Chen *et al.*, *Cancer Res.*, 4345 (2013).
22. H. Dewitte *et al.*, *Theranostics*, 97 (2015).
23. A. E. Prigodich *et al.*, *ACS Nano*, 2147 (2009).
24. P. Wang *et al.*, *Diabetes*, 3247 (2012).
25. M. E. Caldorera-Moore, W. B. Liechty, N. A. Peppas, *Acc. Chem. Res.*, 1061 (2011).

26. A. Chrastina, K. A. Massey, J. E. Schnitzer, *Wiley Interdiscip. Rev. Nanomed. Nanobiotechnol.*, 421 (2011).
27. S. K. Sriraman, B. Aryasomayajula, V. P. Torchilin, *Tissue Barriers*, 2 (2014).
28. G. Storm, S. O. Belliot, T. Daemen, D. D. Lasic, *Adv. Drug Deliv. Rev.*, 31 (1995).
29. M. R. Hamblin, J. L. Miller, T. Hasan, *Cancer Res.*, 5205 (1996).
30. M. Giacca, S. Zacchigna, *J. Control Release*, 377 (2012).
31. J. Park *et al.*, *Cancer Gene Ther.*, 741 (2012).
32. R. R. Sawant *et al.*, *Biomater.*, 33, 3942 (2012).
33. V. Torchilin, *Adv. Drug Deliv. Rev.*, 131 (2011).
34. N. Bertrand, J. Wu, X. Xu, N. Kamaly, O.C. Farokhzad, *Adv. Drug Del. Rev.*, 2 (2014).
35. M. K. Yu, J. Park, S. Jon, *Theranostics*, 3 (2012).
36. G. Sahay, D. Y. Alakhova, A. V. Kabanov, *J Control Release*, 182 (2010).
37. L. Nobs, F. Buchegger, R. Gurny, E. Allémann, *J Pharm. Sci.*, 1980 (2004).
38. A.T. Florence, *J Control Release*, 115 (2012).
39. N. Kamaly, Z. Xiao, P. M. Valencia, A. F. Radovic-Moreno, O. C. Farokhzad, *Chem. Soc. Rev.*, 2971 (2012).
40. N. Ahmed, H. Fessi, A. Elaissari, *Drug Discovery Today*, 17, 928 (2012).
41. S. Ferber *et al.*, *Cancer Lett.*, 81 (2014).
42. N. Schleich *et al.*, *J Control Release*, 82 (2014).
43. M. P. Melancon, R. J. Stafford, C. Li, *J Control Release*, 177 (2012).
44. W. Lu *et al.*, *Cancer Res.*, 6116 (2011).
45. W. Lu *et al.*, *Cancer Res.*, 3177 (2010).
46. Z. Yang *et al.*, *Nanotechnol.*, 165101 (2009).
47. Z. Yang *et al.*, *Biomacromol.*, 3422 (2007).
48. G. Zhang *et al.*, *Biomater.*, 1928 (2009).
49. M. Melancon, W. Lu, C. Li, *Mater. Res. Bull*, 415 (2009).
50. M. Zhou *et al.*, *J Am. Chem. Soc.*, 15351 (2010).
51. S. M. Janib, A. S. Moses, J. A. MacKay, *Adv. Drug Deliv. Rev.*, 1052 (2010).
52. T. F. Massoud, S. S. Gambhir, *Genes Dev.*, 545 (2003).
53. L. Liu *et al.*, *Chem. Commun.* (*Camb*), 6759 (2009).
54. J. M. Bryson *et al.*, *Proc. Natl. Acad. Sci. USA*, 16913 (2009).

55. S. R. Hwang, S. H. Ku, M.K. Joo, S.H. Kim, I.C. Kwon, *MRS Bulletin*, 44 (2014).
56. J. S. Choi *et al.*, *J Control Release*, 445 (2004).
57. B. A. Pfeifer, J. A. Burdick, S. R. Little, R. Langer, *Int. J Pharm.*, 210 (2005).
58. D. G. Anderson, A. Akinc, N. Hossain, R. Langer, *Mol. Ther.*, 426 (2005).
59. S. J. Hwang, N. C. Bellocq, M. E. Davis, *Bioconjug. Chem.*, 280 (2001).
60. T. Kean, S. Roth, M. Thanou, *J Control Release*, 643 (2005).
61. L. Jin, X. Zeng, M. Liu, Y. Deng, N. He, *Theranostics*, 240 (2014).
62. J. A. Wolff, D. B. Rozema, *Mol. Ther.*, 8 (2008).
63. Y. Zhang, A. Satterlee, L. Huang, *Mol. Ther.*, 1298 (2012).
64. S.-D. Li, L. Huang, *J Control Release*, 178 (2010).
65. F. M. Veronese, G. Pasut, *Drug Discov. Today*, 1451 (2005).
66. M. S. Huh *et al.*, *J Control Release*, 134 (2010).
67. J. Yhee *et al.*, in *Chitosan for Biomaterials I*, R. Jayakumar, M. Prabaharan & R. A. A. Muzzarelli (eds.), Springer, Berlin Heidelberg, Vol. 24, 139, 2011.
68. J. H. Ryu *et al.*, *Adv. Drug Deliv. Rev.*, 1447 (2012).
69. D. W. Pack, A. S. Hoffman, S. Pun, P. S. Stayton, *Nat. Rev. Drug Discov.*, 581 (2005).
70. Y. Kim *et al.*, *J Control Release*, 132 (2009).
71. C. Dufès, I. F. Uchegbu, A. G. Schätzlein, *Adv. Drug Deliv. Rev.*, 2177 (2005).
72. P. Kesharwani, K. Jain, N. K. Jain, *Prog. Polym. Sci.*, 268 (2014).
73. A. Agrawal *et al.*, *ACS Nano*, 2495 (2009).
74. A. A. Gabizon, H. Shmeeda, S. Zalipsky, *J Liposome Res.*, 175 (2006).
75. S. Kawakami, M. Hashida. *Drug Metab. Pharmacokinet.*, 142 (2007).
76. T. M. Allen. *Trends Pharmacol. Sci.*, 15, (1994) 215.
77. G. D. Kenny *et al.*, *J. Control. Release*, 111 (2011).
78. T. Kanazawa *et al.*, *Eur. J Pharm. Biopharm.*, 470 (2012).
79. Y. T. Ko, A. Kale, W. C. Hartner, B. Papahadjopoulos-Sternberg, V. P. Torchilin. *J Control Release*, 132 (2009).
80. G. Navarro, R. R. Sawant, S. Essex, C. Tros de Ilarduya, V. P. Torchilin, *Drug Deliv. Transl. Res.*, 25 (2011).
81. A. M. Jhaveri, V. P. Torchilin, *Front Pharmacol.*, 5 (2014).

82. G. A. Husseini, W. G. Pitt, *Adv. Drug Deliv. Rev.*, 1137 (2008).
83. M. C. P. de Lima, S. Simões, P. Pires, H. Faneca, N. Düzgüneş. *Adv. Drug Deliv. Rev.*, 277 (2001).
84. C. G. Hadjipanayis *et al.*, *Cancer Res.*, 6303 (2010).
85. J. N. Bruce *et al.*, *Neurosurg.*, 1272 (2011).
86. Z. Lidar *et al.*, *J Neurosurg.*, 472 (2004).
87. G. Chen *et al.*, *Biomater.*, 1962 (2009).
88. A. Moore, Z. Medarova, A. Potthast, G. Dai, *Cancer Res.*, 1821 (2004).
89. A. H. Schmieder *et al.*, *FASEB J*, 4179 (2008).
90. J. R. McCarthy, R. Weissleder, *Adv. Drug Deliv. Rev.*, 1241 (2008).
91. A. Accardo *et al.*, *Int. J Nanomed.*, 2007 (2012).
92. X. He *et al.*, *Mol. Pharm.*, 430 (2011).
93. W. Xia, P. S. Low, *J Med. Chem.*, 6811 (2010).
94. P. S. Low, W. A. Henne, D. D. Doorneweerd, *Acc. Chem. Res.*, 41, 120 (2007).
95. P. S. Low, S. A. Kularatne, *Curr. Opin. Chem. Biol.*, 256 (2009).
96. W. Lu *et al.*, *Cancer Res.*, 3177 (2010).
97. M. K. Yu, J. Park, S. Jon, *Theranostics* 2, 3 (2012).
98. X. -B. Xiong, H. Uludağ, A. Lavasanifar, *Biomater.*, 30, 242 (2009).
99. M. S. Shim, C. S. Kim, Y. -C. Ahn, Z. Chen, Y.J. Kwon, *J Am. Chem. Soc.*, 132, 8316 (2010).
100. A. K. Gupta, M. Gupta, *Biomater.*, 3995 (2005).
101. C. Richard, M. de Chermont Qle, D. Scherman, *Tumori*, 264 (2008).
102. Q. Wan *et al.*, *Nanoscale*, 744 (2013).
103. J. H. Lee *et al.*, *Angew. Chem. Int. Ed. Engl.*, 4174 (2009).
104. S. Chandra, S. Nigam, D. Bahadur. *J Biomed. Nanotechnol.*, 32 (2014).
105. O. Veiseh, J. W. Gunn, M. Zhang, *Adv. Drug Deliv. Rev.*, 284 (2010).
106. D. Yoo, J. -H. Lee, T. -H. Shin, J. Cheon. *Acc. Chem. Res.*, 863 (2011).
107. C. Wang *et al.*, *J Mater. Chem. B Mater. Biol. Med.*, 4396 (2013).
108. C. A. Hong, Y. S. Nam, *Theranostics* 1211 (2014).
109. P. Ghosh, G. Han, M. De, C. K. Kim, V. M. Rotello, *Adv. Drug Deliv. Rev.*, 1307 (2008).
110. J. Conde *et al.*, *Nanotoxicol.*, 521 (2014).
111. Y. Yu, D. Sun, *Expert Rev. Clin. Pharmacol.*, (2010).
112. P. B. Santhosh, N. P. Ulrih, *Cancer Lett.*, 8 (2013).

113. J. Xie, S. Lee, X. Chen, *Adv. Drug Deliv. Rev.*, 1064 (2010).
114. X. Ren, H. Chen, V. Yang, D. Sun, *Front Chem. Sci Eng.*, 253 (2014).
115. O. Veiseh *et al.*, 8032 (2010).
116. S. Jiang, A. A. Eltoukhy, K. T. Love, R. Langer, D. G. Anderson, *Nano Lett.*, 1059 (2013).
117. J. Xie, S. Lee, X. Chen, *Adv. Drug Deliv. Rev.*, 1064 (2010).
118. X. Gao, Y. Cui, R. M. Levenson, L. W. Chung, S. Nie, *Nat. Biotechnol.*, 969 (2004).
119. Y. -P. Ho, K. W. Leong, *Nanoscale,* 60 (2010).
120. H. Lee, I. -K. Kim, T. G. Park, *Bioconjug. Chem.*, 289 (2010).
121. M. V. Yezhelyev, L. Qi, R. M. O'Regan, S. Nie, X. Gao, *J Am. Chem. Soc.*, 9006 (2008).
122. W. B. Tan, S. Jiang, Y. Zhang. *Biomater.*, 28, 1565 (2007).
123. A. A. Chen, A. M. Derfus, S. R. Khetani, S. N. Bhatia. *Nucleic Acids Res.*, e190 (2005).
124. L. Qi, X. Gao, *ACS Nano,* 1403 (2008).
125. C. Liu *et al.*, *Biomater.*, 3604 (2012).
126. K. -T. Yong *et al.*, *J Am. Chem. Soc.*, 1236 (2013).
127. R. Hardman, *Environ. Health Perspect*, 165 (2006).
128. Q. Zhao *et al.*, *Theranostics*, 113 (2012).
129. C. -K. Lim *et al.*, *Theranostics*, 871 (2012).
130. J. K. Young, E. R. Figueroa, R. A. Drezek, *Ann. Biomed. Eng.*, 438 (2012).
131. M. P. Melancon, M. Zhou, C. Li. *Acc. Chem. Res.*, 947 (2011).
132. D. K. Kirui, S. Krishnan, A. D. Strickland, C. A. Batt, *Macromol. Biosci.*, 779 (2011).
133. A. C. Bonoiu *et al.*, *Proc. Natl. Acad. Sci. USA.*, 5546 (2009).
134. H. Kim, W. J. Kim, *Small,* 117 (2014).
135. H. -C. Huang, S. Barua, D. B. Kay, K. Rege, *ACS Nano,* 2941 (2009).
136. P. Debbage, W. Jaschke, *Histochem, Cell Biol.*, 845 (2008).
137. Z. Medarova, W. Pham, C. Farrar, V. Petkova, A. Moore, *Nat. Med.*, 372 (2007).
138. J. R. Lindner, *Nat. Rev. Drug Disc.*, 527 (2004).
139. S. Hernot, A. L. Klibanov, *Adv. Drug Deliv. Rev.*, 1153 (2008).
140. Y. Liu, H. Miyoshi, M. Nakamura, *J Control Release*, 89 (2006).
141. A. Lawrie *et al.*, *Gene Ther.*, 2023 (2000).

142. F. Kiessling, S. Fokong, P. Koczera, W. Lederle, T. Lammers, *J Nucl. Med.*, 345 (2012).
143. S. R. Sirsi, M. A. Borden, *Theranostics*, 1208 (2012).
144. H. Leong-Poi *et al.*, *Circ Res.*, 295 (2007).
145. S. Zhou *et al.*, *J Exp. Clin. Cancer Res.*, 170 (2010).
146. Y. Endo-Takahashi *et al.*, *Biomater.*, 2807 (2013).
147. H. Ke *et al.*, *Angew. Chem. Int. Ed. Engl.*, 3073 (2011).
148. Z. Cheng, A. Al Zaki, J. Z. Hui, V. R. Muzykantov, A. Tsourkas, *Sci.*, 903 (2012).

CHAPTER 9

NANOTHERANOSTICS IN CARDIOVASCULAR DISEASES

Maya Juenet, Mariana Varna, Cédric Chauvierre and Didier Letourneur*

Inserm, U1148, Cardiovascular Bio-Engineering, X. Bichat Hospital
Université Paris Diderot, Université Paris 13, Sorbonne Paris Cité, France
**didier.letourneur@inserm.fr*

Cardiovascular diseases (CVD) are the primary cause of death in the world. This chapter describes the potential of lipid-based, polymer-based and inorganic nano- and microparticles as new tools for diagnosis and therapy of CVD. The detailed systems are in preclinical development and a few of them have been tested in clinical trials. The developed nano- and microparticles act as carriers for contrast agents and/or drugs, associating ligands to target specific biomarkers at cellular and molecular levels. The particles loaded with contrast agents provide molecular imaging of pathological events. Molecular imaging for all main types of modalities greatly completes morphological information provided by traditional imaging methods.

A targeted and controlled drug release using carriers loaded with thrombolytic drugs for thrombus breakdown helps reducing the injected dose. It addresses therefore current therapeutic limitations by decreasing undesirable side effects. Hence, nanomedicine appears as a suitable tool to fight CVD, allowing for a personalized care and risk management.

1. Introduction

Cardiovascular diseases (CVD) are the major cause of death in the world with 17.3 million deaths per year and represent major medical and economic issues. Among CVD, ischemic heart disease and stroke caused by atherosclerosis are responsible for 12.5 million deaths every year.[1]

Atherosclerosis is a multifactorial and slowly progressing pathophysiological process.[2] It is characterized by the penetration of Low-Density Lipoproteins (LDL) into the intima resulting in the formation of lipid-rich plaques on the internal wall of large and mid-arteries. It is often located at arterial bifurcations where the flow is the most perturbed. Risk factors include hypercholesterolemia, hypertension, diabete, obesity, high fat diet, stress and cigarette smoking. Complications induced by atherosclerotic plaque are either caused by the growing of the plaque itself generating vessel stiffness and occlusion, or by its disruption. In response to plaque disruption, thrombogenic substances are released inducing platelets activation and adhesion to the endothelium and formation of a thrombus composed of fibrin and platelets. The thrombus or part of it can be dislodged, taken by blood flow leading to occlusion of another vessel in the body which could suddenly then generate an acute clinical event (ACE), such as myocardial infarct or ischemic stroke. Significant progress in biological understanding of CVD evolution established a correlation between plaque progression to rupture and expression of specific biomarkers at the molecular scale. Combining targeting of these biomarkers with contrast agents opens the way to an exciting field of research: molecular imaging for personalized care.

Imaging methods performed to assess atherosclerosis development mostly provide morphological information, looking for vessel occlusion at site of plaque (stenosis). Angiography (X-ray Computed Tomography (CT)) with radiocontrast agent and Doppler Ultrasonography (Ultrasound (US) imaging) allow for visualizing lumen size and local flow perturbations on vessel walls. Magnetic Resonance Imaging (MRI) stands as the tool of choice for visualizing cerebral inflow with a good spatial resolution. However, beyond these morphological data, physicians lack tools to better define risks and adapt follow-up treatment. It has indeed been observed that unstable plaques are not necessarily associated with an advanced degree of stenosis and are most often diagnosed further to an ACE.[3] Therefore, a personalized medicine is required to better characterize atherosclerotic lesions and predict their progression. Many biological mechanisms of plaque evolution and molecular markers are now described.[4] For instance the mechanisms contributing to rupture-prone plaques are described to be associated with accumulation of macrophages, presence of foam cells, apoptotic events, hypoxia and new micro vessels development (angiogenesis) (Figure 1).[3]

Different molecular markers have been identified, among which: endothelial targets (PECAM-1, VECAM-1, ICAM-1, E- and P- selectins, integrins $\alpha_v\beta_5$, $\alpha_v\beta_3$, $\alpha_v\beta_1$),[5] macrophage targets (Scavenger receptor class A (SR-A) or integrin MAC-1), inflammation (CD204), fibrous cap and extracellular matrix (collagen types I, III, IV), apoptosis (phosphatidylserine), angiogenesis (VEGFR, integrin $\alpha_v\beta_3$, CD13) and thrombus (activated platelets, activated factor XIII, fibrin).[6] Other pathologies which would benefit from molecular imaging are for instance Abdominal Aortic Aneurysms (AAA). In clinic, the size of the aneurysm is the only criterion to predict its evolution and to assess risk for rupture. However, its expansion rate could be better predicted with complementary information about its activation state.[7]

As regards therapy, the inflammation, the reduction of cholesterol level, the smooth muscle cell proliferation, the angiogenesis or the thrombus were principally treated.[8–12] However, a major issue is the administration of high doses of drugs in order to obtain a therapeutic effect. Injection of high doses may lead to undesirable side effects.[13]

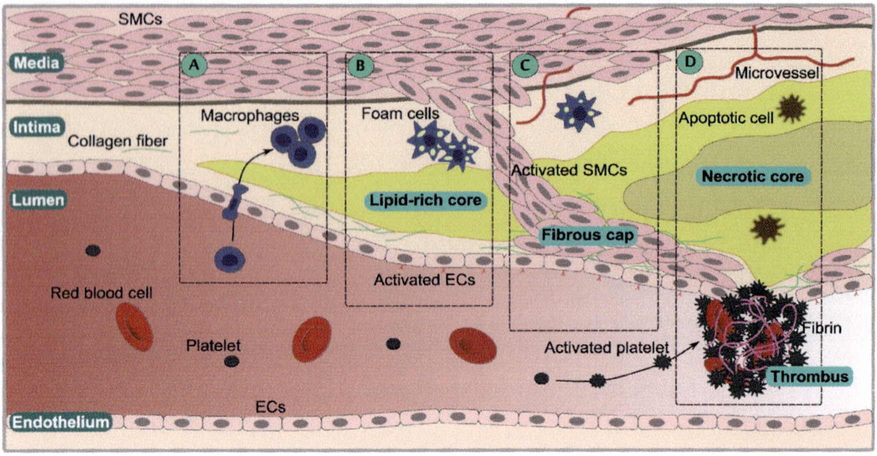

Fig. 1: Atherosclerotic plaque development showing molecular and cellular mechanisms as targets of nano- or microparticles. (A) Lipid accumulation (yellow) in the intima is associated with macrophage infiltration and accumulation. (B) Activated endothelial cells express specific markers such as P- and E-selectins, VECAM-1 and ICAM-1. In the plaque, foam cells and a lipid-rich core are generated. (C) Smooth muscle cells (SMCs) migrate into the intima and become activated, losing their stretching phenotype. A fibrous cap forms made of SMCs and collagen fibers. Remodeling affects intima size outwards the vessel wall. (D) Apoptotic events and necrotic areas appear in a hypoxic environment inducing microvessels development. In case of plaque rupture, the activated endothelium is broken allowing platelet activation through contact with the fibrous cap. A fibrin mesh forms and platelets and red blood cells accumulate at the site of injury.

Directing the drug against a specific biomarker expressed at the surface of activated endothelial cells or in the thrombus could enhance its therapeutic effect. However, this does not prevent drug degradation by enzymes into the blood. For that purpose, nano- and microparticles appear to be the dedicated tools. We choose here to focus on thrombolytic drugs and the usefulness of the different types of carriers to overcome limitations of conventional therapy.

Thrombolytic drugs used in clinical practice are mainly recombinant-based tissue plasminogen activators (rtPA), which are the recombinant forms of tissue plasminogen activator (tPA).[14,15] Other thrombolytic drugs exist but, because of their expensive price, or of allergic reactions development (uPA: urokinase, SK: streptokinase), are not currently administrated. These agents convert inactive plasminogen into active plasmin which digests fibrin in clots. Because of their short half-lives and rapid inactivation by circulating inhibitors such as plasminogen activator inhibitor-1 (PAI-1), it is necessary to administer high doses to obtain a therapeutic response. Major drawbacks of thrombolytic therapy are a low treatment efficacy and intracranial hemorrhages.[88–91] In addition, tPA is able to cross the blood–brain barrier (BBB) due to an abnormal permeability of capillaries within the ischemic zone[16] and to promote neuronal death. tPA also increases matrix metalloproteinases activity which degrade matrix proteins and break down the BBB integrity.

In next sections we describe nano- and microparticles in preclinical development and in clinical use in cardiovascular field. We detail molecular imaging applications as well as the therapeutic opportunities.

2. Design of Particles for CVD

Three main types of particle have been developed for CVD imaging and/or therapy: lipid-based, polymer-based and inorganic particles. They are versatile systems. Their surface can be functionalized by grafting bioactive molecules. In addition, hydrophobic or hydrophilic compounds can be incorporated in the core of the particles during their synthesis.

2.1. *Lipid-based particles*

Lipid-based nanoparticles mostly rely on a phospholipids assembly, mimicking the cellular membrane. Phospholipids are amphiphilic. Under certain conditions, they organize into micelles or liposomes. Different forms of lipid-based systems for molecular imaging were reviewed in details by Mulder *et al.*[17] Micelles show a hydrophobic core and their size is generally less than 50 nm. On the contrary, liposomes are made of a double layer of lipids that surrounds a hydrophilic core. Their size can reach several hundreds of nanometers.

Another lipid-based vector consists in micelle containing hydrophobic nanodroplets. They are named micro-emulsions and are larger than previously described systems (few hundreds of nm). In particular, micro-emulsions made of liquid perfluorocarbon droplets are good candidates for CVD molecular imaging since perfluorocarbons (PFC) are inert, non-toxic and naturally eliminated from the body through the lungs. These chemicals are exclusively composed of atoms of carbon and fluorine. They were extensively studied in the 70s/80s for their capacity to dissolve oxygen in their liquid form and were first tested in clinic as blood substitute[18] and for liquid breathing.[19] Furthermore, they are compatible with US and MRI.[20,21] Natural high-density lipoproteins (HDL) or HDL-like synthetic particles were also investigated as vectors for therapy and diagnosis.[22] There are micelles made of extracted or synthesized lipoproteins, mainly apolipoproteins apo A-I and apo A-II. Their size stands around 5–17 nm. They are naturally entering LDL-rich plaques and show the advantages of being endogenous and entirely biodegradable. According to their biocompatibility and their versatility, lipid-based nanosystems have led to numerous formulations.

2.2. *Polymer-based particles*

Synthetic or natural polymers are also of great interest to design nano- or microparticles more resistant to mechanical constraints than lipid-based ones. Functional agents can be embedded into the polymer matrix during synthesis. Besides core loading, polymer surface generally enhances protein adsorption. Polymer particles are synthesized by different mechanisms, like nanoprecipitation, emulsion-reticulation and ionic gelation. According to the polymer nature and to the synthesis parameters, polymer particles can be tuned in terms of size, porosity and hydrophobicity. Polymers offering good biocompatibility and biodegradability should of course be preferred. Polysaccharides show promising properties for CVD.[23] In particular chitosan and fucoidan present affinity for fibrin and P-selectin respectively. Poly(lactic-co-glycolic acid) (PLGA), a biodegradable FDA-approved polymer, and Polyvinyl alcohol (PVA) have also been formulated into nanoparticles.[24] Natural polymers, such as gelatin, have been considered for therapeutics loading too. Beyond their potential as vectors, polymers and especially polyethylene glycol (PEG), a hydrophilic biocompatible and biodegradable polymer, are also widely used to coat all types of particles in order to prevent their aggregation. In addition, by steric inhibition, PEG delays the opsonic recognition and thus macrophage uptake prolonging the circulation time of nanoparticles into whole blood. Moreover, PEG can be easily modified to attach different ligands for a specific delivery.

2.3. *Inorganic particles*

Inorganic nanoparticles are composed of an inorganic core with imaging properties, generally coated with a polymer shell. The polymer coating improves colloidal stability and particle biocompatibility. This type of particle includes magnetic nanoparticles, metal nanocrystals and quantum dots. Magnetic nanoparticles are usually composed of a paramagnetic iron oxide core, either made of magnetite (Fe_3O_4) or maghemite (γ-Fe_2O_3) or a mixture of both, surrounded by a shell made of dextran or derivatives.[25] Magnetic particles are biodegradable, participating in the iron homeostasis in the body.[26] They can be formulated into ultrasmall superparamagnetic iron oxides (USPIO), which hydrodynamic size is defined as inferior to 50 nm (coating included), or into superparamagnetic iron oxides (SPIO) particles, which hydrodynamic size stands between 50 and a few hundreds of nanometers. Under a uniform and strong magnetic field (generally from 1.5 to 3 T), these nanoparticles are used as contrast agents for MRI. Under local application of a magnet, they are promising candidates for magnetic guided thrombolytic therapy. Metal nanocrystals developed for CVD molecular imaging concern especially gold (Au). This element show good properties for CT, because of its high atomic number and its high K-edge energy. Quantum dots are nanocrystals of semiconductors, such as Cadmium Selenide (CdSe), with a size of a few nanometers. They emit light when illuminated at a given wavelength related to their size and their composition. As they are known to be toxic and carcinogenic, they are only used for preclinical development, along with an appropriate coating to be tolerated by the cells. Alternatively to polymer coating, other coatings developed for inorganic nanoparticles include small molecules as bisphosphonates and phospholipids.

3. Imaging Modalities and Corresponding Contrast Agents

CVD diagnosis may be based on several exams relying on different physical phenomena. The imaging modalities have to be chosen according to the type of pathology and to its location. Molecular imaging particles are in development for all modalities described below (Figure 2).

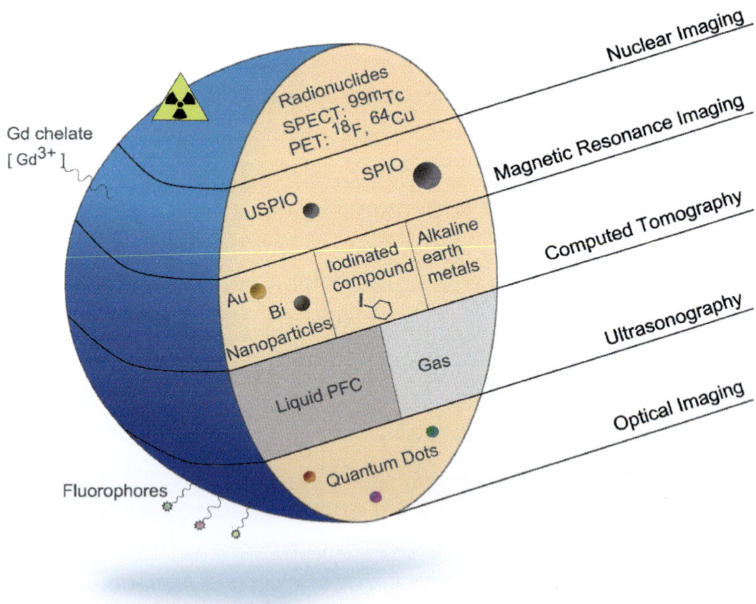

Fig. 2: Illustration of nano- and microparticles for various imaging modalities in preclinical molecular imaging of CVD.

3.1. *Nuclear imaging*

Single-photon emission computed tomography (SPECT) and positron emission tomography (PET) provide functional imaging of the body, highlighting for example cell metabolic activity. These two techniques require the intra-venous (iv) injection of a radionuclide (also called radioactive nuclide or radioisotope). In clinic, most machines perform a CT-scan at the same time to localize in two or three dimensions the accumulation of radionuclides in the body. Nuclear imaging is the most sensitive technique and is therefore at an advanced stage for CVD molecular imaging. In particular, nanoparticle uptake by macrophages has been exploited for atherosclerosis imaging. ^{18}F-fluorodeoxyglucose (FDG) is a commonly used radiopharmaceutical for PET imaging.[27] This glucose analog is trapped into metabolically active macrophages where it accumulates. ^{18}F-FDG imaging has been set up in humans for imaging high-risk plaques[27] and is now employed as an endpoint in most clinical trials[28] testing new therapeutics. ^{18}F-FDG PET scans provide an image 2–3 h after injection. The main limitation is that it does not interact exclusively with macrophages. ^{18}F-FDG unspecific uptake is especially an issue for imaging coronary diseases as myocardial assimilation is very important. Other radioisotopes, such as Technetium-99m (^{99m}Tc) and Copper-64 (^{64}Cu) were associated with molecules for targeting. For instance, radio-labelled ^{99m}Tc-fucoidan proved its efficacy in detecting the intra-arterial thrombi in different models of vessel injury in rats (Figure 3).[29,30] More generally, radiotracers combined with targeting agents forming molecular assembly were reviewed by Stacy *et al.* in case of peripheral vascular disease.[31] Combining these molecular probes into nanoparticles would enable to improve their specificity and avoid their rapid clearance.[32] Nuclear imaging is also frequently used in preclinical development to study biodistribution of newly developed nano- and microparticles.

3.2. *MRI*

MRI relies on the nuclear magnetic resonance of hydrogen atoms of water molecules present in abundance in tissues. Hydrogen nuclei

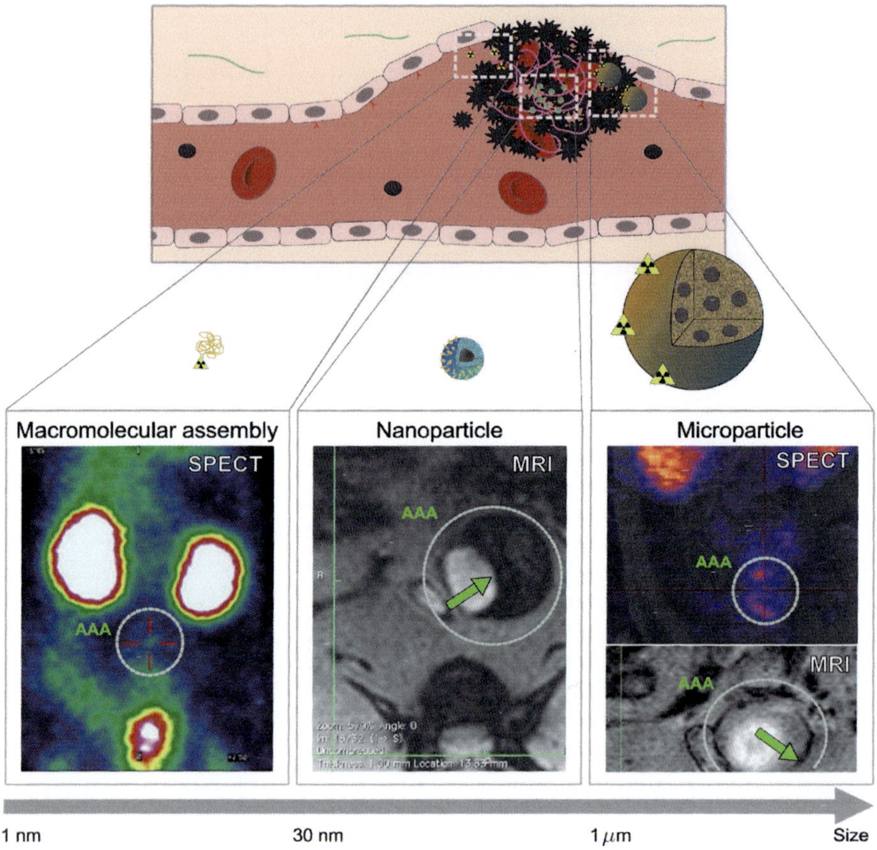

Fig. 3: Illustration of P-selectin targeting using different types of carriers as examples of molecular imaging in preclinical diagnosis of CVD. P-selectin is expressed by activated endothelial cells and activated platelets. All images were taken in rat models of AAA. From left to right: a macromolecular system made of fucoidan radiolabelled with ^{99m}Tc was injected to image intra-arterial thrombus with SPECT.[29] A dextran-coated USPIO grafted with fucoidan allowed to detect thrombus and activated endothelium by MRI.[58] Microparticles made of cross-linked dextran, pullulan and fucoidan were either radiolabelled with ^{99m}Tc for SPECT [59] or contained USPIOs for MRI, [60] and enable thrombus detection.

behave as small magnets exhibiting an intrinsic magnetic moment. A strong and uniform magnetic field is applied to the body via a superconducting magnet, in order to align magnetic moment of all hydrogen atoms. An oscillating magnetic field is then switched on temporarily at a given frequency that makes the magnetic moments deviate from their equilibrium position. This phenomenon is called resonance. When the oscillating field is switched off, magnetic moments return to their equilibrium position at a given rate called relaxation. Two different relaxation times characterize a nucleus; its longitudinal relaxation time (T1) and its transversal one (T2). The relaxation intensity coming from a precise scanned area is directly correlated to the density of hydrogen atoms, varying from one tissue to another. MRI offers a very good spatial resolution (25 μm to 1 mm) and precise morphological localization in the body. Recently, improvements in MRI sequences and parameters (multiparameters-MRI) enable to distinguish plaque components, like necrotic core, fibrous cap and lipid-rich area, without requiring nanoparticles. To complete this information, molecular imaging tools based on MRI contrast agents are developed.

MRI contrast agents are classified in two types according to the way they influence their magnetic environment: Gadolinium chelates (T1-shortening agents) and iron oxide-based particles (T2-shortening agents). Relaxivity is defined as the capacity of contrast agents to modify the relaxation rate of surrounding protons. Gadolinium (III) (Gd^{3+}) complexes are small paramagnetic compounds commonly used in MR angiography as blood pool enhancers. They are usually hydrophilic but can easily be grafted onto lipids.[33] Gadolinium (III)-chelates (Gd-chelates) have been covalently bound to targeting peptides, leading to systems such as the fibrin specific EP-2104R (EPIX Pharmaceuticals, Inc.). This molecular probe has been proved to successfully target thrombus in humans[34] and penetrate plaque in animals.[35] The proof-of-concept was achieved in a phase II clinical trial of feasibility on 52 patients. However, its poor relaxivity limited its translation to clinic. Gd-chelates are now studied to be concentrated into nanostructures. Iron oxides-based contrast agents are USPIOs and SPIOS detailed in the previous section. They show a great potential for molecular imaging as their relaxivity is much higher than that of Gd-chelates. In T2 imaging, iron oxides generate a signal loss (hyposignal).

3.3. *X-ray CT*

Computed Tomography scan (CT-scan) is based on the capacity of tissues to absorb X-rays. One major application of CT-scan for CVD diagnosis is angiography performed with IV injection of radiocontrasts. These radiocontrasts are small iodine-based molecules working as blood pool enhancers. They are strongly radiopaque and enable to draw a map of the vessels with a very good spatial resolution (50–200 μm) in only few minutes. As iodinated compounds may cause severe adverse effects, research is going on to decrease the dose by incorporating them into more complex structures, such as PEGylated nanoemulsions. Additionally, new radiopaque agents are investigated.[36,37] In particular, elements with higher atomic number have a better X-ray attenuation capacity. Furthermore, k-edge imaging with multicolor CT (more commonly referred to as spectral CT) is an emerging technique that provides elemental characterization of a tissue with an enhanced sensitivity, detecting for example calcium phosphate in atherosclerotic lesions. Contrast agents for k-edge imaging should be composed of elements with high k-edge energy. Metal nanoparticles, in particular gold and bismuth are good candidates as they have high atomic numbers and high k-edge energy levels. Although their toxicity has to be studied in depth, they are believed to be better tolerated than iodine-based agents. For preclinical studies with micro-CT, development of alkaline earth-based nanoparticles seems promising, as they generated strong contrast enhancement of vessels.[38,39]

3.4. *Ultrasonograpy*

Ultrasonography (or US imaging) is the least sensitive method but an accessible and lower cost technique that stands as the tool of choice for bedside patient management. An ultrasonic pulse is sent to the body via a transducer. In standard modes, the contrast is based on the ability of tissues to reflect ultrasonic waves according to their acoustic impedance.

Contrast-enhanced ultrasound (CEUS) imaging has been developed in the 1990s. Gas microbubbles (MBs) (1–5 μm) emerged as very good scatters due to their impedance difference with surrounding blood and tissue. They were developed in order to enhance blood pool signal and visualize flow even in the capillaries. Most importantly, they allowed visualizing left ventricle endocardial borders and quantifying myocardial perfusion.[40] The first generation consisted in air bubbles, which dissolve rapidly in blood. Gaseous PFC bubbles appeared to be more stable leading to a longer circulating time and less artefacts. These kinds of systems are stabilized by shell made of lipids, proteins or polymer. Today, three types of MBs are FDA-approved and routinely used in clinic: SonoVue® (Bracco), Definity® (Lantheus Medical Imaging) and Optison™ (GE Healthcare). Their main application is echocardiography for the diagnosis of left ventricular systolic dysfunction which stands as one major type of heart failure. Some PFC show echogenic properties into their liquid form too. Micro-emulsions made of liquid PFC droplets are often stabilized with a lipid coating, but protein and polymer coatings are under investigation. Gas or liquid PFC stand as platforms for molecular imaging tools for US imaging.

3.5. *Fluorescence optical imaging*

Fluorescence optical imaging performed with fluorescence microscopy is of great importance for pre-clinical development. Due to low penetration of light through biological tissues and to the toxicity of some contrast agents, this technique cannot be translated to clinic for CVD. However, it is easily compatible with laboratory practice. Fluorescent compounds (fluorophores) are injected into the animal bloodstream. The tissue of interest is illuminated at an appropriate wavelength depending on the fluorescent elements. The excited compound will emit light back at another wavelength. Optical imaging exhibits a high sensitivity.

Contrast agents are either small fluorescent probes or quantum dots. Quantum dots were described in the previous section. They are known to be toxic and carcinogenic, requiring therefore a coating in order to be tolerated by cells.

4. Nano- and Microparticles for Molecular Imaging

This section reviews several systems with a clinical potential or already in clinical trials for molecular imaging of CVD. All systems described below have been tested in animal models, the most common one being Apolipoprotein E-deficient mouse (ApoE-/-).

4.1. Preclinical development

4.1.1. *Lipid-based particles*

Numerous contrast agents were loaded into lipid-based nanoparticles to image atherosclerotic lesions. The most studied ones have been systems incorporating Gd-diethylene triamine pentaacetic acid (Gd-DTPA) and Gd 1,4,7,10-tetraazacyclododecane-1,4,7,10-tetraacetic acid (Gd-DOTA)- based lipids for MRI.[11] Lipid nanoparticles can concentrate up to several thousands of Gd^{3+} ions per NP.[41,42] Gd-labeled lipids were integrated with success in discoidal reconstituted HDL and native spherical HDL,[43] in fibrin-targeted PFC micro-emulsion,[42] in liposomes and in micelles.[33,44] Surface modification to make these systems specific to a biomarker was further achieved by grafting targeting agents, either directly to lipids or via a PEG spacer. Among others, systems that ensure targeting via an antibody are defined as immuno-micelles or immuno-liposomes. They were shown to significantly increase plaque uptake compared to naked systems. For example, adding an antibody targeted towards the macrophage scavenger receptor improved signal intensity of Gd-loaded micelles from 34% to 79% in atherosclerotic aortas of ApoE-/- mice.[45] More recently, HDL-like particles were functionalized with a peptide via a PEG spacer targeted towards collagen present in the extracellular matrix.[46] As plaque regression is associated with collagen degradation, they were able to assess plaque evolution with MRI in a regression model of mouse atherosclerosis. Biologically active proteins were also grafted for targeting. Van Tilborg *et al.*[44] developed small Gd-loaded PEGylated micelles (15 nm) with covalently bound Annexin A5 to target intra-plaque apoptotic events via phosphatidylserine exposed at cell surface. Their size allows for extravasation and detection of extravascular events. No significant difference in MRI signal compared to untargeted micelles was observed but a heterogeneous distribution of targeted micelles was shown to be more consistent with plaque composition.

Other contrast agents were also successfully loaded into all types of lipid-based nanoparticles. They are detailed by types of particles in the next paragraphs.

4.1.1.1. Liposomes

Insertion of contrast agents into the liposomal bilayer led to imaging tools for US imaging and MRI. As regards US imaging, echogenic liposomes (ELIP) have been developed in the 19's by McPherson's team.[47] A freeze-drying process combined with specific lipids formulation allowed for incorporating air nanobubbles into the bilayer, making it echogenic. Since then, the group has improved the formulation and developed targeted immuno-ELIP, even combined with drug delivery.[48] ELIP show longer circulating time than MBs usually used for US but their echogenic properties still need to be improved.

Gd-chelates were also inserted into the liposomal bilayer instead of being grafted through Gd-labelled lipids. Dellinger *et al.*[49] managed to load a fullerene cage holding Gd. This liposome was functionalized with a peptide to target selectively foam cells by their scavenger receptor CD36 present in atherosclerotic plaques in ApoE-/- mice. Lesions were visualized at 7 T after 30 min post-injection. The toxicity of this system and its activity in clinically relevant conditions have to be further validated. Liposomes that allow in addition incorporation of hydrophilic component in their core for therapy will be described later.

4.1.1.2. Micelles and HDL-like particles

In 2010, Skajaa *et al.*[50] reviewed the potential of HDL-like particles to be loaded with inorganic compounds, such as gold nanocrystals, quantum dots and SPIOs. In particular, Au-HDL combined with spectral CT were tested *in vivo* in ApoE-/- mice. They were shown to accumulate in macrophage-rich plaques and to give a good contrast with micro-CT.[51] Furthermore, combining such systems with multicolor CT allowed distinguishing at once macrophages accumulation and calcification.[52] More recently, Jung *et al.*[53] studied the biodistribution and *in vivo* plaques uptake of SPIO-HDL, showing promising results for the use of such recombinant HDL nanoparticles.

4.1.1.3. Micro-emulsions

Ding *et al.*[54] developed a bimodal platform where quantum dots were dispersed in an iodinated oil (Lipiodol®, Guerbet). Lipophilic nanodroplets were stabilized in water by PEGylated lipids. This system underwent passive uptake by macrophages in a rabbit model of atherosclerosis. Only 2 h after administration, lumen signal was decreased to its value before injection whereas, a significant uptake was observed in macrophages-rich plaques, compared to 24 h–72 h with USPIOs.

Liquid PFC were also incorporated into micelles leading to micro-emulsions. PFC are interesting for molecular imaging due to their intrinsic properties of being visualized by both ultrasound and MRI.[55] Fluor ^{19}F has indeed a non-zero spin. It is present in negligible amount in the body. Therefore, direct imaging of the compound accumulation is possible by MRI, but this technique cannot be easily implemented in clinic. PFC nanodroplets stabilized by lipid shell are much smaller than MBs made of gaseous PFC. Hence they can extravagate into vascular walls. They ensure also a better accessibility to diseased organs, as they are not affected by pulmonary passage.[21] In 1996, Lanza *et al.*[56] established a three step approach using biotin/streptavidin bond to link MBs to thrombus *in vivo* in dogs. The nanodroplets appeared far less echogenic in the circulation but give a strong signal enhancement while accumulating at their targeting site. Since then and beyond their imaging potential, PFC liquids with lipid coating have rather been used as vectors for loading lipophilic therapeutics[57] and amphiphilic targeting agents.[55]

4.1.1.4. Microbubbles

As previously indicated, gaseous PFC were mostly developed as blood pool agents for ultrasound imaging. Integration of targeting moieties in their shell makes them interesting tools for real time therapeutic effect monitoring.[61] Due to their size, they cannot be considered for imaging molecular events happening inside vascular walls. However, in early stage of thrombus formation or in post-ischemic area, ECs are exposed to the flow express specific markers, such as P- or E-selectins and VECAM-1. MBs targeted towards P-selectin through its natural ligand Sialyl Lewis^{X}[62] or through specific anti-P-selectin antibody[63] were evaluated in different animal models of thrombus or ischemia.[64] Correlation with histological results showed that area of signal enhancement, observed on average after 2 h, corresponded to activated endothelium. Other MBs were shown to target successfully glycoprotein IIb/IIIa expressed in thrombi.[65,66] One should be careful of the reliability of *in vitro* and *in vivo* models, as first systems were tested at low shear rate, which is not consistent with arterial pathologies. Furthermore, the synthesis was achieved via a biotin/streptavidin linkage and covalent binding should be investigated to avoid immunogenic potential. Finally lipid-based MBs are easily destroyed in the body. One strategy could be to use polymeric shell.[67]

4.1.2. *Polymer-based particles*

4.1.2.1. Polysaccharide-based particles

Polymer nanoparticles of a few nanometers (13 nm) were obtained by cross-linking short chain dextran with epichlorohydrin.[68] These nanoparticles were radiolabelled with Zirconium-89 (^{89}Zr) via desferoxamine for PET. PET/CT imaging was performed 48 h after injection of 354 ± 13 μCurie/mouse. A significant activity was detected in the aortic root of ApoE-/- mice compared to wild-type controls, which was consistent with the development of atherosclerotic lesions. However, epichlorohydrin raises an issue for translation to clinic as it is not biodegradable. Bonnard *et al.*[59,60] used STMP to cross-link dextran, pullulan and fucoidan to form targeted biodegradable microparticles (MPs). These particles were either loaded with USPIOs (Sinerem®, Guerbet) for MRI[60] or labelled with ^{99m}Tc for SPECT (Figure 3).[59] *In vivo* results were promising, as MPs accumulated onto the affected endothelium in a rat model of AAA. MRI was performed at 7.4 T after injection of an iron dose of 0.56 mg Fe/kg. A contrast uptake was observed after 30 min. Similarly, contrast enhancement in the abdominal aortic region was registered after 30 min with SPECT after injection of radiolabelled MPs (at a dose of 37 MBq/rat). Interestingly, their size (< 4 μm) and their behavior make them mimic rolling of leukocytes, which could be of great importance for drug release.

4.1.2.2. Other polymer particles

Another type of iron oxide MPs, tosyl-activated polystyrene-coated superparamagnetic colloids (Dynabeads®, Life Technologies) with a covalent grafting of P-selectin antibody were shown to accumulate onto activated endothelium.[69] Over several weeks of injection in ApoE-/- mice, the highest accumulation was obtained at the initial stage where the leukocytes were recruited, before apparition of a necrotic core. Although this system is not biodegradable, it remains interesting for basic studies in CVD understanding.

Poly (methyl methacrylate) (PMMA), which is not biodegradable either, was also studied for pre-clinical investigation. Luehmann *et al.*[70] developed PMMA nanoparticles covered with a functionalized PEG shell targeted towards chemokine receptor 5. Nanoparticles were radiolabelled with ^{64}Cu for PET. Nanoparticles were compared to ^{64}CU-chelate directly coupled to the targeting unit. Using a nanoplatform greatly improved ^{64}Cu-chelate imaging potential.

PLGA seems more promising as regards its degradability and biocompatibility. It has been used with success for atherosclerosis as the core matrix of targeted systems[71] even combined with drug release.[72] Zhou *et al.*[72] developed HDL mimicking polymer-lipid nanoparticle platform where iron oxides (Fe_3O_4) were embedded in a PLGA matrix. The polymer core was covered by a shell of chitosan bound to cyclic RGD peptides. The PLGA matrix encapsulated a thrombolytic drug (see Sec. 5). These nanoparticles showed a good affinity for thrombi and induced a hyposignal at site of injury in a rat model of ferric chloride induced thrombus.

Hyafil *et al.*[73] demonstrated that a colloidal suspension of crystalline iodinated particles (N1177, Nanoscan Imaging LCC) allowed detecting high risk plaques with CT in a rabbit model of atherosclerotic lesions. Nanoparticles were obtained by precipitation of an iodinated ester and stabilized by PEG and surfactants. After iv injection, the detection relied on nanoparticle uptake by macrophages.

4.1.3. *Inorganic particles*

4.1.3.1. Magnetic particles for MRI

Most iron oxide-based particles are coated with dextran or derivatives. Dextran-coated USPIO and SPIO undergo spontaneous uptake by macrophages and can therefore be injected to image high-risk plaques. A few systems already reached the clinic (see next section). However, macrophage detection remains non-specific. In consequence, high doses are required and the time from injection to imaging is generally more than 24 h. Therefore, grafting of ligands was investigated to improve the particles specificity. For instance fucoidan has been covalently grafted onto synthesized dextran-coated USPIOs. USPIO-fucoidan led to a strong hyposignal only 1 h after injection in area of thrombus formation in a rat model of AAA (Figure 3). *In vivo* MRI experiments were performed at 4.7 T before and after injection of 0.2 mmol Fe/kg.[58] Iron oxide-based particles were also studied to image thrombus formed in a rat model of myocardial ischemia-reperfusion by adding a clot-binding peptide sequence to a dextran-coated SPIO.[74] Four hours after injection, targeted SPIO generate a significant signal loss in the heart where microthrombi were formed, compared to untargeted systems.

Other coatings have also been investigated to replace dextran. Mannan coating has been set up to enhance macrophage uptake of SPIO and USPIO via mannose receptors.[75] Mannan-coated SPIO and USPIO were significantly more internalized by phagocytic cells than carboxydextran-coated systems in a rabbit model of atherosclerosis (after injection of 0.8 mmol Fe/kg). Muhlen *et al.*[76] constructed another iron oxide-based structure targeted toward the integrin MAC-1 via an anti-CD11b, as CD11b is believed to participate in the phagocytosis of USPIO. The coating consisted in a PVA and a Vinyl alcohol–vinyl amine copolymer. After injection of 1 mg/kg, an uptake was observed in atherosclerotic plaques of ApoE-/-mice but quantification assessment showed no significant difference between control and targeted particles. Another system under investigation consists in a core made of maghemite and magnetite coated with a copolymer of gem-bisphosphonate. Functionalized with a PEG spacer, it allowed for grafting peptides targeted towards VECAM-1.[77,78] This system enabled to decrease the recommended dose of 1 mmol Fe/kg with available unspecific USPIOs to 0.1 mmol Fe/kg at 4.7 T to image atherosclerotic lesions in mice. Most importantly, only 6 h were necessary to obtain a good contrast.

4.1.3.2. Magnetic particles as platforms for PET/CT

Cross-linked iron oxide (CLIO) nanoparticles have been developed as a platform that can concentrate one or several monocrystalline iron oxides.[79] In these systems, the dextran coating is cross-linked via epichlorohydrin and is aminated, what makes the surface easily tunable. As they constitute accessible experimental platforms, such superparamagnetic particles were used by the Weissleder team as PET imaging tools radiolabelled with ^{64}Cu and ^{18}F, to overcome issues relative to ^{18}F-FDG imaging.[80–82] As PET is the most sensitive modality, it enabled to decrease the amount of particles injected (4.5 mg of iron oxide/kg that is less that the recommended dose of current FDA-approved iron oxides-based particles). In addition, the biodistribution of such nanotools depends greatly on the size of the particle which can be tuned and adapted to the radionuclide half-life. Another team showed the potential for such bimodal platform by injecting ^{64}Cu radiolabelled CLIO in several mouse and rat models of CVD.[83]

4.1.3.3. Gold nanoparticles

In addition to Au-HDL described in the lipid-based section, glycol chitosan (GC) coating has also been demonstrated to enhance retention and compatibility of gold nanoparticles (Au-NPs).[84] Furthermore, its affinity for fibrin makes it a coating of choice for thrombus targeting. Injection of 0.5 mg GC-AuNPs/mouse allowed to immediately image the thrombus and monitored the response to thrombolytic therapy in real time.

4.2. *Clinical use*

Apart from MBs detailed in the Sec. 3 used as blood pool enhancers, only polymer-coated USPIO and SPIO have already led to clinical trials for the diagnosis of several pathologies including pelvic and carotid atherosclerosis, AAA and acute ischemic events. Dextran-coated iron oxide-based particles without targeting agents have been shown to spontaneously accumulate in macrophage-rich area allowing to detect inflammatory-like processes expressed in CVD. Pilot studies using iron oxide-based nanoparticles were recently reviewed in details by Cicha *et al.*[85] The main results will be briefly described below. Macrophages detection relies on what is called passive targeting; particles are phagocytized by macrophages via physiological mechanisms. FDA-approved Ferumoxtran-10 (Sinerem, Guerbet/ Combidex, AMAG Pharma) has been proved more than a decade ago to undergo spontaneous uptake by macrophages in high-risk plaques.[86] Ferumoxtran-10 is coated with dextran T10 and shows a long circulating time due to its small hydrodynamic size (30 nm). Kooi *et al.*[86] injected Ferumoxtran-10 to eleven patients suffering from advanced stage carotid stenosis. USPIOs significant uptake by rupture-prone plaques was observed after 24 h by MRI at 1.5 T and validated by histological analysis after endarterectomy. A significant hyposignal in rupture-prone plaques compared to stable plaques was further validated in several clinical trials for carotid atherosclerosis. More recently, Ferumoxtran-10 injection in patients after ischemic stroke suggested inflammatory variability in post-ischemic areas, underlining the need for personalized post-traumatic therapy.[87] This USPIO was also used in the atheroma trial to monitor the effects of atorvastatin therapy for reducing plaque progression.[88] Post-analytical results were not significantly conclusive in predicting statistical risk for ACE. Two other iron oxide-based contrast agents were FDA-approved: SPIO Ferumoxides (Feridex IV, Berlex Laboratories/ Endorem, Guerbet) which size is much larger (50–180 nm) and SPIO Ferucarbotran (Resovist®, Bayer Healthcare) (55–65 nm) coated with carboxymethyldextran.[89] Both were tested for CVD application. A correlation was found between Ferumoxides uptake (observed at 24 h and 36 h after injection) and rapidly progressive AAA expansion, independently from the initial size of the aneurysm.[90]

However, these three types of particles are now totally or partially withdrawn from the market as regards their initial application, what make them less accessible. More recently, ferumoxytol (Feraheme), an USPIO (20–40 nm) coated with polyglucose sorbital carboxymethylether emerged as a promising tool. In the recent NIMINI-2 clinical trial ferumoxytol injection combined with mutiparameters MRI successfully delimited infarction area, as well as the peri-infarct zone in patients suffering from acute myocardial infarction.[91] This is currently confirmed in another clinical trial.[92] One limitation of imaging with these USPIOs is the time required after injection to get a signal in the region of interest. Significant passive accumulation requires 24 h–72 h after injection. Another drawback is the dose of particles required (generally 1–20 mg of iron oxide/kg).[80] As detailed in the previous section, researchers work on increasing the affinity of iron oxides for plaques and activated area by incorporating targeting moieties.

5. Nano- and Microparticles for Thrombolytic Therapy

Another application of nano- and microparticles is based on the delivery of therapeutic drugs. This strategy shows several advantages such as: (i) Protection of active compounds (AC) from enzymatic inhibition in the circulation and degradation. (ii) Increase of circulating time: the circulating time of encapsulated drugs is much higher than that of non-encapsulated drugs. Moreover coating with hydrophilic compounds such as PEG avoids uptake by macrophages and thus increases the circulation time. (iii) The possibility for a targeted delivery which induce the concentration of AC into a specific site (Figure 4).

In this section, we detail the preclinical and clinical applications of thrombolytic drug delivery using nano- and microparticles.

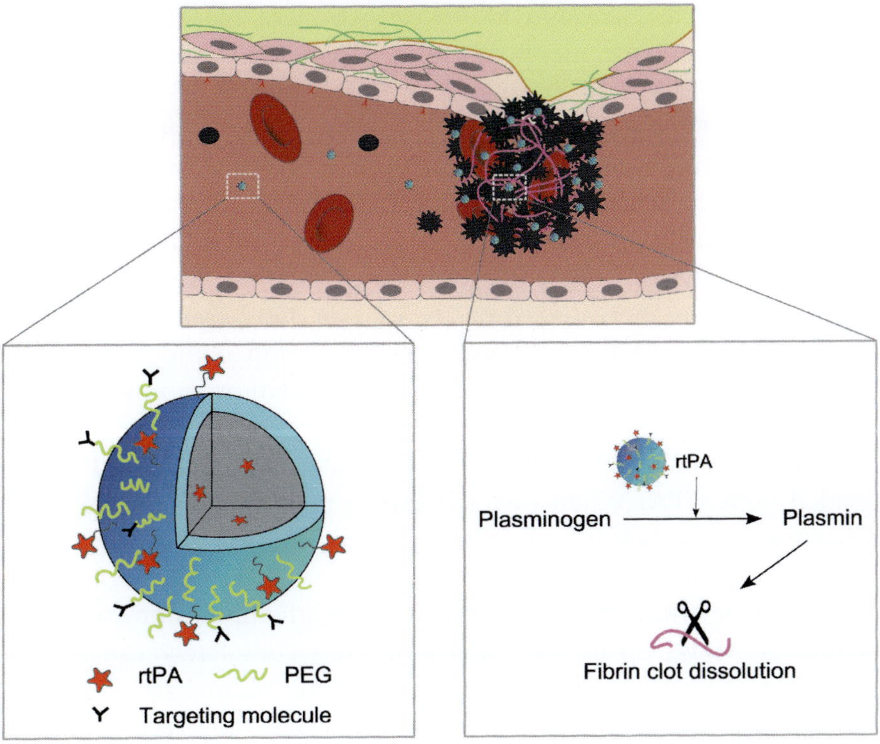

Fig. 4: Schematic representation of thrombolysis induced by nanoparticles. Most of developed nanoparticles loaded with thrombolytic agents (rtPA) are protected with a PEG shell. A targeting molecule can be used in order to enhance accumulation of the particles into the thrombus. Inside the thrombus, the rtPA activates the conversion of plasminogen into plasmin which degrades the fibrin clot.

5.1. *Preclinical development*

5.1.1. *Polymer-based particles*

Among polymer materials, PEGylated polyvinyl-alcohol (PVA) nanocapsules encapsulating streptokinase were developed by Leach *et al.* The same quantity of streptokinase, free or loaded into nanocapsules, was injected into dogs with coronary artery thrombosis. The authors observed that dogs receiving streptokinase loaded in nanocapsules showed an enhanced thrombolytic activity with a reduction of clot size and also a reduction of bleeding complications.[93] This enhancement of thrombolysis was explained by the greater penetration of encapsulated agent into clots compared to non-encapsulated streptokinase.[94] Nanoparticles composed of a polymer mixture made by chitosan and tripolyphosphate and coated with urokinase with a final size of 236 nm, were prepared by Jin *et al.* The authors obtained a high drug encapsulation efficiency of urokinase (94.8 ± 2.1%). When injected into rabbits with jugular thrombosis, an increased capacity of clot lysis compared to free urokinase was observed.[95] One possible reason could be that the encapsulation protects urokinase from degradation and induces also a slow release of the encapsulated drug.

Uesugi *et al.* developed PEGylated gelatin nanoparticles (192 nm) loaded with rtPA. When injected into a rabbit with femoral artery thrombosis, the half-life of rtPA was enhanced by a factor of three, due to its complexation with gelatin. Despite the fact that rtPA activity was 45% lower than the original rtPA, the application of ultrasound (1 MHz, up for 60 min) induced a complete recanalization compared to nanoparticles-rtPA alone. This recanalization can be explained by the fact that the rtPA activity was fully recovered after the dissociation of rtPA from gelatin.[96] Later, the same team tested gelatin nanoparticles (100–150 nm) loaded with rtPA in swine with acute myocardial infarction with a thrombotic occlusion of left coronary artery. They applied trans-thoracic ultrasound (1.0 MHz, 40 min) after administration of either nanoparticles containing rtPA (55,000 UI/kg) or rtPA alone. A recanalization in nine of the ten animals was observed in swine receiving rtPA nanoparticles. When rtPA alone was administered, only one out of ten animals showed complete recanalization (Table 1).[97]

5.1.2. *Magnetic particles*

Magnetic nanoparticles are equally promising candidates for therapy. Under a non-uniform magnetic field obtained with a magnet, the nanoparticles have the tendency to approach the magnet. This property was largely used in order to attract and retain the magnetic

Table 1. Examples of thrombolytic drug delivery using polymer-based (nano) carriers in preclinical models.

Composition/ Coating/Drug	Advantages	Drawbacks	Refs.
Gelatin-zinc acetate/rtPA	Enhanced thrombolytic activity.	45% suppression of rtPA activity when complexed with nanoparticles.	96, 97
Poly vinyl-alcohol/ PEG/streptokinase	Enhancement of thrombolytic activity. High accumulation into clot.		93, 94
Chitosan and tripolyphosphate/ urokinase	Drug encapsulation efficiency of urokinase. Increased thrombolytic efficacy.		95

nanoparticles at a specific site. Thus, cells labelled with magnetic nanoparticles were used in the field of tissue engineering and regenerative medicine for cardiovascular applications.[98] Substitutes of vessels were coated with a uniform layer of endothelial progenitor cells through the use of magnetic forces on the cells labelled by the nanomagnets.[99,100] Another study showed a therapeutic benefit of the magnetic targeting of stem cells in cardiac cell therapy. Autologous cardiac stem cells labelled with magnetic particles were attracted toward the magnet and accumulated in the ischemic area of a mouse's heart.[101]

Magnetic nanoparticles conjugated with thrombolytic agents show interesting theranostic properties (Table 2). Bi *et al.* synthesized dextran coated magnetic nanoparticles conjugated with urokinase, with a final size of 116 nm. These nanoparticles were injected into rats with carotid artery and left jugular vein thrombosis. Using two discal permanent magnets around the site of the thrombus, the nanoparticles were concentrated at the thrombotic site. The thrombolytic activity was 5 times higher in rats receiving urokinase-coated nanoparticles than in rats receiving only urokinase.[102]

Table 2. Examples of thrombolytic drug delivery using magnetic (nano) carriers in preclinical models.

Composition/ Coating/Drug	Advantages	Drawbacks	Refs.
Dextran/urokinase	Enhancement of thrombolytic activity.		102
PEG/rtPA	Reduced amounts of rtPA necessary to obtain the restauration of blood flow.	Low amounts of rtPA loaded.	103
Poly [aniline-co-N-(1-one-butyric acid) aniline]/rtPA	High amount of rtPA loaded; no haematological toxicity.		104
PEG/rtPA	Very low amounts of rtPA necessary to the restoration of blood flow.	Reduced number of animals.	105
Dextran/PEG spacer/ FXIIIa target/rtPA	Thrombus targeted with FXIIIa factor.	Steric hindrance; reduced activity of rtPA.	106

Ma *et al.* used magnetic nanoparticles (246 nm size) coated with polyacrylic acid and covalently coupled with rtPA (PAA–MNP–rtPA), for a targeted thrombolysis. After injection into rats with iliac artery embolisms and concentration into thrombus under external magnetic guidance, the blood flow was restored 75 min later. This effect was obtained with an equivalent of 0.2 mg/kg of rtPA coupled with magnetic nanoparticles. Free rtPA administration of a dose of 0.5 mg/kg did not show any effect in rats, while with a dose of 1 mg/kg, the blood flow restoration occurred within 30 min.[103] Similar results were obtained with rtPA immobilized on chitosan-coated nanoparticles.[107] In order to improve the drug-carrying capacities, magnetic nanoparticles (with a size of 12–14.8 nm) were developed with a shell of poly [aniline-co-N-(1-one-butyric acid) aniline]. The amount of rtPA loaded with this polymer was 50% higher than that obtained previously with PAA–MNP. These magnetic nanoparticles were injected into rats with iliac embolism and guided using an external magnet into the clot. The authors observed a restoration of blood flow within

15–25 min of treatment without hematological toxicity.[104] However, a limitation of this method is that the magnetic field generated by an external magnet decreases with the deep localization into the body, leading to difficulties to target a specific area.

A strategy for improving magnetic force is to use ferromagnetic stents. Along these lines, a recombinant tPA covalently coupled with PEGylated magnetic nanoparticles (rtPA-NP) was tested for the treatment of in-stent thrombosis. The amount of drug loaded on the surface of the nanoparticles was between 63 and 71 μg/mg, with an enzyme activity yield between 41–45%. These nanoparticles were injected to treat thrombosis in pigs with ferromagnetic stents in the coronary artery and an external magnet. The restoration of blood flow was reached with an amount of rtPA-NP corresponding to 0.38 mg of free rtPA. This dose is lower than the dose administered in humans (100 mg for 90 min).[105] However, a limitation of this study is the low number of animals used ($n = 2$) and the fact that the authors did not compared with the animals receiving only rtPA (control group). The McCarthy team designed magnetic nanoparticles for thrombus targeting without an external magnetic field but targeted with a peptide. They used CLIO dextran-coated with a size between 10 and 30 nm and coupled with rtPA. A PEG spacer moiety was added to minimize the steric interactions and to increase the distance between the fibrinolytic drug and the particles. The nanoparticles targeted a component of thrombi named activated factor XIII (FXIIIa) via peptide affinity ligands. These nanoparticles were injected in mice with pulmonary embolisms obtained with human clots. The injection of the same amount of rtPA loaded or not to CLIO showed a similar or slightly lower efficacy as compared with free rtPA. This study represents the proof of principle of thrombus targeted fibrinolytic agent using a peptide without an external magnetic field.[106] Zhou *et al.* developed magnetic nanoparticles loaded with rtPA and a peptide for a specific accumulation in abdominal aorta thrombi in rats.[72]

These studies showed that thrombolytic drugs loaded to magnetic nanoparticles, directed to a specific site with an external magnetic field or with peptides, could enhance thrombolysis with a smaller quantity of the drug and thus circumvent the undesirable side effects.

5.1.3. *Lipid-based particles*

Liposomes are largely used for therapy. Since the work in 1960 by the Bangham team,[108,109] liposome technology continues to be developed and improved. The first liposomes developed were uncoated and rapidly cleared by the reticuloendothelial system. Stealth liposomes, obtained after incorporation of a hydrophilic polymer, such as PEG at the surface, showed an increased circulation time into the body[110] while targeting liposomes can improve the specific delivery of therapeutics.[111] These nanoparticles protect thrombolytic drugs, reducing their side effects.

Leach *et al.* encapsulated streptokinase into naked liposomes and injected them in rabbits with carotid artery thrombosis. The efficacy of encapsulation of streptokinase into liposomes was 30%. They compared the thrombolytic effect of 6000 UI/kg free streptokinase with streptokinase encapsulated into liposomes. Two hours after drug administration, they showed that the thrombolytic effect was improved with liposome-loaded streptokinase.[112] Encapsulation into liposomes protects the drug from premature inactivation into the blood. However, the authors noted some difficulties with the stability of the liposomes and low encapsulation efficacy.

Streptokinase encapsulation into liposomes, with 18% efficacy of entrapment, was carried out by Vaidya *et al.* The authors loaded the liposomes with arginine–glycine–aspartic acid (RGD) peptide. These liposomes, with a size between 100 nm and 200 nm, were injected into rats with carotid thrombosis obtained with a human clot. Thirty minutes after treatment, a higher thrombolytic activity was observed in rats receiving liposomes encapsulating streptokinase compared to streptokinase alone (28% vs 17% respectively). This thrombolytic effect was explained by a higher accumulation of liposomes in the thrombus area.[113]

tPA encapsulated into PEGylated (173 nm) and non-PEGylated (150 nm) liposomes showed an entrapment efficacy of approximately 20%. When injected into rats, encapsulated rtPA showed a prolonged circulation time (21 and 16 fold respectively).[114] Targeted stealth liposomes were developed by Absar *et al.* They loaded rtPA with

PEGylated or non-PEGylated liposomes decorated with a peptide sequence (CQQHHLGGAKQAGDV) of fibrinogen gamma-chain targeting GPIIb/IIIa on activated platelets. The entrapment efficacy of the non-PEGylated liposomes was between 12% and 26%, whereas, for PEGylated liposomes was higher, between 36% and 52%. When injected into rats with inferior vena cava thrombosis, an increased half-life was observed for rtPA loaded into PEGylated and non-PEGylated liposomes (141 min and 103 min respectively). Compared to native rtPA, an enhancement of 35% of thrombolytic activity was observed in rtPA-loaded into the peptide-linked PEGylated liposomes.[115]

In order to target thrombolytic activity, PFC nanoparticles loaded with urokinase were used by different research teams.[116] Marsh *et al.* have developed PFC nanoparticles covalently coupled with an anti-fibrin antibody and urokinase. The nanoparticles had 20 antibody and 200 urokinase molecules attached to their surface for a final size of 240 nm. When injected into dogs with femoral thrombosis, the authors showed that the dissolution of plasma clots was higher in animals receiving urokinase-functionalized PFC nanoparticles compared to the control group receiving irrelevant IgG targeted urokinase nanoparticles (Table 3).[117]

5.1.4. *Sonothrombolysis associated to microbubbles as adjuvant therapy*

In experimental preclinical studies, ultrasound was used as an adjuvant to enhance recanalization rate (sonothrombolysis). Excellent reviews summarized sonothrombolysis in preclinical studies.[124,125] The added value of ultrasound was demonstrated using different types of lipid-based carriers.

ELIP composed by phospholipids bilayer vesicles with both gas and fluid were synthesized by Laing *et al.* These liposomes were loaded with rtPA, with 15% entrapment in the core and 35% associated with the bilayer.[118] In order to compare the thrombolytic activity of these carriers, they injected them into rabbits with an aorta thrombus. Their results showed that encapsulated tPA had an enhanced

Table 3. Examples of thrombolytic drug delivery using lipid-based (nano) carriers in preclinical models.

Composition/Coating/Drug	Advantages	Drawbacks	Refs.
Liposome/PEG/peptide (CQQHHLGGAKQAGDV)/rtPA	Enhanced thrombolytic activity; reduced haemorrhagic risk.		115
PFC/ anti-fibrin antibody/ urokinase	Enhanced thrombolytic activity.	Possible steric inhibition of urokinase activity by the anti-fibrin antibody.	117
ELIP/rtPA	Prolonged circulation time for rtPA; enhanced thrombolytic activity for ELIP/rtPA associated with ultrasound.	Low amounts of rtPA encapsulated.	118
PFC/RGD peptide	High recanalization rate when PFC/RGD peptide is associated with iv rtPA and ultrasound.	Low recanalization rate for PFC and ultrasound.	119
MBs ±ultrasound	Equivalent to rtPA for restoration of blood flow.		120
MBs/±rtPA/ ultrasound	High recanalization rate for MBs/rtPA associated with ultrasound.		121
MBs/urokinase/±ultrasound	High recanalization rate for MBs/ urokinase associated with ultrasound.		122, 123

circulation time into the blood. Moreover, the efficacy for thrombus dissolution of encapsulated rtPA was similar to the free drug. The addition of 5.7 MHz ultrasound for two minutes, significantly enhanced lytic treatment efficacy for both rtPA and rtPA ELIP.[126]

ELIP (with a size <200 nm) grafted or not with RGD peptides were developed by Hagisawa *et al.* When injected into rabbits with iliac artery occlusion, they showed a higher recanalization rate (9 of 10 rabbits) when ultrasound was applied, compared to the animals receiving non-targeted liposomes (2 of 10 rabbits) or receiving rtPA monotherapy (27,500 IU kg^{-1}).[119]

MBs, with a size between 2 and 8 μm, composed by a phospholipid, a polymer or an albumin shell, and air or high molecular weight gas in the core, were already used as contrast agents in echography.[124] Alone or with rtPA, they have been combined with ultrasound in order to enhance recanalization rate.[127] In rats with acute cerebral ischemia, Moumouh *et al.* showed that the treatment with iv rtPA ($n = 5$) or MBs and ultrasound ($n = 5$) were equivalent in the restoration of blood flow.[120] Nedelmann *et al.* have worked on a larger number of rats ($n = 25$ per group) with occlusion of the right middle cerebral artery. They showed that rtPA alone partially improved hemispheric perfusion, while the association of rtPA, MBs and ultrasound completely restored the blood flow.[121] A better recanalization rate was also obtained with urokinase, MBs and transcranial Doppler (TCD) ultrasound (2 MHz) when compared with the results obtained on rabbits receiving only urokinase.[122] Similar results were observed in pigs with coronary thrombotic occlusion.[123]

A smaller quantity of rtPA was necessary to obtain a beneficial effect on rabbits with carotid artery clot when MBs and trans-cutaneous pulsed ultrasound (1MHz) were applied.[128] Several mechanisms have been proposed to explain the phenomenon of ultrasound enhanced thrombolysis including acoustic cavitation,[129–131] thermal effects [132] and micro-streaming.[133]

These preclinical results showed on one hand that sonothrombolysis could be equivalent to the efficacy of thrombolytic drugs. On the other hand, the association of ultrasound, MBs and thrombolytics enhanced the recanalization rate.

5.2. *Clinical use*

Only MBs were tested in clinics for thrombolytic therapy with or without ultrasound (Table 4). MBs and ultrasound, associated or not with thrombolytics, showed encouraging results.[134] Molina *et al.* in their clinical trial, included 111 patients with middle cerebral artery occlusions. Thirty-eight patients received tPA and galactose-based MBs plus 2 h continuous 2 MHz pulsed waves TCD monitoring and another 73 patients received either tPA and ultrasound or only tPA. This study showed that a high recanalization rate was observed in the group with tPA, continuous 2 MHz TCD and MBs when compared with groups receiving tPA and ultrasounds or tPA alone.[135] Later, they showed in the Transcranial Ultrasound in Clinical Sonothrombolysis (TUCSON) trial, conducted on 35 patients receiving either iv tPA, 2MHz TCD and perflutren lipid (MRX-801) or standard iv tPA, that the complete recanalization rates at the end of TCD monitoring were 67% and 46% respectively.[136]

Another clinical trial was carried out by Alexandrov *et al.*, on 15 patients receiving tPA, 2 MHz continuous TCD monitoring and perflutren-lipid-based MBs (n = 12) or only tPA and ultrasound (n = 3). The authors observed a complete recanalization rate in 50% of patients (6/12) while none reached complete recanalization in the control group.[137] Perren *et al.*, evaluated the recanalization rate in 26 patients receiving iv rtPA and phospholipid encapsulated sulfur hexafluoride MBs combined with 60 min of transcranial color-coded duplex (TCCD) ultrasound monitoring (n = 11). They compared with patients receiving only rtPA and ultrasound (n = 15). This study showed a higher recanalization rate in patients receiving MBs (64%) compared to patients without MBs (53%). This could be explained by the fact that the streaming of MBs under ultrasound pulses induces mechanical damages at the surface of the thrombus allowing a higher penetration of rtPA into the thrombus.[138] Pagola *et al.* have determined the time of recanalization rate in patients with stroke with basilar artery occlusion. All 20 patients have received iv tPA with 2 h continuous ultrasound and galactose-basedMBs. They observed a difference between the recanalization rates in these patients. Only

Table 4. Clinical trials in patients with stroke receiving thrombolytic drug associated or not with MBs and/or ultrasound.

Patients (n=)	Therapy procedures	Outcomes	Refs.
111	Group 1: tPA/US 2MHz TCD 2 h monitoring ($n = 73$). Group 2: tPA/US 2MHz TCD 2 h monitoring/Galactose-based MBs ($n = 38$).	Group 1: 38% recanalization rate. Group 2: 55% recanalization rate.	135
15	Group 1: tPA/US 2MHz TCD 2 h monitoring/Perflutren-based MBs ($n = 12$). Group 2: tPA/US 2MHz TCD 2 h monitoring ($n = 3$).	Group 1: complete recanalization rate 6/12. Group 2: none reached complete recanalization rate.	137
35	Group 1: tPA/2MHz TCD/Perflutren lipid microspheres MRX-801 ($n = 23$). Group 2: tPA/Brief TCD assessments ($n = 12$).	Rate of recanalization higher in group 1 without statistical significance.	136
26	Group 1: rtPA/60 min TCCD pulsed-wave monitoring/Phospholipid MBs encapsulating sulfur hexafluoride ($n = 11$). Group 2: rtPA/60 min TCCD pulsed-wave monitoring ($n = 15$).	Group 1: recanalization rate (53%). Group 2: recanalization rate (64%).	138
20	rtPA/2 h TCD monitoring/Galactose-based MBs.	10 patients with progressive recanalization: 10% raised at 1 h, 50% raised at 24 h. 10 patients showed no recanalization.	139
138	Group 1: rtPA/Galactose-based air filled MBs ($n = 91$). Group 2: rtPA/Sulfur hexafluoride-filled MBs ($n = 47$).	Similar recanalization rate at 6 h.	140

Ten patients showed a progressive recanalization rate while ten others did not show any recanalization rate at 24 h.[139] On 138 patients with stroke with middle cerebral artery occlusion, Rubiera *et al.* compared the outcome of patients receiving rtPA, and one of two different types of MBs galactose-based and phospholipid encapsulated sulfur-hexafluoride-based and underwent 2 MHz TCD. The recanalization was similar in both groups despite the different characteristics of microbubbles.[140]

These clinical trials showed that MBs associated with ultrasound could be an interesting tool for increasing recanalization rates in patients with stroke. Another advantage could be the reduction of the drug quantity administered to obtain a beneficial effect, thus limiting intracranial bleeding.

6. Conclusions and Outlook

Molecular imaging with nano- and microparticles provides precise information on the expression of specific biomarkers compared to conventional imaging. This allows an improved understanding and a better management of the CVD. Materials have been validated for the development of nano- and microparticles *in vitro* and in animal models. Despite development of several versatile platforms in preclinical research, only two types of systems have been tested in clinical trials for cardiovascular imaging: MBs and iron oxide-based particles. For therapy, no system loaded with a therapeutic drug exists yet in clinics in the cardiovascular domain. It would be of a great importance to improve existing preclinical systems that are biocompatible, biodegradable and of low toxicity for clinical applications. The actual limitations are linked to the amount of drug encapsulated, the possibility to control the release, and the specific targeting. When these limitations will be overcome a new era will be open in for personalized cardiovascular medicine.

Acknowledgments

This study was supported by Inserm, University Paris 13 and University Paris Diderot, France. This work was also supported in part by the EU project NanoAthero FP7-NMP-2012-LARGE-6-309820, Lefoulon-Delalande scholarship (to MV), IMOVA project (FUI/ OSEO, CG93), and ANR-13-LAB1-0005-01 "FucoChem".

References

1. A. S. Go, D. Mozaffarian, V. L. Roger, E. J. Benjamin, J. D. Berry, W. B. Borden, D. M. Bravata, S. Dai, E. S. Ford, C. S. Fox, S. Franco, H. J. Fullerton, C. Gillespie, S. M. Hailpern, J. A. Heit, V. J. Howard, M. D. Huffman, B. M. Kissela, S. J. Kittner, D. T. Lackland, J. H. Lichtman, L. D. Lisabeth, D. Magid, G. M. Marcus, A. Marelli, D. B. Matchar, D. K. McGuire, E. R. Mohler, C. S. Moy, M. E. Mussolino, G. Nichol, N. P. Paynter, P. J. Schreiner, P. D. Sorlie, J. Stein, T. N. Turan, S. S. Virani, N. D. Wong, D. Woo, M. B. Turner, *Circulation*, e6 (2013).
2. A. J. Lusis, *Nature,* 233 (2000).
3. P. Libby, M. DiCarli, R. Weissleder, *J. Nucl. Med.*, 33S (2010).
4. P. Libby, *J. Lipid Res.*, S352 (2009).
5. E. D. Hood, M. Chorny, C. F. Greineder, S. A. I, R. J. Levy, V. R. Muzykantov, *Biomater.*, 3708 (2014).
6. K. Douma, L. Prinzen, D. W. Slaaf, C. P. Reutelingsperger, E. A. Biessen, T. M. Hackeng, M. J. Post, M. A. van Zandvoort, *Small*, 544 (2009).
7. A. Klink, F. Hyafil, J. Rudd, P. Faries, V. Fuster, Z. Mallat, O. Meilhac, W. J. Mulder, J. B. Michel, F. Ramirez, G. Storm, R. Thompson, I. C. Turnbull, J. Egido, J. L. Martin-Ventura, C. Zaragoza, D. Letourneur, Z. A. Fayad, *Nat. Rev. Cardiol.*, 338 (2011).
8. V. J. Dzau, R. C. Braun-Dullaeus, D. G. Sedding, *Nat. Med.,* 124 (2002).
9. J. E. Feig, B. Hewing, J. D. Smith, S. L. Hazen, E. A. Fisher, *Circ. Res.,* 205 (2014).
10. L. N. Marzec, T. M. Maddox, *Curr. Cardiol. Rep.*, 418 (2013).
11. D. J. Rader, G. K. Hovingh, *Lancet*, 618 (2014).
12. C. Weber, H. Noels, *Nat. Med.*, 1410 (2011).
13. C. R. Sirtori, *Pharmacol. Res.*, 3 (2014).
14. D. Collen, H. R. Lijnen, *Thromb. Haemost.*, 627 (2005).
15. G. Lippi, R. Rossi, L. Ippolito, V. Zobbi, D. Azzi, S. Pipitone, E. J. Favaloro, D. M. Funk, *Semin. Thromb. Hemost.*, 834 (2013).

16. J. Alvarez-Sabin, O. Maisterra, E. Santamarina, C. S. Kase, *Lancet Neurol.*, 689 (2013).
17. W. J. Mulder, G. J. Strijkers, G. A. van Tilborg, A. W. Griffioen, K. Nicolay, *NMR Biomed.*, 142 (2006).
18. N. S. Faithfull, C. E. King, S. M. Cain, *Microvasc. Res.*, 183 (1987).
19. U. Kaisers, K. P. Kelly, T. Busch, *Br. J. Anaesth.*, 143 (2003).
20. J. Chen, H. Pan, G. M. Lanza, S. A. Wickline, *Adv. Chronic Kidney Dis.*, 466 (2013).
21. R. Diaz-Lopez, N. Tsapis, E. Fattal, *Pharm. Res.*, 1 (2010).
22. J. C. Frias, K. J. Williams, E. A. Fisher, Z. A. Fayad, *J. Am. Chem. Soc.*, 16316 (2004).
23. A. K. Silva, D. Letourneur, C. Chauvierre, *Theranostics*, 579 (2014).
24. F. Danhier, E. Ansorena, J. M. Silva, R. Coco, A. Le Breton, V. Preat, *J. Control. Release*, 505 (2012).
25. M. Di Marco, C. Sadun, M. Port, I. Guilbert, P. Couvreur, C. Dubernet, *Int. J. Nanomed.*, 609 (2007).
26. Y. Javed, L. Lartigue, P. Hugounenq, Q. L. Vuong, Y. Gossuin, R. Bazzi, C. Wilhelm, C. Ricolleau, F. Gazeau, D. Alloyeau, *Small*, 3325 (2014).
27. J. M. Tarkin, F. R. Joshi, J. H. Rudd, *Nat. Rev. Cardiol.*, 443 (2014).
28. N. Tahara, H. Kai, M. Ishibashi, H. Nakaura, H. Kaida, K. Baba, N. Hayabuchi, T. Imaizumi, *J. Am. Coll. Cardiol.*, 1825 (2006).
29. F. Rouzet, L. Bachelet-Violette, J. M. Alsac, M. Suzuki, A. Meulemans, L. Louedec, A. Petiet, M. Jandrot-Perrus, F. Chaubet, J. B. Michel, D. Le Guludec, D. Letourneur, *J. Nucl. Med.*, 1433 (2011).
30. P. Saboural, F. Chaubet, F. Rouzet, F. Al-Shoukr, R. B. Azzouna, N. Bouchemal, L. Picton, L. Louedec, M. Maire, L. Rolland, G. Potier, D. Guludec, D. Letourneur, C. Chauvierre, *Mar. Drugs*, 4851 (2014).
31. M. R. Stacy, W. Zhou, A. J. Sinusas, *J. Nucl. Med.*, 2104 (2013).
32. C. J. Anderson, J. W. Bulte, K. Chen, X. Chen, B. A. Khaw, M. Shokeen, K. L. Wooley, H. F. VanBrocklin, *J. Nucl. Med.*, 3S (2010).
33. A. Beilvert, D. P. Cormode, F. Chaubet, K. C. Briley-Saebo, V. Mani, W. J. Mulder, E. Vucic, J. F. Toussaint, D. Letourneur, Z. A. Fayad, *Magn. Reson. Med.*, 1195 (2009).
34. J. Vymazal, E. Spuentrup, G. Cardenas-Molina, A. J. Wiethoff, M. G. Hartmann, P. Caravan, E. C. Parsons, Jr., *Investig. Radiol.*, 697 (2009).

35. M. R. Makowski, S. C. Forbes, U. Blume, A. Warley, C. H. Jansen, A. Schuster, A. J. Wiethoff, R. M. Botnar, *Atherosclerosis*, 43 (2012).
36. J. C. De La Vega, U. O. Hafeli, *Contrast Media Mol. Imaging*, (2014).
37. E. Jin, Z. R. Lu, *Biomater.*, 5822 (2014).
38. H. Boll, S. Nittka, F. Doyon, M. Neumaier, A. Marx, M. Kramer, C. Groden, M. A. Brockmann, *PLoS One*, e25692 (2011).
39. B. Trachet, R. A. Fraga-Silva, A. Piersigilli, A. Tedgui, J. Sordet-Dessimoz, A. Astolfo, C. Van der Donckt, P. Modregger, M. F. Stampanoni, P. Segers, N. Stergiopulos, *Cardiovasc. Res.*, 213 (2015).
40. T. R. Porter, *J. Am. Coll. Cardiol.*, 491 (2000).
41. S. Hak, H. M. Sanders, P. Agrawal, S. Langereis, H. Grull, H. M. Keizer, F. Arena, E. Terreno, G. J. Strijkers, K. Nicolay, *Eur. J. Pharm. Biopharm.*, 397 (2009).
42. S. Flacke, S. Fischer, M. J. Scott, R. J. Fuhrhop, J. S. Allen, M. McLean, P. Winter, G. A. Sicard, P. J. Gaffney, S. A. Wickline, G. M. Lanza, *Circulation*, 1280 (2001).
43. J. C. Frias, Y. Ma, K. J. Williams, Z. A. Fayad, E. A. Fisher, *Nano Lett.*, 2220 (2006).
44. G. A. van Tilborg, E. Vucic, G. J. Strijkers, D. P. Cormode, V. Mani, T. Skajaa, C. P. Reutelingsperger, Z. A. Fayad, W. J. Mulder, K. Nicolay, *Bioconjug. Chem.*, 1794 (2010).
45. V. Amirbekian, M. J. Lipinski, K. C. Briley-Saebo, S. Amirbekian, J. G. Aguinaldo, D. B. Weinreb, E. Vucic, J. C. Frias, F. Hyafil, V. Mani, E. A. Fisher, Z. A. Fayad, *Proc. Natl. Acad. Sci. USA.*, 961 (2007).
46. W. Chen, D. P. Cormode, Y. Vengrenyuk, B. Herranz, J. E. Feig, A. Klink, W. J. Mulder, E. A. Fisher, Z. A. Fayad, *JACC Cardiovasc. Imaging*, 373 (2013).
47. S. M. Demos, H. Alkan-Onyuksel, B. J. Kane, K. Ramani, A. Nagaraj, R. Greene, M. Klegerman, D. D. McPherson, *J. Am. Coll. Cardiol.*, 867 (1999).
48. H. Kim, P. H. Kee, Y. Rim, M. R. Moody, M. E. Klegerman, D. Vela, S. L. Huang, D. D. McPherson, S. T. Laing, *Atherosclerosis*, 252 (2013).
49. A. Dellinger, J. Olson, K. Link, S. Vance, M. G. Sandros, J. Yang, Z. Zhou, C. L. Kepley, *J. Cardiovasc. Magn. Reson.*, 7 (2013).

50. T. Skajaa, D. P. Cormode, E. Falk, W. J. Mulder, E. A. Fisher, Z. A. Fayad, *Arterioscler. Thromb. Vasc. Biol.*, 169 (2010).
51. D. P. Cormode, T. Skajaa, M. M. van Schooneveld, R. Koole, P. Jarzyna, M. E. Lobatto, C. Calcagno, A. Barazza, R. E. Gordon, P. Zanzonico, E. A. Fisher, Z. A. Fayad, W. J. Mulder, *Nano Lett.*, 3715 (2008).
52. D. P. Cormode, E. Roessl, A. Thran, T. Skajaa, R. E. Gordon, J. P. Schlomka, V. Fuster, E. A. Fisher, W. J. Mulder, R. Proksa, Z. A. Fayad, *Radiology*, 774 (2010).
53. C. Jung, M. G. Kaul, O. T. Bruns, T. Ducic, B. Freund, M. Heine, R. Reimer, A. Meents, S. C. Salmen, H. Weller, P. Nielsen, G. Adam, J. Heeren, H. Ittrich, *Circ. Cardiovasc. Imaging*, 303 (2014).
54. J. Ding, Y. Wang, M. Ma, Y. Zhang, S. Lu, Y. Jiang, C. Qi, S. Luo, G. Dong, S. Wen, Y. An, N. Gu, *Biomater.*, 209 (2013).
55. T. D. Tran, S. D. Caruthers, M. Hughes, J. N. Marsh, T. Cyrus, P. M. Winter, A. M. Neubauer, S. A. Wickline, G. M. Lanza, *Int. J. Nanomedicine*, 515 (2007).
56. G. M. Lanza, K. D. Wallace, M. J. Scott, W. P. Cacheris, D. R. Abendschein, D. H. Christy, A. M. Sharkey, J. G. Miller, P. J. Gaffney, S. A. Wickline, *Circulation*, 3334 (1996).
57. P. M. Winter, A. M. Neubauer, S. D. Caruthers, T. D. Harris, J. D. Robertson, T. A. Williams, A. H. Schmieder, G. Hu, J. S. Allen, E. K. Lacy, H. Zhang, S. A. Wickline, G. M. Lanza, *Arterioscler. Thromb. Vasc. Biol.*, 2103 (2006).
58. M. Suzuki, L. Bachelet-Violette, F. Rouzet, A. Beilvert, G. Autret, M. Maire, C. Menager, L. Louedec, C. Choqueux, P. Saboural, O. Haddad, C. Chauvierre, F. Chaubet, J. B. Michel, J. M. Serfaty, D. Letourneur, *Nanomedicine* (*Lond*), 1 (2014).
59. T. Bonnard, G. Yang, A. Petiet, V. Ollivier, O. Haddad, D. Arnaud, L. Louedec, L. Bachelet-Violette, S. M. Derkaoui, D. Letourneur, C. Chauvierre, C. Le Visage, *Theranostics*, 592 (2014).
60. T. Bonnard, J. M. Serfaty, C. Journe, B. Ho Tin Noe, D. Arnaud, L. Louedec, S. M. Derkaoui, D. Letourneur, C. Chauvierre, C. Le Visage, *Acta Biomater.*, 3535 (2014).
61. X. Wang, C. E. Hagemeyer, J. D. Hohmann, E. Leitner, P. C. Armstrong, F. Jia, M. Olschewski, A. Needles, K. Peter, I. Ahrens, *Circulation*, 3117 (2012).

62. F. S. Villanueva, E. Lu, S. Bowry, S. Kilic, E. Tom, J. Wang, J. Gretton, J. J. Pacella, W. R. Wagner, *Circulation*, 345 (2007).
63. B. P. Davidson, B. A. Kaufmann, J. T. Belcik, A. Xie, Y. Qi, J. R. Lindner, *J. Am. Coll. Cardiol.*, 1690 (2012).
64. B. A. Kaufmann, C. L. Carr, J. T. Belcik, A. Xie, Q. Yue, S. Chadderdon, E. S. Caplan, J. Khangura, S. Bullens, S. Bunting, J. R. Lindner, *Arterioscler. Thromb. Vasc. Biol.*, 54 (2010).
65. W. Wu, Y. Wang, S. Shen, J. Wu, S. Guo, L. Su, F. Hou, Z. Wang, Y. Liao, J. Bin, *Investig. Radiol.*, 803 (2013).
66. G. Hu, C. Liu, Y. Liao, L. Yang, R. Huang, J. Wu, J. Xie, K. Bundhoo, Y. Liu, J. Bin, *Thromb. Haemost.*, 172 (2012).
67. S. Fokong, A. Fragoso, A. Rix, A. Curaj, Z. Wu, W. Lederle, O. Iranzo, J. Gatjens, F. Kiessling, M. Palmowski, *Investig. Radiol.*, 843 (2013).
68. M. D. Majmudar, J. Yoo, E. J. Keliher, J. J. Truelove, Y. Iwamoto, B. Sena, P. Dutta, A. Borodovsky, K. Fitzgerald, M. F. Di Carli, P. Libby, D. G. Anderson, F. K. Swirski, R. Weissleder, M. Nahrendorf, *Circ. Res.*, 755 (2013).
69. M. A. McAteer, K. Mankia, N. Ruparelia, A. Jefferson, H. B. Nugent, L. A. Stork, K. M. Channon, J. E. Schneider, R. P. Choudhury, *Arterioscler. Thromb. Vasc. Biol.*, 1427 (2012).
70. H. P. Luehmann, E. D. Pressly, L. Detering, C. Wang, R. Pierce, P. K. Woodard, R. J. Gropler, C. J. Hawker, Y. Liu, *J. Nucl. Med.*, 629 (2014).
71. S. Marrache, S. Dhar, *Proc. Natl. Acad. Sci. U. S. A.*, 9445 (2013).
72. J. Zhou, D. Guo, Y. Zhang, W. Wu, H. Ran, Z. Wang, *ACS Appl. Mater. Interfaces*, 5566 (2014).
73. F. Hyafil, J. C. Cornily, J. E. Feig, R. Gordon, E. Vucic, V. Amirbekian, E. A. Fisher, V. Fuster, L. J. Feldman, Z. A. Fayad, *Nat. Med.*, 636 (2007).
74. Y. Song, Z. Huang, J. Xu, D. Ren, Y. Wang, X. Zheng, Y. Shen, L. Wang, H. Gao, J. Hou, Z. Pang, J. Qian, J. Ge, *Biomater.*, 2961 (2014).
75. K. Tsuchiya, N. Nitta, A. Sonoda, H. Otani, M. Takahashi, K. Murata, M. Shiomi, Y. Tabata, S. Nohara, *Eur. J. Radiol.*, 1919 (2013).
76. C. von zur Muhlen, A. Fink-Petri, J. Salaklang, D. Paul, I. Neudorfer, V. Berti, A. Merkle, K. Peter, C. Bode, D. von Elverfeldt, *Contrast Media Mol. Imaging*, 268 (2010).

77. C. Burtea, S. Ballet, S. Laurent, O. Rousseaux, A. Dencausse, W. Gonzalez, M. Port, C. Corot, L. Vander Elst, R. N. Muller, *Arterioscler. Thromb. Vasc. Biol.*, e36 (2012).
78. M. Michalska, L. Machtoub, H. D. Manthey, E. Bauer, V. Herold, G. Krohne, G. Lykowsky, M. Hildenbrand, T. Kampf, P. Jakob, A. Zernecke, W. R. Bauer, *Arterioscler. Thromb. Vasc. Biol.*, 2350 (2012).
79. L. Josephson, C. H. Tung, A. Moore, R. Weissleder, *Bioconjug. Chem.*, 186 (1999).
80. M. Nahrendorf, H. Zhang, S. Hembrador, P. Panizzi, D. E. Sosnovik, E. Aikawa, P. Libby, F. K. Swirski, R. Weissleder, *Circulation*, 379 (2008).
81. W. J. Mulder, F. A. Jaffer, Z. A. Fayad, M. Nahrendorf, *Sci. Transl. Med.*, 239sr1 (2014).
82. M. Nahrendorf, E. Keliher, B. Marinelli, F. Leuschner, C. S. Robbins, R. E. Gerszten, M. J. Pittet, F. K. Swirski, R. Weissleder, *Arterioscler. Thromb. Vasc. Biol.*, 750 (2011).
83. B. R. Jarrett, C. Correa, K. L. Ma, A. Y. Louie, *PLoS One*, e13254 (2010).
84. D. E. Kim, J. Y. Kim, I. C. Sun, D. Schellingerhout, S. K. Lee, C. H. Ahn, I. C. Kwon, K. Kim, *Ann. Neurol.*, 617 (2013).
85. I. Cicha, C. Garlichs, C. Alexiou, *Eur. J. Nanomed.*, (2014).
86. M. E. Kooi, V. C. Cappendijk, K. Cleutjens, A. G. H. Kessels, P. Kitslaar, M. Borgers, P. M. Frederik, M. Daemen, J. M. A. van Engelshoven, *Circulation*, 2453 (2003).
87. A. Saleh, M. Schroeter, A. Ringelstein, H. P. Hartung, M. Siebler, U. Modder, S. Jander, *Stroke*, 2733 (2007).
88. A. J. Degnan, A. J. Patterson, T. Y. Tang, S. P. Howarth, J. H. Gillard, *Cerebrovasc. Dis.*, 169 (2012).
89. Y. X. Wang, *Quant. Imaging Med. Surg.*, 35 (2011).
90. J. M. Richards, S. I. Semple, T. J. MacGillivray, C. Gray, J. P. Langrish, M. Williams, M. Dweck, W. Wallace, G. McKillop, R. T. Chalmers, O. J. Garden, D. E. Newby, *Circ. Cardiovasc. Imaging*, 274 (2011).
91. A. Yilmaz, S. Rosch, H. Yildiz, S. Klumpp, U. Sechtem, *Circulation*, 1932 (2012).
92. S. R. Alam, A. S. Shah, J. Richards, N. N. Lang, G. Barnes, N. Joshi, T. MacGillivray, G. McKillop, S. Mirsadraee, J. Payne, K. A. Fox,

P. Henriksen, D. E. Newby, S. I. Semple, *Circ. Cardiovasc. Imaging*, 559 (2012).
93. J. K. Leach, E. Patterson, E. A. O'Rear, *Thromb. Haemost.*, 1213 (2004).
94. J. K. Leach, E. Patterson, E. A. O'Rear, *J. Thromb. Haemost.*, 1548 (2004).
95. H. J. Jin, H. Zhang, M. L. Sun, B. G. Zhang, J. W. Zhang, *J. Thromb. Thrombolysis*, 458 (2013).
96. Y. Uesugi, H. Kawata, J. Jo, Y. Saito, Y. Tabata, *J. Control. Release*, 269 (2010).
97. H. Kawata, Y. Uesugi, T. Soeda, Y. Takemoto, J. H. Sung, K. Umaki, K. Kato, K. Ogiwara, K. Nogami, K. Ishigami, M. Horii, S. Uemura, M. Shima, Y. Tabata, Y. Saito, *J. Am. Coll. Cardiol.*, 2550 (2012).
98. E. A. Lee, H. Yim, J. Heo, H. Kim, G. Jung, N. S. Hwang, *Arch. Pharmacal Res.*, 120 (2014).
99. D. Robert, D. Fayol, C. Le Visage, G. Frasca, S. Brule, C. Menager, F. Gazeau, D. Letourneur, C. Wilhelm, *Biomater.*, 1586 (2010).
100. D. Fayol, N. Luciani, L. Lartigue, F. Gazeau, C. Wilhelm, *Adv. Healthc. Mater.,* 313 (2013).
101. K. Cheng, T. S. Li, K. Malliaras, D. R. Davis, Y. Zhang, E. Marban, *Circ. Res.*, 1570 (2010).
102. F. Bi, J. Zhang, Y. Su, Y. C. Tang, J. N. Liu, *Biomater.*, 5125 (2009).
103. Y. H. Ma, S. Y. Wu, T. Wu, Y. J. Chang, M. Y. Hua, J. P. Chen, *Biomater.*, 3343 (2009).
104. H. W. Yang, M. Y. Hua, K. J. Lin, S. P. Wey, R. Y. Tsai, S. Y. Wu, Y. C. Lu, H. L. Liu, T. Wu, Y. H. Ma, *Int. J. Nanomed.*, 5159 (2012).
105. M. Kempe, H. Kempe, I. Snowball, R. Wallen, C. R. Arza, M. Gotberg, T. Olsson, *Biomater.*, 9499 (2010).
106. J. R. McCarthy, I. Y. Sazonova, S. S. Erdem, T. Hara, B. D. Thompson, P. Patel, I. Botnaru, C. P. Lin, G. L. Reed, R. Weissleder, F. A. Jaffer, *Nanomed.* (*Lond*), 1017 (2012).
107. J. P. Chen, P. C. Yang, Y. H. Ma, T. Wu, *Carbohydr. Polym.*, 364 (2011).
108. D. Deamer, A. D. Bangham, *Biochim. Biophys. Acta*, 629 (1976).
109. S. M. Johnson, A. D. Bangham, M. W. Hill, E. D. Korn, *Biochim. Biophys. Acta*, 820 (1971).

110. S. M. Moghimi, J. Szebeni, *Prog. Lipid Res.*, 463 (2003).
111. S. Gurudevan, R. K. Kanwar, R. N. Veedu, S. Sasidharan, R. L. Kennedy, K. Walder, N. Prasad, J. R. Kanwar, *Curr. Gene Ther.*, 322 (2013).
112. J. K. Leach, E. A. O'Rear, E. Patterson, Y. Miao, A. E. Johnson, *Thromb. Haemost.*, 64 (2003).
113. B. Vaidya, G. P. Agrawal, S. P. Vyas, *Eur. J. Pharm. Sci.*, 589 (2011).
114. J. Y. Kim, J. K. Kim, J. S. Park, Y. Byun, C. K. Kim, *Biomater.*, 5751 (2009).
115. S. Absar, K. Nahar, Y. M. Kwon, F. Ahsan, *Pharm. Res.*, 1663 (2013).
116. G. M. Lanza, P. M. Winter, S. D. Caruthers, M. S. Hughes, G. Hu, A. H. Schmieder, S. A. Wickline, *Angiogenesis,* 189 (2010).
117. J. N. Marsh, G. Hu, M. J. Scott, H. Zhang, M. J. Goette, P. J. Gaffney, S. D. Caruthers, S. A. Wickline, D. Abendschein, G. M. Lanza, *Nanomed.* (*Lond*), 605 (2011).
118. S. T. Laing, M. R. Moody, H. Kim, B. Smulevitz, S. L. Huang, C. K. Holland, D. D. McPherson, M. E. Klegerman, *Thromb. Res.*, 629 (2012).
119. K. Hagisawa, T. Nishioka, R. Suzuki, K. Maruyama, B. Takase, M. Ishihara, A. Kurita, N. Yoshimoto, Y. Nishida, K. Iida, H. Luo, R. J. Siegel, *J. Thromb. Haemost.*, 1565 (2013).
120. A. Moumouh, L. Barentin, F. Tranquart, S. Serrierre, I. Bonnaud, J. P. Tasu, *Ultrasound Med. Biol.,* 51 (2010).
121. M. Nedelmann, N. Ritschel, S. Doenges, A. C. Langheinrich, T. Acker, P. Reuter, M. Yeniguen, J. Pukropski, M. Kaps, C. Mueller, G. Bachmann, T. Gerriets, *J. Cereb. Blood Flow Metab.*, 1712 (2010).
122. W. S. Liu, Z. Z. Huang, X. W. Wang, J. Zhou, Thromb. Res., 547 (2012).
123. F. Xie, J. Lof, T. Matsunaga, R. Zutshi, T. R. Porter, *Circulation*, 1378 (2009).
124. M. de Saint Victor, C. Crake, C. C. Coussios, E. Stride, *Expert Opin. Drug Deliv.*, 187 (2014).
125. S. Ricci, L. Dinia, M. Del Sette, P. Anzola, T. Mazzoli, S. Cenciarelli, C. Gandolfo, *Cochrane Database Syst. Rev.*, CD008348 (2012).
126. S. T. Laing, M. Moody, B. Smulevitz, H. Kim, P. Kee, S. Huang, C. K. Holland, D. D. McPherson, Arterioscler. *Thromb. Vasc. Biol.*, 1357 (2011).

127. F. Kiessling, S. Fokong, P. Koczera, W. Lederle, T. Lammers, *J. Nucl. Med.*, 345 (2012).
128. A. T. Brown, R. Flores, E. Hamilton, P. K. Roberson, M. J. Borrelli, W. C. Culp, *Investig. Radiol.*, 202 (2011).
129. E. A. Brujan, *Med. Eng. Phys.*, 742 (2009).
130. E. C. Everbach, C. W. Francis, *Ultrasound Med. Biol.*, 1153 (2000).
131. E. Unger, T. Porter, J. Lindner, P. Grayburn, *Adv. Drug Delivery. Rev.*, 110 (2014).
132. D. V. Sakharov, R. T. Hekkenberg, D. C. Rijken, *Thromb. Res.*, 333 (2000).
133. C. W. Francis, A. Blinc, S. Lee, C. Cox, *Ultrasound Med. Biol.*, 419 (1995).
134. G. Tsivgoulis, W. C. Culp, A. V. Alexandrov, *Ultrasonics*, 303 (2008).
135. C. A. Molina, M. Ribo, M. Rubiera, J. Montaner, E. Santamarina, R. Delgado-Mederos, J. F. Arenillas, R. Huertas, F. Purroy, P. Delgado, J. Alvarez-Sabin, *Stroke*, 425 (2006).
136. C. A. Molina, A. D. Barreto, G. Tsivgoulis, P. Sierzenski, M. D. Malkoff, M. Rubiera, N. Gonzales, R. Mikulik, G. Pate, J. Ostrem, W. Singleton, G. Manvelian, E. C. Unger, J. C. Grotta, P. D. Schellinger, A. V. Alexandrov, *Ann. Neurol.*, 28 (2009).
137. A. V. Alexandrov, R. Mikulik, M. Ribo, V. K. Sharma, A. Y. Lao, G. Tsivgoulis, R. M. Sugg, A. Barreto, P. Sierzenski, M. D. Malkoff, J. C. Grotta, *Stroke*, 1464 (2008).
138. F. Perren, J. Loulidi, D. Poglia, T. Landis, R. Sztajzel, *J. Thromb. Thrombolysis*, 219 (2008).
139. J. Pagola, M. Ribo, J. Alvarez-Sabin, M. Lange, M. Rubiera, C. A. Molina, *Stroke*, 2931 (2007).
140. M. Rubiera, M. Ribo, R. Delgado-Mederos, E. Santamarina, O. Maisterra, P. Delgado, J. Montaner, J. Alvarez-Sabin, C. A. Molina, *Ultrasound Med. Biol.*, 1573 (2008).

CHAPTER 10

STIMULI-RESPONSIVE NANOTHERANOSTICS

Basit Yameen*, Jun Wu*, Cristian Vilos*,†, Andrew Whyte*,‡
David Werstler*,‡, Lori Pollit*,‡ and Omid C. Farokhzad*,§,¶

**Laboratory of Nanomedicine and Biomaterials,*
Department of Anesthesiology, Brigham and Women's Hospital,
Harvard Medical School, 75 Francis St., Boston, MA 02115, USA
†Universidad Andres Bello, Facultad de Medicina,
Center for Integrative Medicine and Innovative Science (CIMIS),
Echaurren 183, Santiago, Chile
‡University of Waterloo, 200 University Avenue West Waterloo,
ON, N2L3G1, Canada
§King Abdulaziz University, Jeddah, Saudi Arabia
¶ofarokhzad@zeus.bwh.harvard.edu

Nanomedicine is emerging as an enabling technology for addressing biomedical related challenges. Encouraging developments have been made particularly in overcoming the limitations associated with the conventional therapeutic and diagnostic agents while treating severe diseases including cancer. Recent research efforts have led to the evolution of nanomedicine from merely performing a therapeutic or diagnostic function to the systems that can perform therapeutic and diagnostic functions simultaneously, referred to as nanotheranostics or theranostics. The theranostic systems are capable of providing real-time feedback on the effectiveness of a particular treatment regimen and can help in adapting the treatment plan at an early stage. The real life impact of a theranostic system can be further augmented by introducing an element of stimuli (endogenous or exogenous) responsive release of the payload. The stimuli responsiveness can enhance the safety and efficacy of a nanomedicine via an on-demand and controlled release of a payload exclusively at the site of action and only when it is deemed necessary, as revealed by the diagnostic feature of the theranostic system. Such a provision of controlled treatment and real-time monitoring is expected to help in adjusting the treatment plan in a personalized manner, particularly, for diseases showing heterogeneity, malignancy, and adaptation. In the present chapter, we provide a comprehensive insight into the biological relevance of stimuli responsive character for developing a theranostic system. We further provide a detailed overview on the recent progress regarding the development of theranostic systems showing responsiveness to a variety of stimuli including pH, temperature, reducing agents, light, magnetic field and enzymes.

1. Introduction

Nanomedicine, a joint venture of the fields of nanotechnology and medicine, is emerging as an enabling technology for addressing biomedical related challenges in therapy and diagnosis of a variety of diseases including cancer, inflammatory diseases, cardiovascular diseases, and diabetes.[1–5] Recent multidisciplinary research efforts have demonstrated the ability of nanomedicine to overcome the limitations (non-specific biodistribution and toxicity, poor solubility, non-optimal pharmacokinetics and pharmacodynamics) of conventional therapeutic and diagnostic agents by formulating them with biocompatible and biodegradable nanocarrier systems. A wide variety of nanocarriers-based on polymeric nanoparticles and micelles, liposomes, dendrimers, (mesoporous) silica nanoparticles, porous silica nanoparticles, iron oxide nanoparticles, gold nanoparticles, carbon nanomaterials and quantum dots (QDs) are being explored for the development of nanomedicines.[6–13] The concept of nanomedicine is of particular interest for reducing the collateral damage of cytotoxic agents by improving the treatment selectivity. In this context, the differential physiopathological nature of certain diseases has been exploited for selectively targeting nanocarriers to the diseased area. For instance, the enhanced permeability and retention (EPR) effect stemming from the leaky nature of microvasculature, observed in tumors and other inflammation causing diseases, has been widely explored to achieve a differentially higher accumulation of nanocarriers at the site of action.[1] The therapeutic outcomes relying on this passive way of disease targeting are not always consistent, which is primarily because of the complex biological processes leading to the EPR effect and disease heterogeneity within a patient or among a group of patients.[1] In addition to the EPR effect-based passive targeting, ligands exhibiting high affinity towards certain receptors or molecules differentially overexpressed in the diseased region are being displayed at the surface of nanocarriers for active targeting. Antibodies, single-chain variable fragments (scFvs), peptides, and aptamers (nucleic acid ligands) represent commonly explored classes of high affinity ligands that are being employed for achieving targeted nanocarriers.[6,14] The positive impact of targeted delivery is supported by the encouraging therapeutic outcomes. For instance, a polymer nanocarrier conjugated to an RNA aptamer that specifically binds to prostate specific membrane antigen (PSMA), an established prostate cancer tumor marker, exhibited 77-fold increase in binding to the PSMA expressing cells.[15] An analogous targeted nanocarrier system loaded with platinum(IV) exhibited significantly superior characteristics, such as IC50 values, compared to cisplatin or non-targeted nanocarriers.[16] In subsequent *in vivo* studies using a prostate cancer model, a single intratumoral injection of docetaxel (DTXL) loaded aptamer conjugated polymer nanocarriers led to a complete tumor reduction in >70% of LNCaP xenograft nude mice with 100% animal survival.[17] This seminal work laid the foundation for the clinical translation of PSMA targeted DTXL loaded polymer nanocarriers where a small molecule S,S-2-[3-[5-amino-1-carboxypentyl]-ureido]-pentanedioic acid (ACUPA) was employed as the PSMA targeting ligand. A systematic optimization of the physicochemical attributes of the targeted nanocarrier system resulted in an extremely effective tumor targeted nanomedicine (BIND-014) with remarkable tumor shrinkage in a human clinical study at doses less than the typical clinical doses of solvent-based DTXL formulation.[18] Despite these encouraging results, there are still some concerns regarding the attenuation of the targeting ability of some ligands in biological media.[19] The difference in the level of receptor expression among different types of cancers and variations among different patients can further counter the impact of an active targeting based treatment.[20] Therefore, a real-time monitoring of a certain treatment plan is essential to assess the treatment effectiveness.

The nanomedicines can either be merely performing a therapeutic function or they can be designed to perform therapeutic and diagnostic functions simultaneously, the latter platforms are referred to as theranostics.[21–23] The diagnostic aspect of a theranostic platform reports on the effectiveness of a certain treatment plan for a patient in a non-invasive manner. Such real-time information on the progress of a treatment can help in adapting the treatment regimen at an early stage for the maximum patient benefit and is laying the foundation for personalized nanomedicine.[24] The concept of personalized nanomedicine is of particular benefit in the treatment of rapidly proliferating diseases showing heterogeneity, malignancy and adaptation. The effectiveness and selectivity of a theranostic platform can be further augmented by designing nanocarriers that are programmed for a stimuli (endogenous or exogenous) triggered release of their payloads in the vicinity of the diseased area. Such multifunctional stimuli responsive theranostic platforms are expected to ensure higher safety via an on demand controlled release of therapeutics exclusively at the site of action as opposed to the non-specific biodistribution of toxic drugs in case of conventional chemotherapy. Besides, the diagnostic element will provide real time feedback on the progress of treatment to help adjust the treatment plan in a personalized manner avoiding the issues of under or over-dosage. In this article, we provide an overview of recent progress in the development of the emerging field of stimuli responsive theranostics by describing the biological relevance of commonly employed stimuli (pH, temperature, reducing agent, photosensitivity, magnetic field or combinations of two or more) and their application in development of different therapeutic and diagnostic combinations.

2. pH Responsive Theranostics

The difference between the extracellular tumor pH and the pH of the bloodstream has been widely explored for selective release of the payload in the tumor vicinity. In addition, the acidic endosomal and lysosomal pH (4.0–6.0) conditions have also been exploited to trigger the intracellular release of payloads from the endocytosed nanocarriers.[25] A pH responsive theranostic system can respond to the change in environmental pH either by switching its constituent material between hydrophilic (swollen) and hydrophobic (collapsed) states as a result of protonation and deprotonation of certain functional groups or by degrading due to the cleavage of pH sensitive functional groups (Table 1). Both response mechanisms result in a payload

Table 1. A list of functional groups commonly employed to generate pH responsive theranostics, their physical effect on the nanoassembly and chemical changes in response to pH variation are also depicted.

Common pH responsive functional groups	Physical effect on nanoassembly	Chemical changes in response to pH variations
Carboxylic acid	Swelling/Collapsing	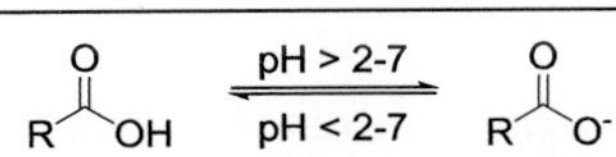
Amine	Swelling/Collapsing	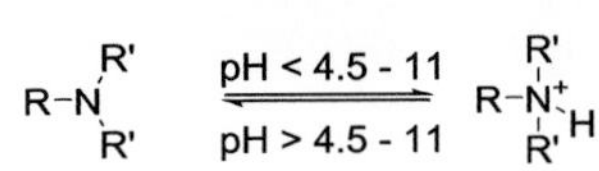
Histidine (imidazole)	Swelling/Collapsing	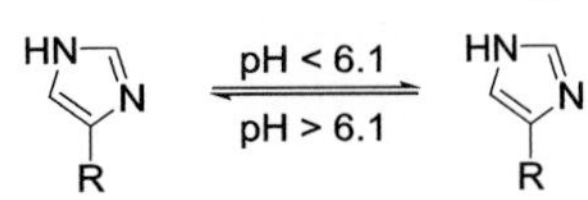
Boronic ester/ boronate ester	Degradation	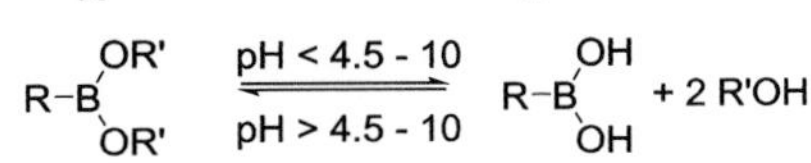
Acetal/Ketal	Degradation	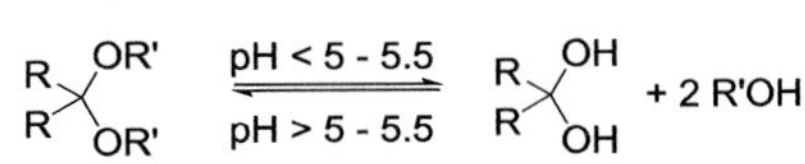
Hydrazone	Degradation	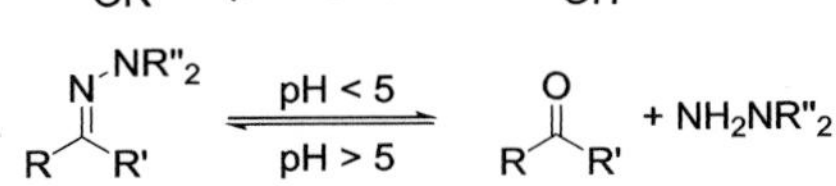

release by destabilizing the physical architecture of the theranostic system. Aromatic or aliphatic amines and carboxylic acid groups are most widely employed to impart a pH responsive swelling/collapsing characteristic to a material while boronate esters, acetals, ketals, hydrozones and imines represent major types of functional groups used to create materials that degrade in response to a change in environmental pH. With a pKa between 2 and 5, carboxylate groups carry negative charge under the physiological conditions, which also protects the nanocarrier systems from protein fouling during the systemic circulation.[26] For polymers bearing pendant carboxylate groups, a change in pH from basic to acidic results in the protonation of carboxylate groups. This makes the polymer chains hydrophobic and leads to a cooperative effect of the collapse of the polymer chains. In a stimuli responsive theranostic system reported by Chiang *et al.*, pH responsive vesicles were prepared from a copolymer containing acrylic acid (AA) and N-isopropylacrylamide (NIPAM).[27] The vesicles were loaded with citric acid coated superparamagnetic iron oxide particles (SPION) and doxorubicin (DOX) (Figure 1(a)). AA and NIPAM constituents gave the vesicles pH and temperature responsiveness. The T_2 relaxation was shown to vary according to pH since the protonation state of carboxylic acid groups in the AA component would change the hydrophilicity of the whole assembly. That in turn changes the amount of water passing through the polymer layer affecting the relaxation time. This theranostic system could be used as a unique type of contrast agent for pH responsive magnetic resonance imaging (MRI) since the acidic nature of the tumor extracellular environment would be sufficient to show a different contrast than healthy tissue. Alongside the ability of the material to be used for diagnostic purposes, a pH responsive DOX release was shown. The DOX was loaded at a slightly basic pH by permeating through the swollen gel layer and binding to the ionized AA through electrostatic interactions. *In vitro* release was seen at a pH 5.0, caused by an increase in the aqueous solubility of the DOX in addition to the decreased ionization of AA moieties. Using the SPIONs magnetic properties and magnetic guidance, the *in vitro* viability of HeLa cells was decreased to 27% compared to the free DOX providing a viability of 34%.

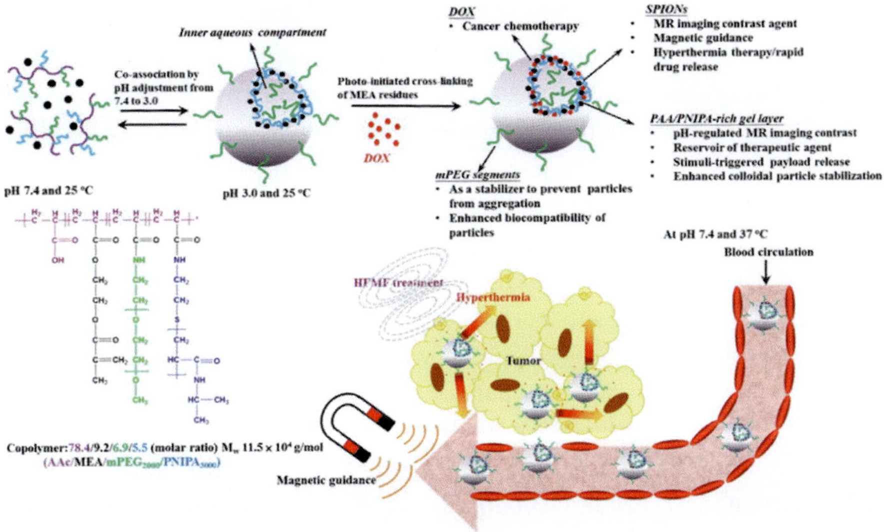

(a)

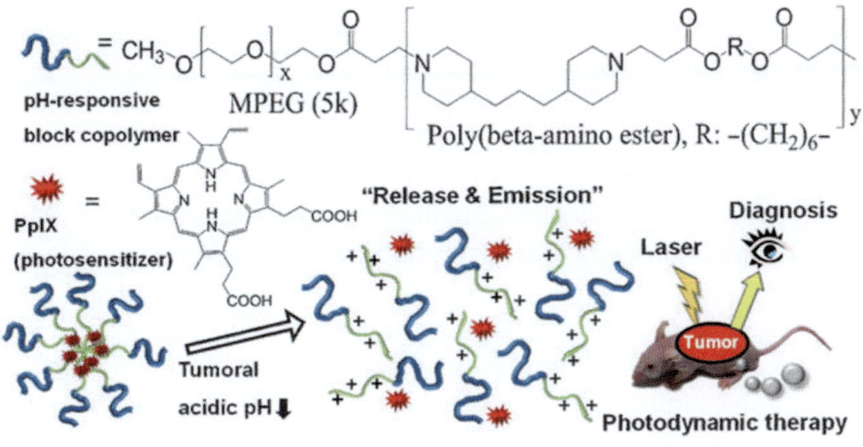

(b)

Fig. 1: (a) A pH and temperature responsive theranostic-based on vesicles derived from a copolymer containing AA and NIPAM and loaded with SPION and DOX. Reprinted with permission from Ref. 27. Copyright American Chemical Society. (b) pH responsive protoporphyrin IX photosensitizer loaded theranostic system for simultaneous non-invasive fluorescence imaging and photothermal therapy. Reproduced with permission from Royal Society of Chemistry.[32]

Contrary to carboxylic acid groups bearing materials, amino group containing materials are hydrophilic when protonated under acidic conditions (Table 1). The polymer chains bearing amino groups are in a swollen state under acidic environments, while they collapse as the pH increases. Depending on the chemical structure, the pKa of the protonated amines can vary from ~ 4.5 to 11, however they are between 6 and 10 for commonly used aliphatic amines.[28] The intrinsic toxicity associated with the amino groups is a matter of concern while fabricating amine-based pH responsive nanocarriers, however, this concern can be mitigated with PEGylation.[29] Amino groups bearing nanocarrier systems can be designed to release the payload precisely at the extracellular acidic pH of the tumor environment. Furthermore, the cationic charge they carry at physiological pH facilitates the cellular uptake through electrostatic interaction with the anionic surface of the cell membrane.[30] Once inside an endosome at a pH of ~5, amines are nearly guaranteed to be ionized which destabilizes the carrier and likely allows for endosomal escape via the proton sponge effect.[31] A wide variety of amine-based systems are under investigation for fabrication of pH responsive theranostic systems capable of releasing the payload at the tumor site. Koo *et al.* created a PEGylated polyester with a pH sensitive tertiary amine in the backbone incorporated as a piperidine-like structure (Figure 1(b)).[32] After loading protoporphyrin IX, a photosensitizer that can be used for diagnosis and treatment, authors demonstrated accelerated release and more singlet oxygen generation at pH 6.4 compared to 7.4. The slightly acidic environment protonates the tertiary amines in the hydrophobic amino ester block making it hydrophilic. The change in the extent of hydration stimulates the demicellization of the block copolymer micelles and releases the cargo. *In vivo* testing in mice with SCC7 tumors showed protoporphyrin accumulation at tumor sites and revealed a substantial number of tumor cells were damaged or destroyed. This damage was seen using the micelles, which provided clear fluorescent imaging of the destroyed tumors.

Besides creating pH responsive theranostics from materials containing either carboxylic or amino groups, efforts have been reported where both carboxylic and amino groups can be used in a single pH responsive system. This approach is seen in the work of Jing *et al.* who created Mn–porphyrin functionalized DOX loaded poly(lactic acid) (PLA) nanoparticles (Mn–porphyrin–DOX NPs).[33] The loading of DOX into the PLA nanoparticles was carried out through a nanoemulsion process and Mn–porphyrin (functioning as a contrast agent) was functionalized to the surface of nanoparticles through amide linkages. These nanoparticles showed pH responsiveness with higher release rates at pH 3.5 than 7.4. The slow release at pH 7.4 was related to the higher electrostatic interaction between the positive amino groups on the DOX and the negative carboxylic acid groups on the PLA. In acidic conditions, the protonation of PLA carboxylate and DOX amino groups reduces the electrostatic interaction between them, which increases the rate of DOX release from the nanocarrier. The cytotoxicity Mn–porphyrin–DOX NPs incubated with HeLa cells exhibited superior anticancer activity in comparison to the free DOX. Analyzing its MRI abilities, Mn–porphyrin–DOX NPs exhibited higher longitudinal relaxivity (r_1 value of 27.8 $mM^{-1} \cdot s^{-1}$ of Mn^{3+}) in water than free Mn–porphyrin (r_1 value of 6.70 $mM^{-1} \cdot s^{-1}$ of Mn^{3+}). The higher r_1 value for Mn–porphyrin–DOX NPs was attributed to covalent grafting of the Mn–porphyrin on the surface of nanoparticles that reduces the tumbling rate of contrast agent and increases its interaction with water. Authors did not report the theranostic effect *in vivo*, however the effectiveness of Mn–porphyrin–DOX NPs for MRI was demonstrated *in vivo* using HT–29 tumor bearing male nude mouse.

The protonation and deprotonation of hydroxyls in response to pH change was employed by Chen *et al.* who used a microemulsion method employing upconversion nanoparticles and boehmite (UCNPs–Al) to create a nanocomposite with mesoporous structure as well as upconversion luminescence.[34] The resulting nanocomposite was positively charged in a low pH environment due to the protonation of UCNPs–Al surface hydroxyl groups found on its surface and negatively charged in the physiological environment due to the deprotonation of these hydroxyl groups. Using the positively charged drug DOX as an example, its electrostatic uptake and retention was facilitated in physiological conditions whereas it was repelled from the carrier at the acidic pH of the tumor. In addition, the positive charge on the surface of UCNPs–Al was also seen to increase cellular uptake. The *in vitro* imaging experiment performed on HeLa cells showed a continually increasing DOX fluorescence inside the cell in a steady continuous manner over 0 h, 30 min, 2 h, 6 h and 12 h at 37°C. This increase in fluorescence was attributed to the sustained release of DOX from UNCPs–Al under the acidic endosomal and lysosomal pH. The upconversion luminescence could also be employed to track the intracellular trafficking of the DOX loaded UCNPs–Al.

In addition to the materials bearing functional groups that exhibit pH responsiveness through the switching of hydration states via protation/deprotonation mechanism, materials with pH responsiveness stemming from the cleavage of pH sensitive covalent linkages (boronate esters, acetals, ketals, hydrozones and imines) are also being explored for fabrication of pH responsive theranostics. Xiao *et al.* conjugated the therapeutic drug DOX onto a unimolecular micelle system through the pH labile hydrazone bond.[35] They designed a hyperbranched amphiphilic block copolymer, H40-poly(L-glutamate-hydrazone-DOX)-b-poly(ethylene glycol) or H40–P(LG–Hyd–DOX)–b–PEG, which underwent micellization in aqueous environments. The conjugate H40–P(LG–Hyd–DOX)–*b*–PEG was functionalized with integrin $\alpha_v\beta_3$-targeting peptide cyclo(Arg–Gly–Asp–D–Phe–Cys) (cRGD) in combination with a macrocyclic chelator for ^{64}Cu (1,4,7-triazacyclononane-N,N′,N″-triacetic acid) for non-invasive positron emission tomography (PET) imaging. *In vitro* tests showed that the DOX was released faster at low pH conditions found at tumor sites than at pH 7.4. The faster DOX release at the low pH was attributed to the cleavage of the pH labile hydrazone linkage. Compared to the non-targeted micelles, the cRGD conjugated H40–P(LG–Hyd–DOX)–b–PEG micelles exhibited a greater uptake in the U87MG human glioblastoma cells due to integrin $\alpha_v\beta_3$-mediated endocytosis. PET scans on U87MG tumor-bearing mice also showed a much higher accumulation of the targeted H40–DOX–cRGD–^{64}Cu micelles in the tumor as compared to the non-targeted micelles. This example highlights that the synergy of active and passive targeting with the ability of pH triggered DOX release and efficient PET imaging can lay a foundation for clinical translation of this pH responsive theranostic system.

Another pH responsive approach to drug delivery utilizes the fact that lipids are capable of restructuring under differing pH environments. This strategy is often demonstrated with DOTAP (1,2-dioleoyl-3-trimethylammonium-propane) that transforms from a sphere to a rod-like micelle then to a disk when moving from physiological to acidic pH. Huang *et al.* used this idea to open and close a 'valve-like' device, more specifically, a cationic lipid-embedded poly(acrylic acid) (PAA) DOX loaded gel layer encapsulating a chitosan/SPION (lipid/gel coated CSN_{DOX}).[36] Additionally, ω-cholesterol PEG-folate was attached to prevent aggregation, improve the systemic stability, and to impart the active targeting characteristic to the resulting assembly. It was seen that the DOTAP within the gel layer restructured at a physiological pH through a hydrophobically-driven assembly (with their non-polar tails) while their positive head groups electrostatically interacted with the ionized (deprotonated) AA residues. At a pH of 5.4, the DOTAP transformed from sphere structures to rod-like structures. Due to the changes in the electrostatic interaction between the DOTAP species and AA residues in different assemblies, a decrease in density of the cross-linked gel layer was seen which consequently increased the release of the drug embedded within the gel layer. The MRI was also seen to be pH responsive with lipid/gel coated CSN_{DOX} exhibiting higher transverse relaxivity (r_2) values at pH 7.4 (252 mM^{-1} s^{-1}) as compared to the r_2 values at pH 5.4 (183 mM^{-1} s^{-1}). The pH dependent r_2 values were related to the change in the crosslinking density of the gel layer at different pH values and different clustering of the SPION because of protonation/deprotonation of the chitosan chains. *In vitro* tests showed improved folate lipid/gel-coated CSN_{DOX} targeting with drug accumulation in the nucleus, facilitated by both acidic pH of endosomes/lysosomes.

3. Reduction Responsive Theranostics

It has been established that the intracellular concentration (~2–10 mM) of glutathione (GSH) reducing agent is higher than the extracellular concentration (~2–10 μM).[37] Tumor cells tend to have 7–10 fold higher GSH levels than that of normal cells.[38] Such a significant difference in the extracellular and intracellular concentrations of GSH reducing agent has been exploited as an endogenous stimulus to trigger the release of a payload from reduction responsive nanocarriers. Disulfide (–SS–) bonds have been identified as bioreducible functional groups that cleave exclusively under the intracellular reducing environment.[39–41] A variety of –SS– bond bearing polymers and hybrid materials are being investigated as potential candidates for the development of reduction responsive theranostics. Cho *et al.* conjugated graphene oxide (GO) to photosensitizer chlorine 6 through the bioreducible –SS– linker (GO–SS–Ce6) (Figure 2(a)).[42] Experiments performed in A549 human lung cancer cell line confirmed that the GO–SS–Ce6 was only fluorescent and phototoxic in a reducing environment where the Ce6 was cleaved from the GO. Strong fluorescence was detected from the cells treated with GO–SS–Ce6 proving that the intracellular GSH was capable of cleaving the Ce6 from the GO, activating its fluorescence and phototoxic effect. Less fluorescence was observed in the cells treated with the pure Ce6, which suggested that the attachment to GO also enhanced cellular uptake of Ce6. In addition to photodynamic therapy and imaging provision described for the GO–SS–Ce6 theranostic system, this report also highlights that the high surface area of GO makes it a practical drug carrier system.

Besides employing materials containing bioreducible –SS– bonds for the development of reduction responsive theranostics, the high intracellular reducing agent concentration is also being exploited to selectively activate cytotoxicity of certain compounds that are otherwise inert in their oxidized state. This idea was examined in the work of Yuan *et al.* where the axial positions of a Pt(IV) prodrug were functionalized with integrin $\alpha_v\beta_3$ targeted cRGD tripeptide and an apoptosis sensor (Figure 2(b)).[43] The apoptosis sensor was made from tetraphenylsilole (TPS) fluorophore with aggregation-induced emission (AIE) properties and a caspase–3 enzyme specific Asp–Glu–Val–Asp (DEVD) peptide. It was demonstrated that when the prodrug was reduced to Pt(II) within the cancer cell, it resulted in cell

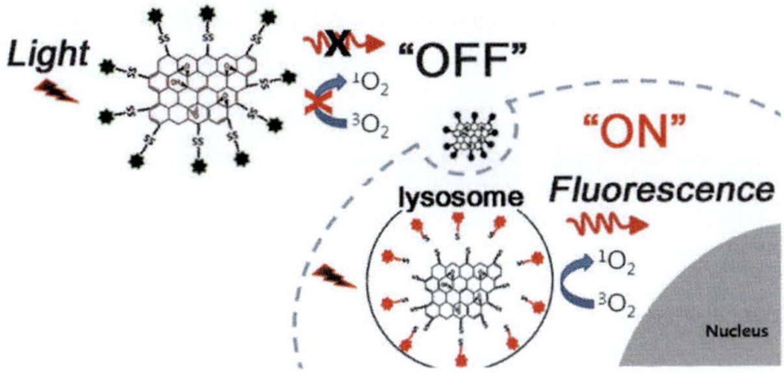

(a)

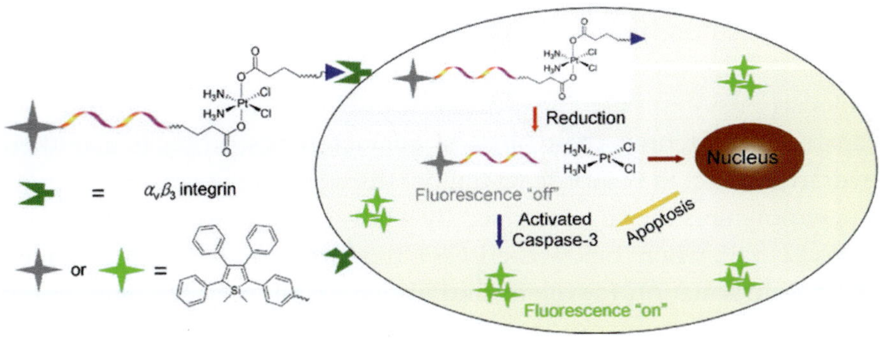

(b)

Fig. 2: (a) Ce6 conjugated to GO via –SS– bond as redox responsive theranostic platform. Fluorescence imaging and photodynamic therapy aspect of the system were only active under the intracellular reduction environment. Reproduced with permission from Royal Society of Chemistry.[42] (b) Pt(IV) prodrug functionalized with integrin $\alpha_v\beta_3$ targeted cRGD tripeptide and an apoptosis sensor. The prodrug is only activated under the reducing intracellular environment. Reproduced with permission from.[43] Copyright American Chemical Society.

death and triggered the caspase-3 enzyme to cut the DEVD peptide, consequently enhancing the fluorescence intensity, which can be observed in fluorescence imaging. *In vitro* tests were conducted by incubating the prodrug with U87–MG human glioblastoma, which showed the fluorescence of the U87–MG cells continually increased with higher cellular death for a 6 h period, where it reached its maximum. The correlation between cytotoxicity and apoptosis-induced fluorescence change was also proven in vitro with U87–MG cells where the apoptotic sensor itself showed no toxic effects, proving the reduced Pt(II) was the cytotoxic component and induced the change in fluorescence. This work highlights a reduction responsive theranostic system that can provide real-time feedback on the effectiveness of a treatment regimen in a non-invasive manner.

4. Thermoresponsive Theranostics

Temperature is classified as an exogenous stimulus that can facilitate triggered release of the payload in a spatiotemporal manner leading to the investigation of controlled and localized release using thermoresponsive nanocarriers.[44–46] The most common thermoresponsive nanocarrier systems are constituted by polymeric components that are capable of switching their physical characteristics, in particular their hydration state, in response to temperature change in a narrow range. These polymers are characterized by a lower critical solution temperature (LCST), where below the LCST they are hydrated with extended chain conformation (swollen) and above LCST they are dehydrated with collapsed chain conformation.[47] When assembled into a nanocarrier system, these thermoresponsive polymers are capable of triggering the payload release due to a change in their hydration state either in response to the intrinsic increase in temperature in the diseased region or in response to externally applied heat. The ideal range for a temperature responsive nanocarrier should release its cargo is between 37 to 42°C.[37] Temperature variations are found when moving from normal tissues to tumors or other inflammation causing diseases with a natural increase of temperature from 37°C to 40°C. However, larger temperature change can also be artificially induced by applying heat from an external source. Zhu *et al.* designed a hybrid nanogel Bi_2O_3@PVA that exploits the natural temperature increase at the tumor site to activate Bi_2O_3 QDs that facilitate dark-field and fluorescence dual-modal imaging (Figure 3).[48] Moreover, this temperature change stimulates a volume phase transition creating swelling/de-swelling that allows for controlled drug release. In addition, this volume change also affects the photoluminescence response of the nanogel. The swelling of the nanogels creates elastic tension within

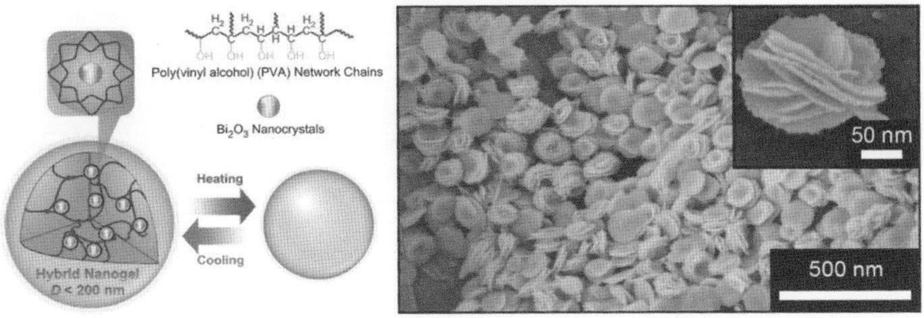

(a) (b)

Fig. 3: (a) Schematic illustration of temperature-responsive Bi_2O_3 in PVA hybrid nanogel-based theranostic system and (b) their SEM images. Reproduced with permission of Elsevier.[48]

the polymer that is transferred to the QDs thereby forming surface quenching states, while deswelling decreases the tension within the polymer network and increases the photoluminescence intensity. This shows an indirect dependence of the photoluminescence on temperature allowing for the temperature to be determined through imaging. *In vitro* tests were done on melanoma cells $B1_6F_{10}$ from mice where dark field imaging was demonstrated using contrast provided by the light scattered by the QDs. The fluorescence under physiological conditions was also applied for imaging purposes. Unfortunately, not all theranostic systems can be stimulated by this minor 3°C temperature increase and for systems that require a temperature greater than 40°C, an alternate arrangement of heat supply is required.

A theranostic system that required a minimum temperature of 44°C to respond was created by Zhang *et al.* who consequently employed high-intensity focused ultrasound (HIFU) to achieve the required temperature specifically at the site of action.[49] This group created a highly stable solid–liquid–gas tri phase transition medium, using L–menthol (LM), which was loaded into hollow mesoporous silica nanoparticles. *In vitro* release tests confirmed that at 37°C, the LM was in its solid state and prevented the release of the loaded compounds in the porous silica. After surpassing 44°C, the LM melted and released the contained drugs. These results were validated by similar results obtained for *in vivo* tests in liver VX2 tumors. *In vivo* experiments were also conducted with hollow mesoporous silica nanoparticles–L–menthol (HMSN–LM) showing no toxic effects without increased temperature, therefore demonstrating biosafety of the carrier. Furthermore, the hollow mesoporous silica nanoparticles filled with solid LM acted as a good ultrasound contrast agent in tumor tissues for improved imaging.

5. Light Responsive Theranostics

The idea of nanocarrier systems capable of payload release in response to exposure to radiation is very appealing. The payload release occurring exclusively in response to light would ensure greater safety against non-specific release in the normal tissues. The release rate of light responsive theranostics can be further tuned by varying certain factors such as wavelength, intensity or duration of exposure. The choice of radiations of the right wavelength is very critical. Shorter wavelength radiations (gamma rays or X-rays) offer high energy and are being used to treat cancer in the form of radiotherapy, [50] however, such strong radiations can damage the healthy cells negating the possibility of their use as a stimulus. There are a variety of chemical functionalities that respond to UV radiations[51] but the energy of these radiations can also be harmful for the human tissues.[52] The two major concerns regarding the use of radiation with shorter wavelengths (gamma rays, X-rays, and UV radiation) as a stimulus are their harmful nature due to high energy, and their limited penetrating depth due to light scattering and higher absorption by the biological components.[53] It has been observed that radiations of longer wavelengths penetrate deeper into the human tissue with relatively less scattering and are attractive for designing light responsive theranostics.[54] Near-Infrared (NIR) radiations offer distinct advantages over their high energy counterparts and are capable of penetrating deeper into the tissues. In addition, it is less harmful to healthy cells compared to lower wavelength radiation. However, there is an upper limit on the wavelength when using NIR that is around 950 nm, above this limit water and lipids will start absorbing the incoming radiation.[53] NIR radiations are also commonly used for their upconversion and photothermal properties. Some materials are capable of absorbing more than one photon in the infrared region which allows for absorption of more energy. This process, called upconversion, is often used in NIR responsive systems since a single photon often does not provide enough energy to cause a chemical change. Upconversion allows for the absorption of more energy while still retaining the advantages of NIR, namely deeper tissue penetration and its less harmful nature. A possible disadvantage of NIR is that a two photon process is not nearly as efficient. Lux *et al.* created two different polymers with the same backbone but different terminal groups.[55] Both terminal groups could respond to UV radiation (through one photon process) and NIR (through two photon process) where the backbone consisted of quinone–methide structure. The quinone–methide backbone is unique as once the end group is cleaved from incoming radiation, the backbone degrades into its monomers in a domino-like fashion. After forming nanoparticles with nile red encapsulated, it was observed that when using UV radiation the release of nile red was a burst release while NIR radiation gave a much more gradual release. NIR radiation is commonly employed for photothermal conversion, which converts the NIR energy into heat. This phenomenon is frequently achieved using gold nanorods, which at certain diameter can respond to incoming NIR and generate heat. The generated heat can be exploited as a stimulus to trigger payload release from a temperature responsive nanocarrier system. NIR-triggered payload release can also be facilitated by the disintegration of bonds (that linked the payload to the carrier) known as photocleaving or the decay of a capping agent (that blocked the payload exit) due to photothermal effect. Frequently, the theranostic agents that use NIR heat-triggered drug release also take advantage of the heat to stimulate photohyperthermia or enable photodynamic therapies. This was seen in the work of Zhang *et al.* who created mesoporous silica-coated gold nanorods that utilized two-photon imaging as well as hyperthermia (Figure 4).[56] The heat produced also weakens the electrostatic interactions between silica and the loaded therapeutic drug (DOX) showing NIR responsive drug release. An enhanced release was observed after the protonation of surface silanol groups

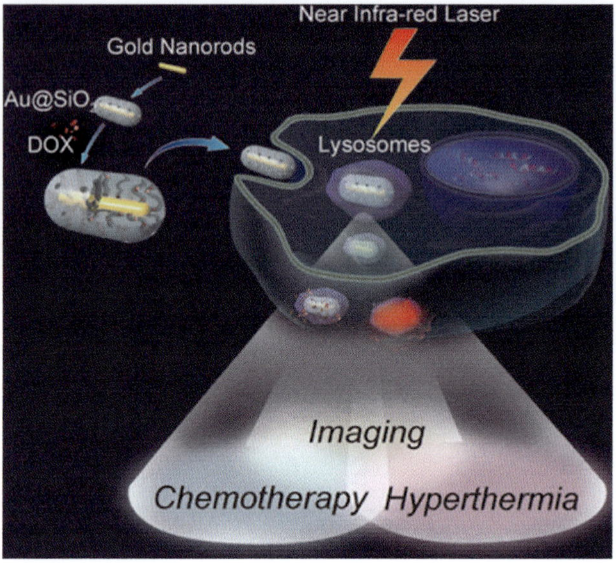

Fig. 4: Illustration of NIR responsive Au@SiO_2-based theranostic system. Reproduced with permission of John Wiley & Sons.[56]

due to the lower pH which further reduced the electrostatic interaction between the silica and DOX.

In another example, DOX was seen to have an increased release rate through illumination using NIR in a polyvinyl pyrrolidone (PVP)-coated rubidium tungsten bronze (Rb–TB) nanorod (Figure 5).[57] The photothermal effect of the Rb–TB nanorods disturbed the physical adsorption of the DOX on the PVP, therefore the payload. These particles provided photoacoustic tomography and X-ray computed tomography (CT) as diagnostic methods. The release of DOX from Rb–TB–DOX was tested *in vitro* at differing pH values; after 7 h around 15% and 21% of the DOX was released at pH 7.4 and 5.0, respectively. However after NIR irradiation, the cumulative release was approximately 41% and 63% after the same allotted time. *In vivo* tests, nude mice with Pance-1 tumors were treated with Rb–TB or Rb–TB–DOX, and underwent stimulating hyperthermia at temperatures reaching 50°C. The Rb–TB–DOX showed impressive tumor growth inhibition with the combination of chemotherapy and phototherapy.

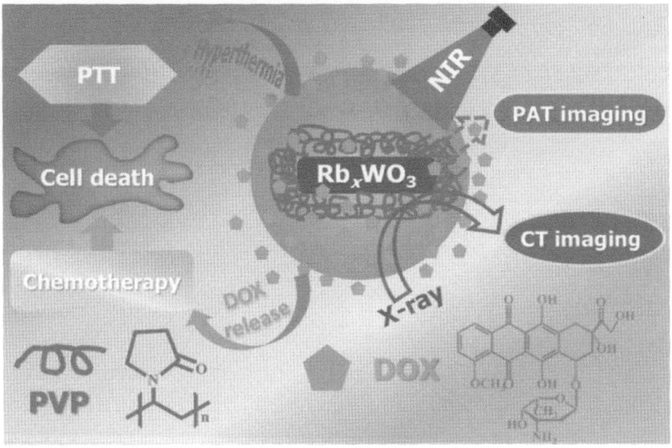

Fig. 5: Schematic description of Rb_xWO_3 nanorods as NIR light-responsive theranostic system capable of chemo-photothermal therapy and dual-modal PAT/CT imaging. Reproduced with permission of John Wiley & Sons.[57]

In addition, strong photoacoustic signals were observed in the tumor area allowing for efficient PAT imaging. Combined with Rb–TB used as a contrast agent for CT imaging, it provided a means for high spatial resolution imaging regardless of depth for the entire body.

A similar NIR responsiveness was achieved by Li *et al.* who created polyhedral Fe_3O_4@Au core-shell nanoparticles taking on a trisoctaheral form made from truncated octahedral Fe_3O_4.[58] The Au trisoctahedral nanoshell provides surface plasmon absorption, functioning as an NIR-responsive nanomaterial providing NIR-responsive chemo-and photothermal effects. A mesoporous SiO_2 nanoshell was also added for biocompatibility and to provide a high surface area for loading drugs. For the drug release, double-stranded complementary oligonucleotides (covering the mesoporous openings holding DOX), were heated by NIR light, unwinding the duplex DNA and uncapping the pores allowing the DOX to be released. The magnetic properties of iron oxide nanoparticles were used for magnetic attraction to increase cellular uptake and acted as a good MRI T_2 contrast agent. HeLa cells were used for *in vitro* tests showing increased targeting with the application of a magnetic field and consequently, increased

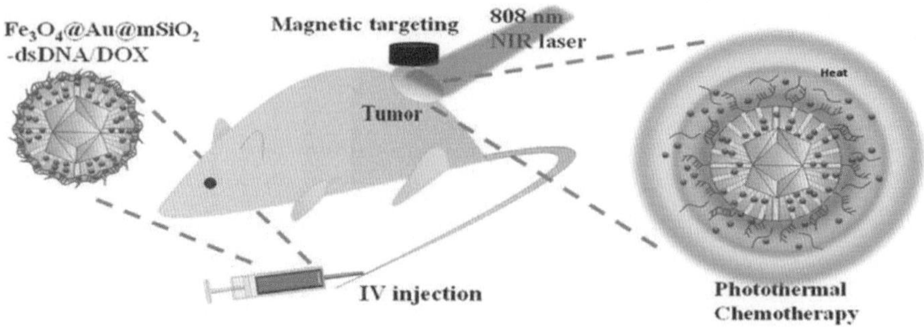

Fig. 6: Illustration of DOX loaded NIR responsive Fe_3O_4@Au@mSiO_2 theranostic system with duplex DNA blocking the non-specific release of the payload. Adapted and reproduced with permission from Ref. 58. Copyright American Chemical Society.

cell death. It was also seen that DOX alone provided higher survival rate for the cells, than when it was combined with photothermal therapeutics showing a synergistic photothermal and chemotherapy effect. *In vivo* MRI, after the nanoparticles have been injected into mice (Figure 6), had a significantly reduced contrast signal in healthy tissues, as the imaging agents were localized in the tumor by the magnetic field. However, no such reduction was observed with normal tissues in mice that were not exposed to a magnetic field. This proves that the magnetic field caused the nanoparticles to quickly accumulate in the tumor, improving the negative contrast effect at a specific location.

6. Magnetic Field Responsive Theranostics

Magnetic field possesses the potential to be the clinically most effective and relevant stimulus. Magnetic hyperthermia is a treatment method that usually uses magnetite (Fe_3O_4) nanoparticles referred to as SPIONs coated with a biologically compatible material. When an alternating magnetic field (AMF) is applied, the SPIONs generate heat attributed to magnetic hysteresis loss and Néel relaxation.[37] In a magnetically responsive system, either a payload or generated heat is responsible to provide the intended therapeutic effect. In the former scenario, the application of AMF is expected to release the payload in response to the generated heat. Hayashi *et al.* created a polypyrrole coupled to PEG with folic acid. DOX and Fe_3O_4 were loaded into the polypyrrole core which exhibited a glass transition temperature of 44°C. Using an alternating current magnetic field (ACMF), they showed that the core temperature could increase sufficiently to cause DOX to leak out of the nanostructures (Figure 7). Mice with

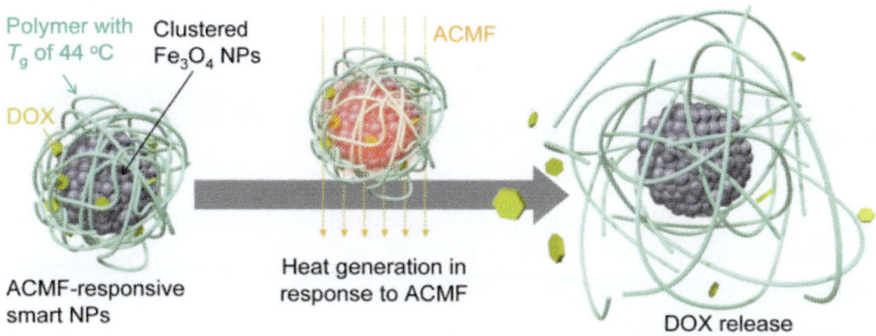

(a)

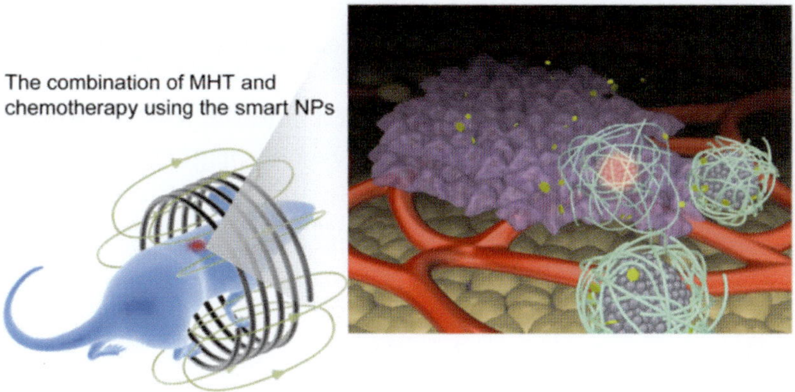

(b)

Fig. 7: (a) ACMF responsive DOX release from a theranostic system derived from a combination of Fe_3O_4 nanoparticles and thermoresponsive polymer. (b) Cancer treatment via a combination of magnetic hyperthermia and chemotherapy. Reproduced with permission from Ivyspring International Publisher.[59]

xenograft tumors from RPMI8226 multiple myeloma cell line were injected with the nanocarrier system followed by an exposure to ACMF. The combination of traditional chemotherapy and magnetic hyperthermia, induced by their nanoparticle system, showed zero tumor volume after 12 days of treatment. In contrast, the two treatments separately showed only a decrease in tumor volume.

In the similar vein, Chen *et al.* designed a triple stimuli responsive theranostic system with SPIONs and paramagnetic manganese oxide loaded onto GO (FeMnGO) nanosheets through a double redox technique.[60] This system provides imaging and drug release that is responsive to pH, redox environments and external magnetic fields. The Fe_3O_4 NPs demonstrate a quick response to an externally applied AMF, which consequently can be used for magnetic hyperthermia where a temperature up to 72°C can be acquired. The system also contained paramagnetic manganese oxide nanoparticles attached onto the GO, which disintegrates (as Mn^{2+}) in a weakly acidic and reducing environment allowing for pH and reduction triggered MRI. This was tested *in vivo* in mice by intratumor injection of the FeMn–GO followed by application of a magnetic field showing that the skin temperature can be raised from 37.8°C to 47°C. In addition, the tumor was stained with hematoxylin and eosin after the hyperthermia. This allowed for the visualization of dead cells proving the effectiveness of the treatment. Without displaying any heating in standard water conditions, no toxicity is observed, and the toxic treatment can be restricted to the desired location. Overall, magnetically responsive nanoparticles show significant promise and with various systems in clinical trials they represent the most clinically advanced stimuli responsive nanostructures.

7. Enzyme Responsive Theranostics

The use of biocatalytic action of enzymes as a stimulus for theranostic systems has also been studied. Researchers have exploited the fact that enzyme activity at the site of a tumor differs from healthy areas, in addition to certain enzymes only being present inside tumors for internal release specificity. For example, certain proteases are found solely inside the cells and therefore a carrier including a peptide sequence sensitive to protease cleavage with targeting ligands provides an effective means to deliver imaging and drug agents inside specified cells.[61] Li *et al.* created an amino-functionalized mesoporous silica-coated QD with a covalently attached cell-penetrating peptide (CPP) sequence (Figure 8).[62] The CPP contains an oligocationic TAT sequence (CRRRQRRKKR) for nucleus targeting, an PGFK linker that can be cleaved by cathepsin B protease, and an oligoanionic-inhibitory domain (EEEEEE) that balances the charge distribution of the peptides. This system allows for nuclear-targeted delivery, specified release of DOX, and real-time imaging through the QDs fluorescence. It was seen that DOX release was hindered without cathepsin B at both pH 5.5 and at pH 7.4, and more significant amounts were released in the presence of enzyme. It is worth noting that at pH 5.5, there was more DOX released than at 7.4 with the same concentration of enzyme, due to the increased activity of cathepsin B enzyme activity in acidic conditions.

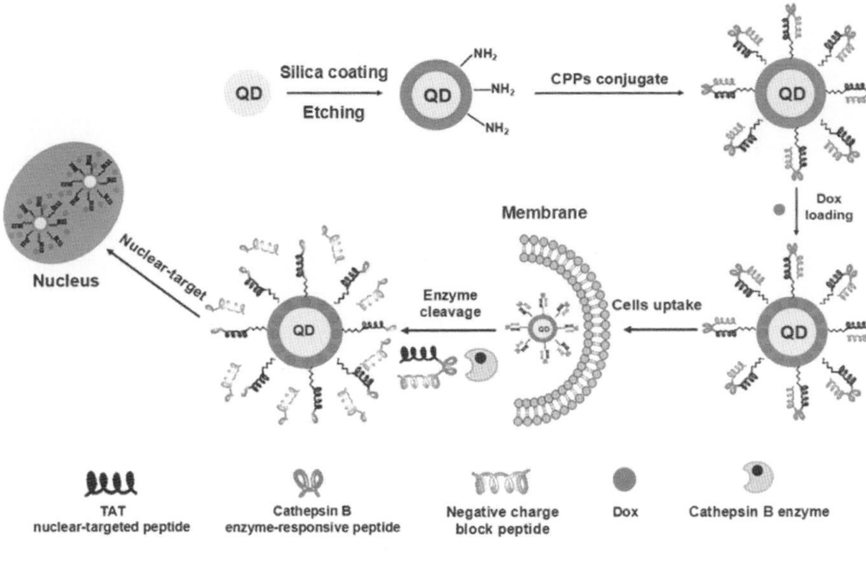

Fig. 8: DOX loaded QDs@mSiO_2 nanoparticles-based Enzyme responsive nucleus targeted theranostic system. Adapted and reproduced with permission of John Wiley & Sons.[62]

8. Dual-Stimuli Responsive Theranostics

It is important to recognize that not all stimuli responsive systems are exclusive from one another. This idea was seen in the work of Wang *et al.* who created magnetic graphene-based compounds combining pH and photothermal responsive release along with dual-targeting chemothermal therapy and MRI, in addition to incorporating interleukin-13-based peptide (IP) modification for targeting glioma and PEG for stealth character. DOX was loaded electrostatically into the mesoporous silica and attached through a π–π stacking interaction with the GO. Lower pH reduced the electrostatic interaction between the DOX and silica, and an increase in temperature further accelerated the release by reducing the hydrophobic interaction between the DOX and graphene. *In vitro* toxicity tests showed that the chemo-photothermal therapy had the greatest toxicity when compared to the chemotherapy or photothermal therapy alone. Experiments in an animal model with glioma showed an increased MRI contrasts in the brain because of the IP modification and the magnetic exposure. These findings suggest that the IP and magnetic targeting increased the uptake of contrast agent at the tumor site. This mechanism of magnetic graphene-based mesoporous silica with IP and PEG can be used for MRI, dual-targeting and chemo-photothermal glioma therapy with both pH and temperature sensitive drug release.

Ultrasound and NIR stimuli were both used in the work of Ke *et al.* with the creation of gold-nanoshelled microcapsules (GNS–MCs) made with ultrasound-responsive polymeric microcapsules that can improve the contrast for ultrasound imaging.[64] In addition, they incorporated the NIR-absorbing gold nanoshells adsorbed onto the microcapsule surface for photohyperthermia. The ultrasound contrast behavior was tested *in vivo* with New Zealand white rabbits and provided greatly enhanced imaging of the rabbit only seconds after injection of the GNS–MCs, with the effects lasting longer than 5 min, which is a therapeutically sufficient length of time. In addition, no harm was done to any of the rabbit's bodily functions. The NIR induced thermal effect was tested through subjecting quartz cells containing various GNS–MC concentrations to NIR radiations.

Temperature increases were apparent with increasing exposure time and increasing concentrations (capable of reaching 42°C to kill the cell). Photothermal effects were tested on HeLa cells and with a sufficient concentration and laser illumination, less than 20% of the HeLa remained viable. Lastly, Zhang *et al.* designed a device where upconverting nanocomposites were enclosed in a mesoporous silica shell that used the polymer poly[(N-isopropylacrylamide)-co-(methacrylic acid)] (P(NIPAm-co-MAA)) to act as a blocker to prevent loaded drugs from being released from the pores.[65] It was tested *in vitro* that the carrier itself provided no cytotoxic effects on L929 cells, and therefore is a suitable drug delivery vesicle. With the loaded DOX, the release rate was seen to be pH and temperature sensitive. *In vitro* drug release was also tested, and with a temperature above the LCST, the polymer collapsed and opened the silica pores allowing the DOX to escape. At a lower pH, the pH-sensitive poly(methacrylic acid) (PMAA) component was altered, thereby diminishing the electrostatic forces between the PMAA and drug causing it to be released faster. The drug was also released through NIR irradiation, which was caused by the heat-induced polymer collapse. In addition, these nanocomposites allowed upconversion luminescence imaging under NIR irradiation making them a multi-stimulated theranostic system.

9. Conclusions

The ability to activate a theranostic system exclusively in response to an endogenous or exogenous stimulus promises enhanced safety and selectivity of nanomedicines used in the treatment of severe diseases such as cancer. A variety of stimuli responsive materials are being evaluated for the development of stimuli responsive theranostics. Several recent research articles are reporting encouraging *in vitro* and animal model results. However, for most of the new stimuli responsive materials, compliance to the requirements of the regulatory agencies is needed before conducting clinical trials. This requires a detailed evaluation of the new materials describing their toxicity, circulation half-life, and pharmacokinetics/pharmacodynamics. While an acidic tumor environment is the most widely exploited stimulus, further studies are required to delineate the specific advantages of one stimulus over the other. The materials responding to endogenous stimuli might be advantageous due to the inherent nature of stimuli, while exogenous stimuli may perform better for the diseases showing heterogeneity. The concept of stimuli responsive theranostics is at its infancy; however, a successful stimuli responsive theranostics system can augment the effectiveness of nanomedicines by proving a spatiotemporal control over the release of therapeutics and can further help in achieving the ambitious goals of personalized nanomedicine.

Acknowledgments

This work was supported by the National Cancer Institute (NCI) (Grant U54-CA151884), the National Heart, Lung and Blood Institute (NHLBI) Program of Excellence in Nanotechnology (PEN) (Contract No. HHSN268201000045C), the National Institute of Biomedical Imaging and Bioengineering (NIBIB) R01 Grant (EB015419-01) and the David Koch–Prostate Cancer Foundation Award in Nanotherapeutics. C.V. acknowledges the support from Center for the Development of Nanoscience and Nanotechnology (Grant FB0807) and the Postdoctoral Program of Becas-Chile/ CONICYT.

Conflict of Interest

In compliance with the Brigham and Women's Hospital and Harvard Medical School institutional guidelines, O.C.F. discloses his financial interest in BIND Biosciences, Selecta Biosciences and Blend Therapeutics, three biotechnology companies developing nanoparticle technologies for medical applications. BIND, Selecta and Blend did not support the research in this study, and currently these companies have no rights to any technology or intellectual property developed as part of this research.

References

1. N. Bertrand, J. Wu, X. Xu, N. Kamaly, O. C. Farokhzad, *Adv. Drug Del. Rev.*, 2 (2014).
2. N. Kamaly, G. Fredman, M. Subramanian, S. Gadde, A. Pesic, L. Cheung, Z. A. Fayad, R. Langer, I. Tabas, O. C. Farokhzad, *Pnas*, 6506 (2013).
3. B. Godin, J. H. Sakamoto, R. E. Serda, A. Grattoni, A. Bouamrani, M. Ferrari, *Trends Pharmacol. Sci.*, 199 (2010).
4. E. M. Pridgen, F. Alexis, T. T. Kuo, E. Levy-Nissenbaum, R. Karnik, R. S. Blumberg, R. Langer, O. C. Farokhzad, *Sci. Transl. Med.*, 167 (2013).
5. J. Wu, N. Kamaly, J. Shi, L. Zhao, Z. Xiao, G. Hollett, R. John, S. Ray, X. Xu, X. Zhang, P. W. Kantoff, O. C. Farokhzad, *Angew. Chemie Int. Ed.*, 8975 (2014).
6. N. Kamaly, Z. Xiao, P. M. Valencia, A. F. Radovic-Moreno, O. C. Farokhzad, *Chem. Soc. Rev.*, 2971 (2012).
7. R. Mout, D. F. Moyano, S. Rana, V. M. Rotello, *Chem. Soc. Rev.*, 2539 (2012).
8. M. Elsabahy, K. L. Wooley, *Chem. Soc. Rev.*, 2545 (2012).
9. E. C. Dreaden, A. M. Alkilany, X. Huang, C. J. Murphy, M. A. El-Sayed, *Chem. Soc. Rev.*, 2740 (2012).
10. J. Khandare, M. Calderón, N. M. Dagia, R. Haag, *Chem. Soc. Rev.*, 2824 (2012).
11. Z. Li, J. C. Barnes, A. Bosoy, J. F. Stoddart, J. I. Zink, *Chem. Soc. Rev.*, 2590 (2012).
12. J. L. Vivero-Escoto, R. C. Huxford-Philips, W. Lin, *Chem. Soc. Rev.*, 2673 (2012).
13. N. Lee, T. Hyeon, *Chem. Soc. Rev.*, 2575 (2012).
14. J. Shi, Z. Xiao, N. Kamaly, O. C. Farokhzad, *Acc. Chem. Res.*, 1123 (2011).
15. O. C. Farokhzad, S. Jon, A. Khademhosseini, T. -N. T. Tran, D. A. LaVan, R. Langer, *Cancer Res.*, 7668 (2004).
16. S. Dhar, F. X. Gu, R. Langer, O. C. Farokhzad, S. J. Lippard, *PNAS*, 17356 (2008).
17. O. C. Farokhzad, J. Cheng, B. A. Teply, I. Sherifi, S. Jon, P. W. Kantoff, J. P. Richie, R. Langer, *PNAS*, 6315 (2006).

18. J. Hrkach, D. V. Hoff, M. M. Ali, E. Andrianova, J. Auer, T. Campbell, D. D. Witt, M. Figa, M. Figueiredo, A. Horhota, S. Low, K. McDonnell, E. Peeke, B. Retnarajan, A. Sabnis, E. Schnipper, J. J. Song, Y. H. Song, J. Summa, D. Tompsett, G. Troiano, T. V. G. Hoven, J. Wright, P. LoRusso, P. W. Kantoff, N. H. Bander, C. Sweeney, O. C. Farokhzad, R. Langer, S. Zale, *Sci. Transl. Med.*, 128 (2012).
19. A. Salvati, A. S. Pitek, M. P. Monopoli, K. Prapainop, F. B. Bombelli, D. R. Hristov, P. M. Kelly, C. Aberg, E. Mahon, K. A. Dawson, *Nature Nanotech.*, 137 (2013)
20. Z. Cao, R. Tong, A. Mishra, W. Xu, G. C. L. Wong, J. Cheng, Y. Lu, *Angew. Chem. Int. Ed.*, 6494 (2009).
21. V. Bagalkot, X. Gao, *ACS Nano.*, 8131 (2011).
22. A. Z. Wang, V. Bagalkot, C. C. Vasilliou, F. Gu, F. Alexis, L. Zhang, M. Shaikh, K. Yuet, M. J. Cima, R. Langer, P. W. Kantoff, N. H. Bander, S. Jon, O. C. Farokhzad, *Chem. Med. Chem.*, 1311 (2008).
23. S. Mura, P. Couvreur, *Adv. Drug Del. Rev.*, 1394 (2012).
24. J. H. Ryu, S. Lee, S. Son, S. H. Kim, J. F. Leary, K. Choi, I. C. Kwon, *J. Control. Release.*, 477 (2014).
25. B. Yameen, W. I. Choi, C. Vilos, A. Swami, J. Shi, O. C. Farokhzad, *J. Control. Release*, 485 (2014)
26. N. T. K. Thanh, L. A. W. Green, *Nano Today.*, 485 (2010).
27. W.-H. Chiang, V. T. Ho, H. -H. Chen, W. -C. Huang, Y. -F. Huang, S. -C. Lin, C. -S. Chern, H. -C. Chiu, *Langmuir.*, 6434 (2013).
28. A. Matsumoto, R. Yoshida, K. Kataoka, *Biomacromol.*, 1038 (2004).
29. H. Lv, S. Zhang, B. Wang, S. Cui, J. Yan, *J. Control. Release*, 100 (2006).
30. E. L. McConnell, M. D. Short, A. W. Basit, *J. Control. Release*, 154 (2008).
31. W. J. Kim, S. W. Kim, *Pharm. Res.*, 657 (2009).
32. H. Koo, H. Lee, S. Lee, K. H. Min, M. S. Kim, D. S. Lee, Y. Choi, I. C. Kwon, K. Kim, S. Y. Jeon, *Chem. Comm.*, 5668 (2010).
33. L. Jing, X. Liang, X. Li, Y. Yang, Z. Dai, *Acta Biomaterialia.*, 9434 (2013).
34. Y. Chen, K. Ai, Y. Liu, L. Lu, *Appl. Mat. Inter.*, 655 (2014).
35. Y. Xiao, H. Hong, A. Javadi, J. W. Engle, W. Xu, Y. Yang, Y. Zhang, T. E. Barnhart, W. Cai, S. Gong, *Biomater.*, 3071 (2012).

36. Y.-F. Huang, W.-H. Chiang, W.-C. Huang, H.-H. Chen, M.-Y. Shen, S.-C. Lin, C.-S. Chern, H.-C. Chiu, *J. Mat. Chem. B*, 4988 (2014).
37. S. Mura, J. Nicolas, P. Couvreur, *Nat. Mater.*, 991 (2013).
38. S. Ganta, H. Devalapally, A. Shahiwala, M. Amiji, *J. Control. Release*, 187 (2008).
39. G. Zhang, J. Liu, Q. Yang, R. Zhuo, X. Jiang, *Bioconjug. Chem.*, 1290 (2012).
40. S. Son, R. Namgung, J. Kim, K. Singha, W. J. Kim, *Acc. Chem. Res.*, 1100 (2012).
41. R. Cheng, F. Feng, F. Meng, C. Deng, J. Feijen, Z. Zhong, *J. Control. Release*, 2 (2011).
42. Y. Cho, Y. Choi, *Chem. Comm.*, 9912 (2012).
43. Y. Yuan, R. T. K. Kwok, B. Z. Tang, B. Liu, *J. Am. Chem. Soc.*, 2546 (2014).
44. J. Hu, G. Zhang, Z. Ge, S. Liu, *Prog. Polym. Sci.*, 1096 (2014).
45. T. Ta, T. M. Porter, *J. Control. Release*, 112 (2013).
46. E. G. Kelley, J. N. L. Albert, M. O. Sullivan, T. H. Epps, III, *Chem. Soc. Rev.*, 7057 (2013).
47. M. T. Calejo, S. A. Sande, B. Nyström, *Expert Op. Drug Del.*, 1669 (2013).
48. H. Zhu, Y. Li, R. Qiu, L. Shi, W. Wu, S. Zhou, *Biomater.*, 3058 (2012).
49. K. Zhang, H. Chen, F. Li, Q. Wang, S. Zheng, H. Xu, M. Ma, X. Jia, Y. Chen, J. Mou, X. Wang, J. Shi, *Biomater.*, 5875 (2014).
50. G. Delaney, S. Jacob, C. Featherstone, M. Barton, *Am. Cancer Soc.*, 1129 (2005).
51. R. Tong, H. D. Hemmati, R. Langer, D. S. Kohane, *J. Am. Chem. Soc.*, 8848 (2012).
52. M. K. G. Jayakumar, N. M. Idris, Y. Zhang, *Proc. Natl. Acad. Sci. USA.*, 8483 (2012).
53. A. M. Smith, M. C. Mancini, S. Nie, *Nat. Nanotech.*, 710 (2009).
54. L. Fodor, Y. Ullman, M. Elman, *Aesthetic Applications of Intense Pulsed Light*, Springer-Verlag London Limited, 11, 2011.
55. C. D. G. Lux, C. L. McFearin, S. Joshi-Barr, J. Sankaranarayanan, N. Fomina, A. Almutairi, *ACS Macro Lett.*, 922 (2012).
56. Z. Zhang, L. Wang, J. Wang, X. Jiang, X. Li, Z. Hu, Y. Ji, X. Wu, C. Chen, *Adv. Mat.*, 1418 (2012).

57. G. Tian, X. Zhang, X. Zheng, W. Yin, L. Ruan, X. Liu, L. Zhou, L. Yan, S. Li, Z. Gu, Y. Zhao, *Small.*, 4160 (2014).
58. W.-P. Li, P.-Y. Liao, C.-H. Su, C.-S. Yeh, *J. Am. Chem. Soc.*, 10062 (2014).
59. K. Hayashi, M. Nakamura, H. Miki, S. Ozaki, M. Abe, T. Matsumoto, W. Sakamoto, T. Yogo, K. Ishimura, *Theranostics.*, 834 (2014).
60. Y. Chen, P. Xu, Z. Shu, M. Wu, L. Wang, S. Zhang, Y. Zheng, H. Chen, J. Wang, Y. Li, J. Shi, *Adv. Funct. Mat.,* 4386 (2014).
61. R. de la Rica, D. Aili, M. M. Stevens, *Adv. Drug Del. Rev.,* 967 (2012).
62. J. Li, F. Liu, Q. Shao, Y. Min, M. Costa, E. K. L. Yeow, B. Xing, *Adv. Health. Mat.,* 1230 (2014).
63. Y. Wang, R. Huang, G. Liang, Z. Zhang, P. Zhang, S. Yu, J. Kong, *Small.*, 109 (2014).
64. H. Ke, J. Wang, Z. Dai, Y. Jin, E. Qu, Z. Xing, C. Guo, X. Yue, J. Liu, *Theranostic Agents.*, 3073 (2011).
65. X. Zhang, P. Yang, Y. Dai, P. Ma, X. Li, Z. Cheng, Z. Hou, X. Kang, C. Li, J. Lin, *Adv. Funct. Mat.*, 4067 (2013).

CHAPTER 11

ADVANCING THE PRACTICAL CLINICAL UTILITY IN PERSONALIZED MEDICINE: CAPABILITIES AND LESSONS LEARNED FOR PHARMACOLOGY AND PHARMACEUTICS

Ioannis S. Vizirianakis[*,‡], Christina Karavasili[†],
Elsa P. Amanatiadou[*] and Dimitrios G. Fatouros[†]

[*]Department of Pharmacology,
School of Pharmacy,
Aristotle University of Thessaloniki GR-54124, Greece
[†]Department of Pharmaceutical Technology,
School of Pharmacy,
Aristotle University of Thessaloniki,
Thessaloniki GR-54124, Greece
[‡]ivizir@pharm.auth.gr

Although, the wide exploitation of genomic information represents a revolutionary approach as well as a major task in health and pharmaceutical care after the completion of human genome project, the roadmap in order the society to get maximum benefits on a broader basis and practical clinical utility terms seems, however, still very challenging and questionable. Practically, an efficient direction toward achieving the concept of personalized medicine interventions worldwide means that all the main components contributing to the clinical setting and medicines administration process have to be appropriately revisited and formulated. This dynamics covers the existed infrastructure in the regulatory environment, the cost-risk-benefit issues in healthcare, the monitoring methodologies of diseases and therapeutics, the societal-ethical concerns, the pharmacovigilance database structure, the clinical pharmacology guidelines, the education of health practitioners and the curricula in medicine and pharmacy, the illnesses management protocols, as well as the drug prescription process. In this chapter, specific attempts aiming to formulate personalized medicine concepts of practical clinical utility in modern pharmacology and pharmaceutics will be critically presented and discussed.

1. Introduction

Undoubtedly nowadays, the research capabilities for practical clinical translation of the genomics knowledge accumulated from diverse sources increase over the time. Moreover, the nanotechnological breakthroughs achieved thus far, efficiently enter into the clinical setting thus permitting their implementation in the everyday healthcare practice. As a matter of fact, practitioners face a reality where a revolutionary perception on how drugs and therapy are delivered moves toward individualized patient care by increasing the precision of evidence-based medicine interventions and improving the safety and efficacy clinical outcomes. Such a direction, formulates the idea for the structure of an interdisciplinary healthcare environment. Importantly in such common scientific ground, the contribution of various scientific advancements coming from different disciplines will enrich the medical and pharmacy sectors by enabling personalized (precision) medicine decisions for most, if not all, patients worldwide. Although, the prospects of personalized medicine interventions look very promising, the roadmap in order the society to get maximum benefits on a broader basis and practical clinical utility terms it seems, however, very challenging and still questionable. Unanimously, such speculation is more intensive in stressfully demanding solutions in the case of multi-factorial and complex polygenic illnesses, like cancer, by negatively impacting any progress gained thus far. Practically, the latter concern refers to both researchers and clinicians, since society is waiting for them to effectively establish new practices in the clinical setting on how e.g., the health and pharmaceutical care regulatory environments, the cost-benefit issues, the risk-benefit concepts, the drug safety and efficacy monitoring profiles, the pharmacovigilance database structure, just to mention a few, could be better served in real time to comply with the use of personalized medicine interventions worldwide and for any disease. Alternatively and *vice versa*, the skepticism applies upon working to develop personalized medicine decisions, on how for example these powerful medical approaches will implement and comply with the already established clinical practice guidelines for disease management protocols and drug prescription (Rx) dosage schemes? Fortunately, such existed hindering issues in the arena of personalized medicine environment has been started to be efficiently addressed both in research and the clinics and it is expected to fulfill more effectively and in some way specific societal expectations in the years to come [for more detailed information see Refs. 1–9].

Another, however, very crucial issue related to personalized medicine era is the public concern about the economic impact of all these therapeutic directions. Indeed, besides clinical validation and utility, the creation of suitable economics models to assess the pharmacoeconomic value of personalized medicine interventions will obviously help decision makers to positively approach and evaluate budget management and healthcare infrastructure for the benefit of patients worldwide. Especially as an example, the latter refers to the field of personalized cancer therapy where the companion molecular diagnostics and the application of personal genome sequencing are entering the clinical practice in a manner of keeping hope to revolutionize oncology therapy. To this end, the lack of such pharmacoeconomic models hindering the proper implementation of innovative pharmacological interventions and cancer genomics into guidelines for everyday oncology therapy protocols has been recently defined.[6–12] Importantly moreover, the proper education of future healthcare practitioners still represents one of the crucial factors upon trying to implement in real-time and in practical clinical utility terms the personalized medicine decisions for routine healthcare and Rx. To fill the gap for interdisciplinary-oriented revised and structured curricula, a recently edited book has been published covering research and educational needs in the era of personalized medicine.[1] In such a way, this chapter will present and discuss personalized medicine concepts of practical clinical utility by covering specific tasks in modern pharmacology and pharmaceutics aiming to critically address specific issues of the skepticism outlined above.

2. Quantitatively Assessing Pharmacological Response Variability and Clinical Phenotype Heterogeneity for Individual Patients

Nowadays, pharmacogenomics (PGx) holds great promise in guiding individualized prescription of delivered drugs to achieve maximum efficacy and safety in the clinical setting. Thus, it is important of being able to quantitatively correlate drug effects in the body with predictive biomarkers and gene expression molecular signatures of prognostic, diagnostic, and even of therapeutic value. However, the knowledge accumulated thus far in pharmacology clearly proposes that various factors contribute to patient response heterogeneity phenotypes seen in drug administration/delivery (see Figure 1). In particular, such variables are either patient-related or drug-related. But importantly, the response of an organism to therapeutics administration can be seen as the interplay between genes and drugs with the contribution of environmental/epigenetics factors to also play a crucial role in achieving the final pharmacological phenotype. In such a way, by

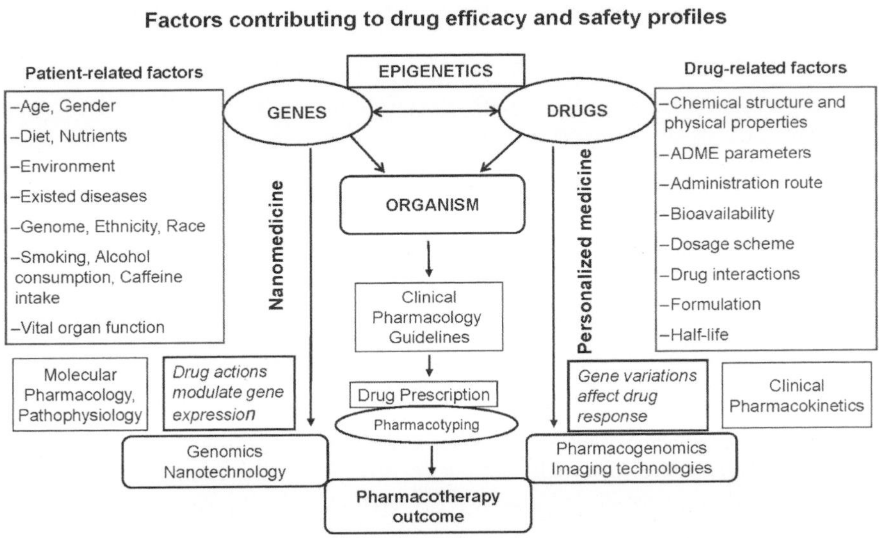

Fig. 1: Outline of scientific advancements contributing to pharmacotherapy outcome focusing on the factors being capable to modulate drug efficacy and safety profiles. (See text for details).

trying to understand the impact of genetic polymorphism on drug response heterogeneity and drug interactions obviously enables personalized medicine decisions.[13–18] Alternatively, one can argue that such an approach necessitates the direction of enriching the translational capacity in genomic medicine to contribute into specific pharmacokinetic/pharmacodynamic (PK/PD) parameters and generate data applicable for any specific drug either under development or already in the market. Nowadays, various predictive PGx biomarkers for drugs belonging to several pharmacological classes have been approved and are already included in drug labeling by the regulatory agencies.[13,18–24] However, the inference and the broader integration of such predictive PGx biomarkers into modern pharmacology and the clinical setting are still quite challenging.

It is interesting to note that major pharmaceutical companies through revising their internal R&D infrastructures by conducting comprehensive longitudinal analysis proceed toward increasing productivity, pipeline quality efficiency and success in their new drug development projects.[25] It might be then possible by moving toward better assessing pharmacological response variability and clinical phenotype heterogeneity, in terms of personalized medicine decisions through the establishment of predictive PD/PK models, to also help achieve such goals and launch "smarter" innovative therapeutics with improved safety and efficacy profiles in the clinical setting. Consequently, the driving forces powered by nanotechnology-based applications in healthcare keep promise for pharmacology in developing therapeutics and diagnostics with improved PK/PD behavior in the body. The latter, also implies better drug efficacy and safety profiles and outcome in the clinical setting. Complementary to this, the concepts for precise (personalized) innovative medical interventions for individual patients could be more effective addressed through the targeted delivery of medicines into desired sites, the limitation of distribution in other organs/tissues of the organism and the limitation of systemic toxicity.[26–30] Toward facilitating the broader utility of personalized medicine, the availability of quantitative markers for treatment clearly necessitates the capacity of *in vivo* molecular imaging techniques to assesses drug PK/PD actions in real-time. The latter, contribute in advancing the productivity in drug development and also ensuring improved efficacy and safety outcomes in drug delivery.[31,32] Moreover, the laboratory medicine protocols implemented with cost-affordable sophisticated constructs of lab-on-chip tools and devices, nano-biosensors and imaging probes keep the promise in real-time: (a) to enhance the sensitivity of diagnosis; (b) the selectivity of clinical methodologies (e.g., normal vs injured tissues); and also (c) to monitor therapy outcome for individual patients.[27–29,33–38] The recent application of personal genome sequencing approaches in the clinical setting and drug delivery further ensures the movement of PGx and personalized medicine in establishing PTx upon Rx (see also Figure 2). Overall, this direction initially starting from the combined research efforts of nanotechnology and PGx and through secondly the nanomedicine and personalized medicine advancements, it finally leads to the emergence of personalized nanomedicine as the new era where the challenges of achieving practical clinical utility in healthcare could be better served and broadly expanded all over the world (see also Figure 3).[39]

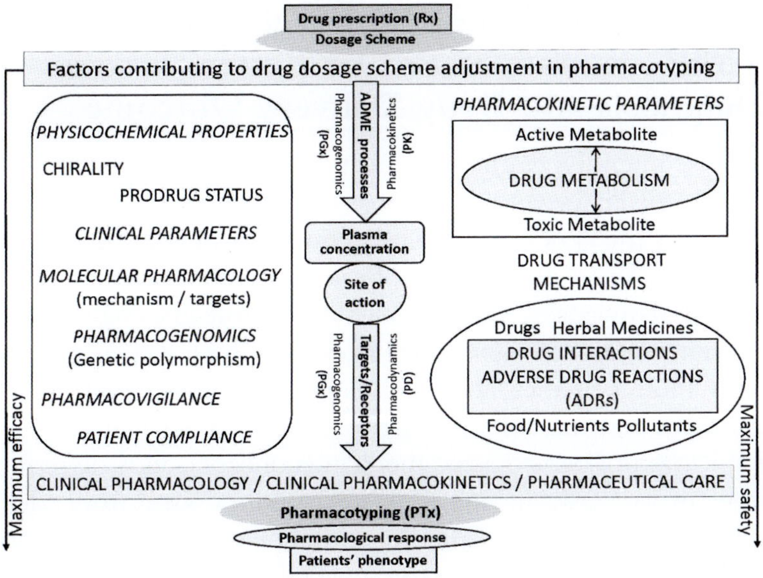

Fig. 2: Presentation of the proposed interdisciplinary collaboration to achieve personalized drug therapy decisions for pharmacotyping (PTx) in routine clinical practice and pharmacotherapy (see text for details).

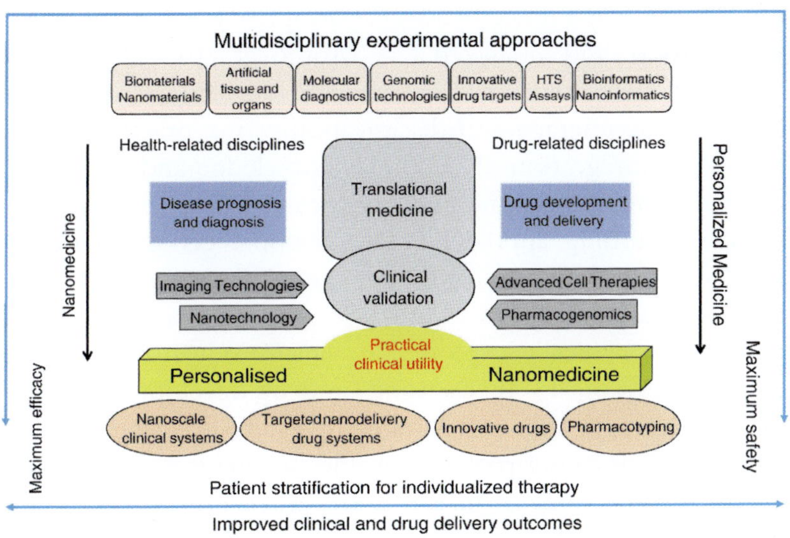

Fig. 3: The interdisciplinary nature of the methodology and experimentation contributing to personalized nanomedicine era is diagrammatically presented (see text for details). (The figure was taken with permission from Ref. 39).

3. The Intersection of Nanotechnology with Genomics to Ensure Better Disease Diagnosis and Drug Delivery Outcome

The disease phenotypes and the effects of drugs are influenced by the uniqueness of an organism; alternatively, the genetic make-up and consequently the genetic variability define individuality as a major factor contributing to illness pathophysiology and therapeutics clinical phenotypes. Nowadays, the genomics and nanotechnological advancements complemented with the achievements in molecular pharmacology and bioinformatics are formulating the new ground in drug development and the clinical practice. This new environment implies the application of personalized medicine concepts, an issue representing the major task in modern therapeutics and drug delivery. Unanimously in the latter case, the enrichment of disease pathophysiology knowledge, the empowerment of clinical diagnosis profiles and the improvement of drug delivery outcome are expected to happen.[13,19] As a matter of fact, therapeutic issues related to the propensity of illnesses susceptibility and the pharmacological variability of drug actions in a given population (lower efficacy and/or safety contributing to the emergence of adverse drug reactions; ADRs) are better understood and analyzed.[20,21] Moreover, the elaboration of sophisticated nano-structured systems and devices and their application in pharmacotherapy and disease monitoring practice has clearly facilitated the integration of genomics knowledge and nanomedicine tools in laboratory medicine and healthcare.[22,23] Molecular medicine techniques including approaches like personal genome sequencing, gene expression-signature profiling, genotyping and haplotyping analysis, molecular diagnostics use, and predictive biomarkers assessment are now clinically exploited to ensure advanced therapeutics outcomes (see Table 1). By focusing on drug development and pharmacology, this approach necessitates to establish specific molecular signatures and signaling pathway profiles in quantitatively evaluating drug effects and behavior in the body. Alternatively, the predictive biomarkers applied to assess the outcome upon drug administration in a given individual, or even for a specific group of patients should have a measurable value on drugs clinical parameters.[14,40,41]

Table 1. PGx predictive biomarkers to assess the safety and efficacy clinical profiles of individual marketed anticancer drugs.[a,b,c]

Drug	Gene	Safety/Efficacy profile
Anastozole	*ER*	Lower efficacy; No response in cancer patients with tumor *ER*-negative expression.
Capecitabine	*DPYD*	Lower safety; ADRs; Orodigestive neutropenia.
Cetuximab	*EGFR*	Lower efficacy; No response in cancer patients with tumor *EGFR*-negative expression.
	K-RAS	Lower efficacy; No response in cancer patients with tumor specific *K-RAS* mutations.
Cisplatin	*TPMT*	Lower safety; ADRs; Cytotoxicity associated with hearing loss in children.
Crizotinib	*ALK*	Efficacy; Indication only in patients bearing ALK gene rearrangement positive tumors (*EML4-ALK* translocation).
Dabrafenib	*BRAF*	Efficacy; Indicated only in melanoma patients with BRAF V600E mutation.
	G6PD	Safety; ADRs; Toxicity in G6PD deficient patients.
Dasatinib	Ph^+	Efficacy; Indicated only for Ph^+ tumors.
Erlotinib	*EGFR*	Lower efficacy; No response in cancer patients with tumor *EGFR*-negative expression.
Everolimus	*Her2/Neu*	Efficacy; Indicated in HER2 protein overexpression negative in breast cancer women.
	ER	Efficacy; Indicated for breast cancer women bearing ER positive tumors ($ESR1^+$).
Exemestane	*ER*	Lower efficacy; No response in cancer patients with tumor *ER*-negative expression.
Imatinib	Ph^+	Efficacy; Indicated only for Ph^+ tumors.
	PDGFR	Efficacy; Indicated in myelodysplastic-myeloproliferative syndromes with *PGFRR* gene rearrangements.
	FIP1L1-PDGFRA	Efficacy; Assessment of *FIP1L1-PDGFRA* translocation-fusion kinase in tumors.
	c-kit	Lower efficacy; No response in cancer patients with absence of tumor activating *c-Kit* mutations.
Irinotecan	*UGT1A1*	Lower safety; ADRs; Diarrhea, Increased risk for severe neutropenia in high doses of irinotecan.
Lapatinib	*Her2/Neu*	Efficacy; Indicated for over-expressing *Her2/Neu* advanced or metastatic breast cancer.

(*Continued*)

Table 1. (*Continued*)

Drug	Gene	Safety/Efficacy profile
Letrozole	*ER*	Lower efficacy; No response in cancer patients with tumor *ER*-negative expression.
Nilotinib	*Ph*⁺	Efficacy; Indicated only for *Ph*⁺ tumors.
	UGT1A1	Safety; Increased risk of hyperbilirubinemia in patients with UGT1A1*28 genotype.
6-Mercapto-purine	*TPMT*	Lower safety; ADRs; Neutropenia.
Panitumumab	*EGFR*	Lower efficacy; No response in cancer patients with tumor *EGFR*-negative expression.
	K-RAS	Lower efficacy; No response in cancer patients with tumor specific *K-RAS* mutations.
Pertuzumab	*HER2/Neu*	Efficacy; Indicated only for *HER2/Neu*⁺ breast cancer.
Tamoxifen	*ER*	Lower efficacy; No response in cancer patients with tumor *ER*-negative expression.
	CYP2D6	Lower efficacy; Loss of therapeutic benefit for PMs and/or upon co-administration with CYP2D6 inhibitors; lower plasma levels of active metabolite endoxifen achieved.
		Safety; ADRs; Risk for venous thromboembolism in breast cancer women also bearing factor V Leiden (FVL) mutations.
	FV F2	Safety; ADRs; Risk for venous thromboembolism in breast cancer women also bearing factor II (prothrombin) mutations.
Thioguanine	*TPMT*	Lower safety; ADRs; Neutropenia.
Trastuzumab	*HER2/Neu*	Lower efficacy; No response in cancer patients with tumor *HER2/Neu*-negative expression.
Vemurafenib	*BRAF*	Efficacy; Indicated only in melanoma patients whose tumors has a mutation at amino acid 600 of the B-raf protein (V600E and/or V600K BRAF mutations).

[a] Used with permission from Ref. 2.

[b] See also the table of PGx biomarkers in drug labeling at the FDA website at: http://www.fda.gov/drugs/scienceresearch/researchareas/pharmacogenetics/ucm083378.htm (Accessed on December 27, 2014).

[c] Additional data can be seen in "The Pharmacogenomics Knowledge Base (PharmGKB)" website at: https://www.pharmgkb.org/ (Accessed on December 27, 2014).

Abbreviations: ADRs: adverse drug reactions; *G6PD*: Glucose-6-phosphate dehydrogenase deficiency; PM: poor metabolizers: ER: estrogen receptor; *TMTP*: thiopurine methyltransferase gene; *DPYD*: dihydropyrimidine dehydrogenase gene; *Ph*: Philadelphia chromosome; FV: Factor V; F2: Factor II (prothrombin).

Both research and clinical efforts focusing on the assessment of PK/PD and pharmacovigilance data of delivered drugs have evidently shown that genetic polymorphism of drug metabolizing enzymes and transporters indeed play an important role in disposition, therapeutic efficacy and emergence of ADRs of several marketed therapeutics.[13–17] Moreover, drug interaction studies have univocally suggested that transporters often work together with drug-metabolizing enzymes to modulate drug absorption and elimination processes. The latter, is also relevant in trying to understand drug response heterogeneity and drug interactions upon new drug development as well. And for sure, it is a critical issue even upon working toward enabling personalized medicine decisions. Alternatively, one can argue that such an approach necessitates the direction of enriching the translational capacity in genomic medicine to contribute into specific PK/PD parameters and generate data applicable for any specific drug either under development or already in the market. Nowadays, various predictive PGx biomarkers for drugs belonging to several pharmacological classes have been approved and are already included in drug labeling by the regulatory agencies.[13,19–23] However, the inference and the broader integration of such predictive PGx biomarkers into modern pharmacology and the clinical setting are still quite challenging.

4. Nano and Genomics Technologies Advancing Translational Medicine Capabilities in both Pharmaceutical and Medical Sectors

By considering the genomics and nanotechnological advances happened in previous decades that cover major breakthroughs ranging from ultra-high-throughput screening methodologies to more thoroughly understanding of disease pathophysiology it might be anticipated that productivity in the drug-related eras would be at an all-time increased rate.[25] For the latter alternatively, one can argue that the success is closely related with the reduction of early attritions upon drug development. By lowering the attrition rate, the likelihood of successful launch of new medicines to the market is increasing.

Importantly and besides to the positive contribution in minimizing failures in organizational R&D structures, that capability also correlates with the efficiency by which the prediction of pharmacological response variability and clinical phenotype heterogeneity has been succeeded in personalized medicine therapeutic interventions. To this end, it is interesting to note that major pharmaceutical companies through revising their internal R&D infrastructures by conducting comprehensive longitudinal analysis proceed toward increasing productivity, pipeline quality efficiency and success in their new drug development projects. It might be possible by moving toward better assessing pharmacological response variability and clinical phenotype heterogeneity, in terms of personalized medicine decisions through the establishment of predictive PD/PK models, to also help achieve such goals and launch "smarter" innovative therapeutics with improved safety and efficacy profiles in the clinical setting.[2,23]

5. Advancing Personalized Medicine Decisions Toward Individualized Drug Delivery and Prescription: Concepts and Opportunities

The long-term aim of clinical pharmacology for delivering lower doses of medicines into the body to minimize the risk of toxicity is now better served through the implementation of PGx and nanotechnology-enabled therapeutics in everyday clinical practice. This means, the efficient clinical translational capacity of drug-related genomic information and also the development of well-suited nanodelivery systems allowing a better and desired PK/PD behavior of administered medicines in the body.[12,13,26–30] The limitation, therefore, of any impact from inter-individual variation in PK processes is thus served, especially in cases of therapeutics where increased drug heterogeneity response seen in clinical practice applies. Moreover, powerful nanotheranostics devices further empower imaging capabilities in laboratory medicine and contribute toward the development of systems and strategies, where upon monitoring control of diseases both the diagnosis profile and the therapy outcome are simultaneously served to benefit personalized medicine.[26] To facilitate broader utility of personalized medicine, the availability of quantitative markers for treatment clearly necessitates the capacity of *in vivo* molecular imaging techniques to assesses drug PK/PD actions in real-time to advance the productivity in drug development and to ensure improved efficacy and safety outcomes in drug delivery.[31,32] Moreover, as it has been already mentioned, the development of smart nanoprobes with enhanced imaging and payloads capabilities to therapeutically target *in vivo* specific cells or normal and damaged tissues, further contribute to diagnosis with increased sensitivity and specificity.[27–29,33,34,42] In addition, the development biosensor-driven lab-on-chip tools and devices cost-affordably implement laboratory medicine in handling sample mixing, transport, integration, detection and data processing.[35–38] The latter, implemented with the use of personal genome sequencing methodologies in clinical practice for each individual in a cost affordable manner, further ensures personalized medicine decisions and PTx implementation in everyday clinical practice (see Figure 2). But in any case, it has to be kept in maximum awareness the main task of improving the effectiveness of translational genomics to achieve such major benefits for the larger possible part of the population by taking lessons from the past, applying promising innovative scientific directions and seeking new solutions.[43–45]

Intra-patient variability in satisfactory therapeutic response has imposed a multi-level stimulation on the therapeutic community, to effectively confront and surpass the 'panacea' effect of a drug platform to the whole patient population. Deriving from the very distinct genotypic and phenotypic identity of each person, patient individuality (idiosyncrasy) demands tailored treatment approaches, especially in cancer therapy.[46,47] On this basis, the development of targeted drug delivery systems on the nano-scale level has outperformed the limitations of conventional systems, regarding both the PD and PK drug behavior. Controlled release profiles, prolonged circulation times and enhanced site-specific drug accumulation, combined with enhanced drug absorption and adjusted metabolism and elimination from the body advocate nano-technological achievements a competitively flourishing field on therapeutic, diagnostic or combinational perspectives.[48]

Development of drug delivery systems amenable to tailoring their PD and/or PK properties, therefore enhancing therapeutic efficacy and limiting toxicity, is of utmost importance. Customization of the aforementioned properties is achieved mainly by functionalization processes of the delivery platforms leading to prolonged circulation times, site-specific targeting and enhanced target uptake.[49] Nano-sized vectors of different materials origin (both organic and inorganic as well as synthetic and bio-inspired) and unique properties have been exhaustively utilized since the onset of nanotechnological evolution.[49–51]

6. Targeted Nanotechnological Drug Delivery Platforms Applied in Therapeutics

Owing to their unique structural geometries, carbonaceous materials including carbon nanotubes and its building block congener graphene have been extensively exploited as biocompatible vehicles of many biological and drug molecules.[52] Cell specific drug targeting, especially in cancer therapy, which is highly desirable in order to minimize peripheral toxicity, was achieved through conjugation with ligand molecules recognizing specific cellular-receptor targets.[53–57] In another approach covalent functionalization of siRNA on single-walled carbon nanotubes achieved selective cancer gene silencing, with minor cell toxicity.[58] Receptor-mediated internalization of doxorubicin loaded carbon nanovectors was combined with NIR irradiation to amplify treatment efficacy.[59]

Poly(amidoamine) (PAMAM) and poly(propylene imine) (PPI) dendrimers comprise a branched class of polymers[60] widely undergone conjugation to induce targeted drug delivery. Sialic acid and mannose binding for macrophage dual targeting in HIV infections,[61] N-acetylgalactosamine association for liver drug accumulation,[62] mitochondrial TSPO targeting[63] and biotin conjugation[64] of dendrimeric vectors both hybridized with FITC as imaging agent and aptamer hybridization for combined chemo-immunotherapy[65] constitute promising platforms as far as specific targeting, enhanced cellular uptake and therapeutic efficacy are concerned.

Gold nanoparticles have been also evaluated for their significance in targeted drug delivery,[66] as suggested by liver cell specific biopolymer[67] and cyclodextrin-hyaluronic acid grafted particles.[68] The synergistic effect of targeted drug delivery and hyperthermia induced by NIR light or radiofrequency was exploited achieving lowering of the therapeutic drug dose,[69] successful photo-thermal ablation of target cells[70,71] and on demand biomolecule release at the site of interest.[72]

Liposomal nanovectors stabilized through pegylation to assure prolonged residence in systemic circulation demonstrated liver specificity and hepatoprotective efficacy,[73] enhanced tumor targeting and metastasis inhibition effect through chlorotoxin modification,[74] dual functionalization with a cell recognizing and a cell penetrating ligand to enhance target accumulation and uptake,[75] while *in vivo* gene silencing potency for inflammation-activated endothelia was still to be further evaluated.[76] A multifunctional thermosensitive liposomal formulation achieved magnetically guided gene and drug co-delivery and thermally triggered drug release against *in vitro* and *in vivo* gastric cancer.[77] Albumin-based lyophillosomes conjugated with Hkc-4 antibody were found to be successfully internalized in target tumor cells.[78]

Preliminary studies exhibited the potential clinical utility of silica nanorattles with antibody functionalization for tumor targeting.[79] In another study organically modified silica (ORMOSIL) achieved neuronal penetration without cell deteriorating effects, which combined to their porous structure paved the way for safe brain delivery applications.[80] Lipid-based silica nanoparticles (protocells) were found to hold remarkably greater loading capacity and stability producing a highly efficient gene silencing effect.[81] Furthermore, magnetically guided nanoparticles[82,83] also combining the synergistic effects of magnetically induced hyperthermia,[84,85] field-controlled drug release[86] or even magneto-mechanical cell-receptor stimulation[87] constitute a diligently growing field utilizing their manifold applicability in nanotherapeutics.

Micellar polymeric doxorubicin loaded formulations exhibiting nuclear-specific accumulation *via* peptide functionalization[88] and controlled drug release[89] exerted dominant oncolytic action compared to free doxorubicin. Polymeric nanoparticles have been successfully employed in cell targeting through ligand association to achieve enhanced PD. Folate conjugation resulted in improved safety compliance and favorable localized accumulation in tumor cells when compared to an already marketed product,[90] while Interleukin-13 attachment enhanced nanoparticles uptake from glioblastoma cells, compared to plain nanoparticles, suppressing tumor cell proliferation.[91] Oxalate transferin (Tf) binding on nanoparticulate vehicles improved cellular association in Tf receptor (TfR) over expressing cells, which together with the application of native Tf-formulations in clinical trials, pave a successful path towards selective delivery of chemotherapeutics.[92] The synergistic effects of simultaneous drug and gene delivery were exploited in a redox-responsive delivery platform competent to targeted (epidermal growth factor receptor) therapeutic delivery and enhanced apoptotic efficacy against pancreatic adenocarcinoma.[93]

7. Targeted Nanodelivery Systems in Diagnostics and Imaging

Innovative approaches in the development of multifunctional imaging moieties has enabled significant advances in the field of diagnosis, steadily introduced in actual clinical practice through computed tomography (CT), Positron Emission Tomography (PET), Magnetic Resonance Imaging (MRI), ultrasound and optical imaging applications.[94] The employment of contrast imaging agents is fundamental, allowing for direct visualization, while at the same time their functionalization into multi-component platforms directs towards more personalized approaches.[95] Nanoparticle design with targeting potency needs to be accompanied by favorable PD/PK properties, showing prolonged circulation times, advanced targeted accumulation and internalization and less toxicity.[94,96,97]

Iron oxide nanoparticles have been widely accepted as imaging elements,[98] being adept at participating in multi-component structures, thus providing the synergy effect of individual components.

A gold-iron oxide hetero-structure, functionalized with anti-EGFR antibody molecules, has been developed serving as trimodal probe for PET, MRI and optical imaging, exhibiting both high affinity and uptake towards EGFR-positive tumors.[99]

Gadolinium-iron oxide nanoparticles with surface zwitterionic modification have been evaluated as MRI contrast agents demonstrating effective tumor targeting in an ovarian tumor xenograft model, with potentially favorable circulation times and elimination through renal clearance.[100] A multi-functionalized nanoparticulate system combined the ligand selectivity of anti-plectin-1 monoclonal antibody for pancreatic ductal adenocarcinoma, the minimizing effect against non-specific binding provided by BSA-conjugation and the bimodal fluorescent and MR imaging activity of a near-infrared fluorescence dye and super-paramagnetic iron oxide respectively.[101]

Target-sensitive gold nanospheres with specific selectivity were developed for photothermal optical coherence tomography applications enabling high resolution in-depth molecular imaging.[102] Polymeric formulations encapsulating manganese oxide nanocrystals demonstrated pH responsive bright contrast generation on MRI[103] and indium-111 coupled bioconjugated micelles reported high gastric tumor accumulation under nuclear imaging.[104] Metastatic tumor imaging via specific integrin recognition on the tumor-associated vascular bed has been achieved by chain-shaped iron-oxide nanoparticles employing fluorescence molecular tomography and MRI.[105]

8. Theranostic Applications

The advent of more personalized perspectives in patient treatment to eliminate PD and PK impediments and adequately respond to individual's requirements has introduced theranostics in clinical utility. The simultaneous real time monitoring of disease status and delivery of the therapeutic agent through a targeted multifunctional delivery system comprise the theranostic approach of personalized medicine.[106] Those multipurpose systems, commonly prepared via conjugation of different functionalities, provide a better insight and understanding of PK through direct visualization, enabling clinicians to tailor individual's therapy and advance therapeutic outcomes.[107]

Nanographenes with target specificity have been pharmacokinetically evaluated through PET imaging, radiolabeled either with ^{66}Ga or ^{64}Cu.[108,109] Silica materials have been involved in the development of theranostic systems as well, exhibiting breast or pancreatic tumor selectivity through specific bioconjugation, with integration of a near-infrared imaging modality[110] or acting as optical biodiagnostic probes in photodynamic therapy with the agent hypocrellin A.[111]

Gold nanomaterials have been extensively utilized as multimodal probes, demonstrating both tumor selectivity via surface functionalization, which in turn produces high anti-tumor activity and imaging capability.[112] Doxorubicin coupled methionine-nanoclusters[113] and folic acid-nanorods[114] suggested successful delivery of their therapeutic cargo with target specificity, enabling simultaneous monitoring of biodistribution by NIR imaging and multi-photon microscopy, respectively.

Biocompatible iron oxide nanoparticles have been comprehensively appraised for both their imaging and drug delivery capabilities. MRI was employed in the visualization of doxorubicin,[115,116] gemcitabine,[117] epirubicin[118] and taxol[119] loaded magnetic nanoparticles, which demonstrated target specificity through surface functionalization, thus improving receptor-mediated uptake from tumor cells and in some cases pH responsive drug release. Fluorescent magnetic nanoparticles adapted to mesenchymal stem cells were evaluated for their hyperthermia therapeutic effect in gastric cancer, caused under the application of an external magnetic field, while simultaneously acting as dual-modality contrast agents in fluorescence and MRI.[120]

Fluorescence was also employed in the imaging of magnetically guided iron oxide nanoparticles, which produced a faster tumor regression effect compared to those administered without the application of an external magnetic field.[121] Furthermore; optical imaging of iron oxide nanoparticles enabled the monitoring of biodistribution and targeted accumulation of a nanoparticulate system in a breast tumor xenograft model.[122]

9. Innovative Drug Delivery Vehicles to Enhance Safety and Efficacy Outcomes in Healthcare

Bioinspiration has qualified innovation in drug delivery, integrating biomimetic/natural platforms adequately engineered as multifunctional vectors. Amongst them, erythrocyte-based carriers have been employed in theranostic applications by cause of their biocompatibility, biodegradability and extended circulation times, accompanied by enhanced PD and clinical utility potentiality.[123]

Magnetic-field guided theranostic red blood cells grafted with functional molecules of manifold purposes, combined chemo- and photothermal therapy to successfully suppress tumor growth after intravenous administration.[124] Drug loaded erythrocytes were subjected to surface conjugation demonstrating site specificity,[125] introduced themselves as a novel therapeutic approach for asparagine auxotrophic malignancies[126] and also in pulmonary drug delivery configured as nanoerythrocytes.[127] The exploitation of red blood cells as transport vectors of nanoparticles expanded their *in vivo* circulation lifetime[128] and site specific accumulation via antibody conjugation, also improving blood PK behavior.[129]

Cancer cell-membrane functionalized nanoparticles[130] and virus-like immunogenic nanoparticles[131] have been reported as vaccination mediators for tumor and influenza multi-strain mediated immune response, respectively. Bio-imitation of cell-derived structures has been adopted not only in the development of immune responsive vectors, but also in drug delivery applications, with bacterial orientating vehicles exhibiting site specific anti-tumor efficacy.[132] Ferritin nanocages comprise another bioinspired platform division with multimodal functionality, enabling a more accurate loading regulation.[133]

10. Conclusions

The limited knowledge that still exists to more thoroughly understand disease pathogenesis and the underlying mechanisms of complex and multi-factorial (polygenic) illnesses (e.g., cancer, autoimmune disorders, degenerative diseases) represent a major obstacle toward: (a) increase the productivity of innovative medicines with improved efficacy and safety profiles; and (b) achieve precision in disease prognosis, diagnosis and therapy clinical environment. As a matter of fact, the development and the broader application of cost-affordable personalized medicine interventions for most, if not all, patients are being questioned and restricted. Although many studies have been carried out, there are very few drug products on the pharmaceutical market delivered as nanotherapeutics confirming the difficulty of formulating active compounds into such formulations. The most successful examples are a PEGylated liposome-doxorubicin product called Doxil®, the liposomal amphotericin B (Ambisome) and the albumin-stabilized paclitaxel (Abraxane). However, the increasing number of clinical trials using nanotherapeutics toward achieving better prognosis and diagnosis outcomes[134] emphasizes the potential of the emerging field of nanomedicine that positively contributes to personalized medicine decisions. Such an attempt however, besides focused research orientation, stresses toward the organization and establishment of interdisciplinary education trends for future healthcare practitioners in the era of pharmacology, drug therapy, personalized medicine and clinical practice.[1,2] Moving forward, the future advancements in nanotechnology, genomics, informatics and materials sciences is evidently expected to contribute in achieving broader personalized medicine decisions of practical clinical utility in both drug delivery and therapeutics.

References

1. I. S. Vizirianakis (ed.,), in *Personalized Medicine: Advances in Nanotechnology, Drug Delivery and Therapy*, Pan Stanford Publishing, Singapore, 2014.
2. I. S. Vizirianakis, *World J. Pharmacol.,* 110 (2014).
3. N . Chatterjee, B. Wheeler, J. Sampson, P. Hartge, S. J. Chanock, J. H. Park, *Nat. Genet.,* 400 (2013).
4. R. Mirnezami, J. Nicholson, A. Darzi, *N. Engl. J. Med.*, 489 (2012).
5. J. J. McCarthy, *Mol. Genet.Genomic Med.*, 455 (2014).
6. J. Mendelsohn, *J. Clin. Oncol.*, 1094 (2013).

7. F. Ciardiello, D. Arnold, P. G. Casali, A. Cervantes, J. Y. Douillard, A. Eggermont, A. Eniu, K. McGregor, S. Peters, M. Piccart, R. Popescu, E. Van Cutsem, C. Zielinski, R. Stahel, *Ann. Oncol.*, 1673 (2014).
8. L. A. Garraway, J. Verweij, K. V. Ballman, *J. Clin. Oncol.,* 1803 (2013).
9. D. Rosenblum, D. Peer, *Cancer Lett.*, 126 (2014).
10. J. C. O'Donnell, *Value Health*, S1 (2013).
11. L. Annemans, K. Redekop, K. Payne, *Value Health*, S20 (2013).
12. J. D. Miller, K. A. Foley, M. W. Russell, *Am. Health Drug Benefits*, 153 (2014).
13. I. S. Vizirianakis, *Clin. Pharmacokinet.,* 807 (2007).
14. R. Kaddurah-Daouk, R. M. Weinshilboum, *Clin. Pharmacol. Ther.*, 154 (2014).
15. S. F. Zhou, J. P. Liu, B. Chowbay, *Drug Metab, Rev.*, 89 (2009).
16. J. W. Lee, F. Aminkeng, A. P. Bhavsar, K. Shaw, B. C. Carleton, M. R. Hayden, C. J. Ross, *Clin. Genet.*, 21 (2014).
17. M. Pirmohamed, *Drug Discov. Today*, 852 (2011).
18. K. M. Hillgren, D. Keppler, A. A. Zur, K. M. Giacomini, B. Stieger, C. E. Cass, L. Zhang, *Clin. Pharmacol. Ther.*, 52 (2013).
19. G. S. Ginsburg, H. F. Willard, *Transl. Res.,* 277 (2009).
20. M. Pirmohamed, *Annu. Rev. Genomics Hum. Genet.*, 349 (2014).
21. I. S. Vizirianakis, *Pharmacogenomics*, 701 (2005).
22. K. Braeckmans, S. C. De Smedt, M. Leblans, R. Pauwels, J. Demeester, *Nat. Rev. Drug Disc.*, 447 (2002).
23. I. S. Vizirianakis (ed.), in *Personalized Medicine: Advances in Nanotechnology, Drug Delivery and Therapy*, Pan Stanford Publishing, Singapore, 893, 2014.
24. I. S. Vizirianakis, *Nanomedicine*, 11 (2011).
25. D. Cook, D. Brown, R. Alexander, R. March, P. Morgan, G. Satterthwaite, M. N. Pangalos, *Nat. Rev. Drug Discov.*, 419 (2014).
26. S. Mura, P. Couvreur, *Adv. Drug Deliv. Rev.*, 1394 (2012).
27. J. H. Ryu, H. Koo, I. C. Sun, S. H. Yuk, K. Choi, K. Kim, I. C. Kwon, *Adv. Drug Deliv. Rev.*, 1447 (2012).
28. A. Daka, D. Peer, *Adv. Drug Deliv. Rev.*, 1508 (2012).
29. M. Wieland, M. Fussenegger, *Adv. Drug Deliv. Rev.*, 1477 (2012).
30. A. L. Petersen, A. E. Hansen, A. Gabizon, T. L. Andresen, *Adv. Drug Deliv. Rev.,* 1417 (2012).

31. V. Ntziachristos, D. Razansky, *Chem. Rev.*, 2783 (2010).
32. A. L. Petersen, A. E. Hansen, A. Gabizon, T. L. Andresen, *Adv. Drug Deliv. Rev.*, 1417 (2012).
33. M. Janowski, J. W. Bulte, P. Walczak, *Adv. Drug Deliv. Rev.*, 1488 (2012).
34. P. Debbage, *Curr. Pharm. Des.*, 153 (2009).
35. S. M. Moghimi, P. P. Wibroe, S. Y. Helvig, Z. S. Farhangrazi, A. C. Hunter, *Adv. Drug Deliv. Rev.*, 1385 (2012).
36. I. A. Cree, *J. Control. Release*, 405 (2013).
37. W. Sadee, *Pharmacogenomics*, 675 (2011).
38. M. Huang, A. Shen, J. Ding, M. Geng, *Trends Pharmacol. Sci.*, 41 (2014).
39. I. S. Vizirianakis, D. G. Fatouros, *Adv. Drug Deliv. Rev.*, 1359 (2012).
40. A. D. Roses, A. M. Saunders, M. W. Lutz, N. Zhang, A. R. Hariri, K. E. Asin, D. G. Crenshaw, K. Budur, D. K. Burns, S. K. Brannan, *Curr. Opin. Pharmacol.*, 81 (2014).
41. D. L. Hertz, H. L. McLeod, *J. Hum. Genet.*, 346 (2013).
42. I. S. Vizirianakis, *Curr. Drug Deliv.*, 73 (2004).
43. C. Huttenhower, O. Hofmann, *PLoS Comput. Biol.*, e1000779 (2010).
44. I. S. Vizirianakis, M. Chatzopoulou, I. D. Bonovolias, I. Nicolaou, V. J. Demopoulos, A. S. Tsiftsoglou, *J. Med. Chem.*, 6779 (2010).
45. K. Ahn, J. Luo, A. Berg, D. Keefe, R. Wu, *Trends Pharmacol. Sci.*, 306 (2010).
46. Y. F. Lu, D. B. Goldstein, M. Angrist, G. Cavalleri, *Cold Spring Harb Perspect Med.*, a008581 (2014).
47. D. Frank, C. Tyagi, L. Tomar, Y. E. Choonara, L. C. du Toit, P. Kumar, C. Penny, V. Pillay, *Int. J. Nanomedicine.*, 589 (2014).
48. M. Hamidi, A. Azadi, P. Rafiei, H. Ashrafi, *Crit. Rev. Ther. Drug Carrier Syst.*, 435 (2013).
49. D. Mishra, J. R. Hubenak, A. B. Mathur, *J. Biomed. Mater. Res. A.*, 3646 (2013).
50. O. C. Farokhzad, R. Langer, *Adv. Drug Deliv. Rev.*, 1456 (2006).
51. X. Q. Zhang, X. Xu, N. Bertrand, E. Pridgen, A. Swami, O. C. Farokhzad, *Adv. Drug Deliv. Rev.*, 1363 (2012).

52. N. A. Fonseca, A. C. Gregório, A. Valério-Fernandes, S. Simões, J. N. Moreira, *Cancer Treat Rev.*, 626 (2014).
53. J. Liu, L. Cui, D. Losic, *Acta Biomater.*, 9243 (2013).
54. A. A. Bhirde, V. Patel, J. Gavard, G. Zhang, A. A. Sousa, A. Masedunskas, R. D. Leapman, R. Weigert, J. S. Gutkind, J. F. Rusling, *ACS Nano.*, 307 (2009).
55. J. M. Berlin, T. T. Pham, D. Sano, K. A. Mohamedali, D. C. Marcano, J. N. Myers, J. M. Tour, *ACS Nano.*, 6643 (2011).
56. H. Wang, W. Gu, N. Xiao, L. Ye, Q. Xu, *Int. J. Nanomedicine.*, 1433 (2014).
57. J. Li, A. Pant, C. F. Chin, W. H. Ang, C. Ménard-Moyon, T. R. Nayak, D. Gibson, S. Ramaprabhu, T. Panczyk, A. Bianco, G. Pastorin, *Nanomedicine.*, 1465 (2014).
58. G. Bartholomeusz, P. Cherukuri, J. Kingston, L. Cognet, R. Lemos, T. K. Leeuw, L. Gumbiner-Russo, R. B. Weisman, G. Powis, *Nano Res.*, 279 (2009).
59. P. Jeyamohan, T. Hasumura, Y. Nagaoka, Y. Yoshida, T. Maekawa, D. S. Kumar, *Int. J. Nanomedicine.*, 2653 (2013).
60. D. Shcharbin, A. Janaszewska, B. Klajnert-Maculewicz, B. Ziemba, V. Dzmitruk, I. Halets, S. Loznikova, N. Shcharbina, K. Milowska, M. Ionov, A. Shakhbazau, M. Bryszewska, *J. Control Release.*, 40 (2014).
61. V. Gajbhiye, N. Ganesh, J. Barve, N. K. Jain, *Eur. J. Pharm. Sci.*, 668 (2013).
62. S. H. Medina, V. Tekumalla, M. V. Chevliakov, D. S. Shewach, W. D. Ensminger, M. E. El-Sayed, *Biomaterials*, 4118 (2011).
63. N. Denora, V. Laquintana, A. Lopalco, R. M. Iacobazzi, A. Lopedota, A. Cutrignelli, G. Iacobellis, C. Annese, M. Cascione, S. Leporatti, M. Franco, *J. Control Release.*, 1111 (2013).
64. W. Yang, Y. Cheng, T. Xu, X. Wang, L. P. Wen, *Eur. J. Med. Chem.*, 862 (2009).
65. I. H. Lee, S. An, M. K. Yu, H. K. Kwon, S. H. Im, S. Jon, *J. Control Release.*, 435 (2011).
66. M. R. Papasani, G. Wang, R. A. Hill, *Nanomedicine.*, 804 (2012).
67. M. Ganeshkumar, T. Ponrasu, M. D. Raja, M. K. Subamekala, L. Suguna, *Spectrochim. Acta A Mol. Biomol. Spectrosc.*, 64 (2014).

68. N. Li, Y. Chen, Y. M. Zhang, Y. Yang, Y. Su, J. T. Chen, Y. Liu, *Sci. Rep.*, 4164 (2014).
69. M. Raoof, S. J. Corr, C. Zhu, B. T. Cisneros, W. D. Kaluarachchi, S. Phounsavath, L. J. Wilson, S. A. Curley, *Nanomedicine.*, 1121 (2014).
70. A. S. Monem, N. Elbialy, N. Mohamed, *Int. J. Pharm.*, 1 (2014).
71. M. S. Mohamed, S. Veeranarayanan, A. C. Poulose, Y. Nagaoka, H. Minegishi, Y. Yoshida, T. Maekawa, D. S. Kumar, *Biochim. Biophys. Acta.*, 1657 (2014).
72. R. Huschka, A. Barhoumi, Q. Liu, J. A. Roth, L. Ji, N. J. Halas, *ACS Nano.*, 7681 (2012).
73. X. Zhang, Q. Zhang, Q. Peng, J. Zhou, L. Liao, X. Sun, L. Zhang, T. Gong, *Biomaterials.*, 6130 (2014).
74. C. Qin, B. He, W. Dai, Z. Lin, H. Zhang, X. Wang, J. Wang, X. Zhang, G. Wang, L. Yin, Q. Zhang, *Biomaterials.*, 5908 (2014).
75. L. Mei, L. Fu, K. Shi, Q. Zhang, Y. Liu, J. Tang, H. Gao, Z. Zhang, Q. He, *Int .J. Pharm.*, 26 (2014).
76. N. G. Leus, H. W. Morselt, P. J. Zwiers, P. S. Kowalski, M. H. Ruiters, G. Molema, J. A. Kamps, *Int. J. Pharm.*, 121 (2014).
77. Z. Peng, C. Wang, E. Fang, X. Lu, G. Wang, Q. Tong, *PLoS One.*, e92924 (2014).
78. E. van Bracht, S. Stolle, T. G. Hafmans, O. C. Boerman, E. Oosterwijk, T. H. van Kuppevelt, W. F. Daamen, *Eur. J. Pharm. Biopharm.*, 80 (2014).
79. S. Sundarraj, R. Thangam, M. V. Sujitha, K. Vimala, S. Kannan, *Toxicol. Appl. Pharmacol.*, 232 (2014).
80. F. Barandeh, P. L. Nguyen, R. Kumar, G. J. Iacobucci, M. L. Kuznicki, A. Kosterman, E. J. Bergey, P. N. Prasad, S. Gunawardena, *PLoS One.*, e29424 (2012).
81. C. E. Ashley, E. C. Carnes, K. E. Epler, D. P. Padilla, G. K. Phillips, R. E. Castillo, D. C. Wilkinson, B. S. Wilkinson, C. A. Burgard, R. M. Kalinich, J. L. Townson, B. Chackerian, C. L. Willman, D. S. Peabody, W. Wharton, C. J. Brinker, *ACS Nano.*, 2174 (2012).
82. S. Jiang, A. A. Eltoukhy, K. T. Love, R. Langer, D. G. Anderson, *Nano Lett.*, 1059 (2013).
83. S. Pilakka-Kanthikeel, V. S. Atluri, V. Sagar, S. K. Saxena, M. Nair, *PLoS One.*, e62241 (2013).

84. S. Balasubramanian, A. R. Girija, Y. Nagaoka, S. Iwai, M. Suzuki, V. Kizhikkilot, Y. Yoshida, T. Maekawa, S. D. Nair, *Int. J. Nanomedicine.*, 437 (2014).
85. B. Clares, R. A. Biedma-Ortiz, E. Sáez-Fernández, J. C. Prados, C. Melguizo, L. Cabeza, R. Ortiz, J. L. Arias, *Eur. J. Pharm. Biopharm.*, 329 (2013).
86. R. Guduru, P. Liang, C. Runowicz, M. Nair, V. Atluri, S. Khizroev, *Sci. Rep.*, 2953 (2013).
87. B. Hu, A. J. El Haj, J. Dobson, *Int. J. Mol. Sci.*, 19276 (2013).
88. Y. Y. Li, L. Li, H. Q. Dong, X. J. Cai, T. B. Ren, *Mater. Sci. Eng. C Mater. Biol. Appl.*, 2698 (2013).
89. S. K. Hira, A. K. Mishra, B. Ray, P. P. Manna, *PLoS One.*, e94309 (2014).
90. F. Tavassolian, G. Kamalinia, H. Rouhani, M. Amini, S. N. Ostad, M. R. Khoshayand, F. Atyabi, M. R. Tehrani, R. Dinarvand, *Int. J. Pharm.*, 123 (2014).
91. H. Gao, S. Zhang, Z. Yang, S. Cao, X. Jiang, Z. Pang, *Int. J. Pharm.*, 8 (2014).
92. R. Y. Chiu, T. Tsuji, S. J. Wang, J. Wang, C. T. Liu, D. T. Kamei, *J. Control Release.*, 33 (2014).
93. J. Xu, A. Singh, M. M. Amiji, *BMC Cancer.*, 75 (2014).
94. R. Toy, L. Bauer, C. Hoimes, K. B. Ghaghada, E. Karathanasis, *Adv Drug Deliv. Rev.*, 79 (2014).
95. N. Han, Y. Y. Yang, S. Wang, S. Zheng, W. Fan, *Curr. Drug. Metab.*, 661 (2013).
96. A. Sharma, N. Jain, R. Sareen, *Biomed Res Int.*, 960821 (2013).
97. N. Anton, T. F. Vandamme, *Pharm. Res.*, 20 (2014).
98. X. Zhao, H. Zhao, Z. Chen, M. Lan, *J. Nanosci. Nanotechnol.*, 210 (2014).
99. M .Yang, K. Cheng, S. Qi, H. Liu, Y. Jiang, H. Jiang, J. Li, K. Chen, H. Zhang, Z. Cheng, *Biomaterials.*, 2796 (2013).
100. Z. Zhou, L. Wang, X. Chi, J. Bao, L. Yang, W. Zhao, Z. Chen, X. Wang, X. Chen, J. Gao, *ACS Nano.*, 3287 (2013).
101. X. Wang, X. Xing, B. Zhang, F. Liu, Y. Cheng, D. Shi, *Int J Nanomedicine.*, 1601 (2014).
102. M. C. Skala, M. J. Crow, A. Wax, J. A. Izatt, *Nano Lett.*, 3461 (2008).

103. M. F. Bennewitz, T. L. Lobo, M. K. Nkansah, G. Ulas, G. W. Brudvig, E. M. Shapiro, *ACS Nano.*, 3438 (2011).
104. C. C. Cheng, C. F. Huang, A. S. Ho, C. L. Peng, C. C. Chang, F. D. Mai, L. Y. Chen, T. Y. Luo, J. Chang, *Int. J. Nanomedicine.*, 1385 (2013).
105. P. M. Peiris, R. Toy, E. Doolittle, J. Pansky, A. Abramowski, M. Tam, P. Vicente, E. Tran, E. Hayden, A. Camann, A. Mayer, B. O. Erokwu, Z. Berman, D. Wilson, H. Baskaran, C. A. Flask, R. A. Keri, E. Karathanasis, *ACS Nano.*, 8783 (2012).
106. J. Barar, Y. Omidi, *Bioimpacts.*, 3 (2014).
107. Z. Cheng, A. Al Zaki, J. Z. Hui, V. R. Muzykantov, A. Tsourkas, *Science.*, 903 (2012).
108. H. Hong, Y. Zhang, J. W. Engle, T. R. Nayak, C. P. Theuer, R. J. Nickles, T. E. Barnhart, W. Cai, *Biomaterials.*, 4147 (2012).
109. H. Hong, K. Yang, Y. Zhang, J. W. Engle, L. Feng, Y. Yang, T. R. Nayak, S. Goel, J. Bean, C. P. Theuer, T. E. Barnhart, Z. Liu, W. Cai, *ACS Nano.*, 2361 (2012).
110. B. M. Barth, R. Sharma, E. I. Altinoğlu, T. T. Morgan, S. S. Shanmugavelandy, J. M. Kaiser, C. McGovern, G. L. Matters, J. P. Smith, M. Kester, J. H. Adair, *ACS Nano.*, 1279 (2010).
111. L. Zhou, J. H. Liu, F. Ma, S. H. Wei, Y. Y. Feng, J. H. Zhou, B. Y. Yu, J. Shen, *Biomed Microdevices.*, 655 (2010).
112. C. Gui, D. X. Cui, *Cancer Biol. Med.*, 221 (2012).
113. H. Chen, B. Li, X. Ren, S. Li, Y. Ma, S. Cui, Y. Gu, *Biomaterials.*, 8461 (2012).
114. B. Book Newell, Y. Wang, J. Irudayaraj, *Eur. J. Med. Chem.*, 330 (2012).
115. Y. Liu, K. Yang, L. Cheng, J. Zhu, X. Ma, H. Xu, Y. Li, L. Guo, H. Gu, Z. Liu, *Nanomedicine.*, 1077 (2013).
116. T. Chen, M. I. Shukoor, R. Wang, Z. Zhao, Q. Yuan, S. Bamrungsap, X. Xiong, W. Tan, *ACS Nano.*, 7866 (2011).
117. G. Y. Lee, W. P. Qian, L. Wang, Y. A. Wang, C. A. Staley, M. Satpathy, S. Nie, H. Mao, L. Yang, *ACS Nano.*, 2078 (2013).
118. S. H. Jalalian, S. M. Taghdisi, N. Shahidi Hamedani, S. A. Kalat, P. Lavaee, M. Zandkarimi, N. Ghows, M. R. Jaafari, S. Naghibi, N. M. Danesh, M. Ramezani, K. Abnous, *Eur. J. Pharm. Sci.*, 191 (2013).

119. S. Santra, S. D. Jativa, C. Kaittanis, G. Normand, J. Grimm, J. M. Perez, *ACS Nano.*, 7281 (2012).
120. J. Ruan, J. Ji, H. Song, Q. Qian, K. Wang, C. Wang, D. Cui, *Nanoscale Res. Lett.*, 309 (2012).
121. A. Fu, R. J. Wilson, B. R. Smith, J. Mullenix, C. Earhart, D. Akin, S. Guccione, S. X. Wang, S. S. Gambhir, *ACS Nano.*, 6862 (2012).
122. S. P. Foy, R. L. Manthe, S. T. Foy, S. Dimitrijevic, N. Krishnamurthy, V. Labhasetwar, *ACS Nano.*, 5217 (2010).
123. P. D. Patel, N. Dand, R. S. Hirlekar, V. J. Kadam, *Current Pharmaceutical Design*, 63 (2008).
124. C. Wang, X. Sun, L. Cheng, S. Yin, G. Yang, Y. Li, Z. Liu, *Adv. Mater.*, 4794 (2014).
125. N. Sternberg, R. Georgieva, K. Duft, H. Bäumler, *J Microencapsul.*, 9 (2012).
126. V. Agrawal, J. H. Woo, G. Borthakur, H. Kantarjian, A. E. Frankel, *Protein Pept Lett.*, 392 (2013).
127. N. Gupta, B. Patel, Ahsan F, *Pharm. Res.,* 1553 (2014).
128. E. Chambers, S. Mitragotri, *Exp. Biol. Med.* (*Maywood*), 958 (2007).
129. A. C. Anselmo, V. Gupta, B. J. Zern, D. Pan, M. Zakrewsky, V. Muzykantov, S. Mitragotri, *ACS Nano.*, 11129 (2013).
130. R. H. Fang, C. M. Hu, B. T. Luk, W. Gao, J. A. Copp, Y. Tai, D. E. O'Connor, L. Zhang, *Nano Lett.*, 2181 (2014).
131. D. P. Patterson, A. Rynda-Apple, A. L. Harmsen, A. G. Harmsen, T. Douglas, *ACS Nano.*, 3036 (2013).
132. V. Gujrati, S. Kim, S. H. Kim, J. J. Min, H. E. Choy, S. C. Kim, S. Jon, *ACS Nano.*, 1525 (2014).
133. X. Lin, J. Xie, G. Niu, F. Zhang, H. Gao, M. Yang, Q. Quan, M. A. Aronova, G. Zhang, S. Lee, R. Leapman, X. Chen, *Nano Lett.*, 814 (2011).
134. I. F. Uchegbu, A. Siew, *J. Pharm. Sci.,* 305 (2013).

EDITORS' BIOGRAPHIES

Simona Mura is currently Associate Professor within the framework of the « *CNRS-Higher Education chairs* » program, in the group of Pr. Patrick Couvreur (Institut Galien Paris-Sud, UMR CNRS 8612) at the University Paris-Sud, Châtenay-Malabry. She gained the degree in Pharmaceutical Chemistry and Technology in 2005. In 2009, she was awarded her PhD in Chemistry and Technology of Drug at the University of Cagliari, Italy, working on the design and *in vitro* evaluation of novel vesicular systems for the topical delivery of drugs. In 2008 she joined the group of Pr. Elias Fattal (UMR CNRS 8612) at the University Paris-Sud, Châtenay-Malabry, France, as Post-doctoral research assistant to study the lung toxicity of biodegradable nanoparticles designed for pulmonary administration of drugs. She possesses a strong background in the formulation/characterization and *in vitro* evaluation of drug delivery systems and a solid knowledge in the field of *in vivo* cancer animal models. Her research focuses on the development of valuable and easy to handle *in vitro* and *in vivo* models to investigate nanoscale systems for drug delivery, aiming to achieve their faster bench-to-bedside translation.

Patrick Couvreur is Full Professor of Pharmacy at the Paris-Sud University, a member of the Institut Universitaire de France and holder of the chair of "Innovation Technologique" (2009–2010) at the prestigious « Collège de France ». He is also the recipient of an "ERC Advanced Grant" (2010–2015). Pr Patrick Couvreur's contributions in the field of drug delivery and targeting are highly recognized around the world with around 500 peer review research publications (H-index 76 and over 22,000 citations). His research on Nanomedicine is interdisciplinary, at the interface between Physico-Chemistry of Colloids, Polymer Chemistry, Material Science, Molecular and Cellular Biology and Experimental Pharmacology. Patrick Couvreur's research has led to the founding of two start-up companies (Bioalliance, which entered the stock market in 2005 and Medsqual) and to the development of a nanomedicine, currently in phase III clinical trials. The major scientific contribution of Patrick Couvreur to the Pharmaceutical Sciences is also recognized by numerous international (incl. among others, the prestigious "Host Madsen Medal" 2007 given by FIP, the European Pharmaceutical Scientist Award 2011, given by EUFEPS, the European Inventor Award 2013, given by the European Patent Office and the Speiser Award 2014) and national awards (incl. among others, the "Prix Galien 2009" and the "Médaille de l'Innovation" 2012 of the CNRS). His appointment as a member of eight academies (Académie des Sciences, Académie des Technologies, Académie de Médecine and Académie de Pharmacie in France, as well as, the Académie Royale de Médecine in Belgium, the Real Academia de Farmacia in Spain, the US National Academy of Medicine and the US National Academy of Engineering) is another recognition of his major scientific and scholarly contributions.

CONTRIBUTORS

Amanatiadou Elsa P. Department of Pharmacology, School of Pharmacy, Aristotle University of Thessaloniki, Thessaloniki GR-54124, Greece

Andresen Thomas Lars Department of Micro- and Nanotechnology; Center for Nanomedicine and Theranostics, Technical University of Denmark, 2800 Lyngby, Denmark

Borden Mark A. Department of Mechanical Engineering, University of Colorado Campus Box 427, 1111 Engineering Drive, Boulder, CO 80309, USA

Bort Guillaume Institut Galien Paris-Sud, UMR 8612, CNRS, Univ. Paris-Sud, Université Paris-Saclay, Faculté de Pharmacie, 5 rue JB Clément, 92296 Châtenay-Malabry, France

Carme Sabin Institute Light & Matter UMR5306 Team FENNEC, Lyon University 2, rue V. Grignard, 69622 Villeurbanne, France

Chauvierre Cédric Inserm, U1148, Cardiovascular Bio-Engineering, X. Bichat Hospital, Université Paris Diderot, Université Paris 13, Sorbonne Paris Cité, France

Couvreur Patrick Institut Galien Paris-Sud, UMR 8612, CNRS, Univ. Paris-Sud, Université Paris-Saclay, Faculté de Pharmacie, 5 rue JB Clément, 92296 Châtenay-Malabry, France

Deshpande Madhura Center for Pharmaceutical Biotechnology and Nanomedicine, Northeastern University, Boston, Massachusetts 02115, USA

Doan Bich-Thuy Paris Sorbonne Cité, Paris Descartes University, Faculty of Pharmacy, Chimie ParisTech, Team Vectors for Targeted Therapy and Molecular Imaging, CNRS UMR 8258, INSERM U1022, 4 avenue de l'Observatoire, 75270 ParisCedex 06, France

Dove Jacob D. Department of Mechanical Engineering, University of Colorado Campus Box 427, 1111 Engineering Drive, Boulder, CO 80309 USA

Farokhzad Omid C. Laboratory of Nanomedicine and Biomaterials, Department of Anesthesiology, Brigham and Women's Hospital, Harvard Medical School, 75 Francis St., Boston, MA 02115, USA.; King Abdulaziz University, Jeddah, Saudi Arabia

Fatouros Dimitrios G. Department of Pharmaceutical Technology, School of Pharmacy, Aristotle University of Thessaloniki, Thessaloniki GR-54124, Greece

Hansen Anders E. Department of Micro- and Nanotechnology; Center for Nanomedicine and Theranostics, Technical University of Denmark, 2800 Lyngby, Denmark

Henriksen Jonas R. Department of Chemistry; Center for Nanomedicine and Theranostics, Technical University of Denmark, 2800 Lyngby, Denmark

Juenet Maya Inserm, U1148, Cardiovascular Bio-Engineering, X. Bichat Hospital, Université Paris Diderot, Université Paris 13, Sorbonne Paris Cité, France

Karavasili Christina Department of Pharmaceutical Technology, School of Pharmacy, Aristotle University of Thessaloniki, Thessaloniki GR-54124, Greece

Laurent Sophie Department of General, Organic and Biomedical Chemistry, NMR and Molecular Imaging Laboratory, University of

Mons, 19 Avenue Maistriau, 7000 Mons, Belgium; Center for Microscopy and Molecular Imaging (CMMI), 8 Rue Adrienne Boland, 6041 Gosselies, Belgium

Le Duc Geraldine ID17 Biomedical Beamline, European Synchrotron Radiation Facility, 6 Rue Jules Horowitz, 38000 Grenoble, France

Letourneur Didier Inserm, U1148, Cardiovascular Bio-Engineering, X. Bichat Hospital, Université Paris Diderot, Université Paris 13, Sorbonne Paris Cité, France

Lux François Institute Light & Matter UMR5306 Team FENNEC, Lyon University 2, rue V. Grignard, 69622 Villeurbanne, France

Mignet Nathalie Paris Sorbonne Cité, Paris Descartes University, Faculty of Pharmacy, Chimie ParisTech, Team Vectors for Targeted Therapy and molecular Imaging, CNRS UMR 8258, INSERM U1022, 4 avenue de l'Observatoire, 75270 ParisCedex 06

Muller Robert Department of General, Organic and Biomedical Chemistry, NMR and Molecular Imaging Laboratory, University of Mons, 19 Avenue Maistriau, 7000 Mons, Belgium; Center for Microscopy and Molecular Imaging (CMMI), 8 Rue Adrienne Boland, 6041 Gosselies, Belgium

Mura Simona Institut Galien Paris-Sud, UMR 8612, CNRS, Univ. Paris-Sud, Université Paris-Saclay, Faculté de Pharmacie, 5 rue JB Clément, 92296 Châtenay-Malabry, France

Murray Todd W. Department of Mechanical Engineering, University of Colorado, Campus Box 427, 1111 Engineering Drive, Boulder, CO 80309, USA

Petersen Anncatrine L. Department of Micro- and Nanotechnology; Center for Nanomedicine and Theranostics, Technical University of Denmark, 2800 Lyngby, Denmark

Pollit Lori Laboratory of Nanomedicine and Biomaterials, Department of Anesthesiology, Brigham and Women's Hospital, Harvard Medical School, 75 Francis St., Boston, MA 02115, USA. University of Waterloo, Canada

Richard Cyrille Paris Sorbonne Cité, Paris Descartes University, Faculty of Pharmacy, Chimie ParisTech, Team Vectors for Targeted Therapy and molecular Imaging, CNRS UMR 8258, INSERM U1022, 4 avenue de l'Observatoire, 75270 Paris Cedex 06, France

Sancey Lucie Institute Light & Matter UMR5306 Team FENNEC, Lyon University 2, rue V. Grignard, 69622 Villeurbanne, France

Sriraman Shravan Kumar Center for Pharmaceutical Biotechnology and Nanomedicine, Northeastern University, Boston, Massachusetts 02115, USA

Stanicki Dimitri Department of General, Organic and Biomedical Chemistry, NMR and Molecular Imaging Laboratory, University of Mons, 19 Avenue Maistriau, 7000 Mons, Belgium

Tillement Olivier Institute Light & Matter UMR5306 Team FENNEC, Lyon University 2, rue V. Grignard, 69622 Villeurbanne, France

Torchilin Vladimir Center for Pharmaceutical Biotechnology and Nanomedicine, Northeastern University, Boston, MA 02115, USA; Department of Biochemistry, Faculty of Science, King Abdulaziz University, Jeddah 21589, Saudi Arabia

Vander Elst Luce Department of General, Organic and Biomedical Chemistry, NMR and Molecular Imaging Laboratory, University of Mons, 19 Avenue Maistriau, 7000 Mons, Belgium; Center for Microscopy and Molecular Imaging (CMMI), 8 Rue Adrienne Boland, 6041 Gosselies, Belgium

Varna Mariana Inserm, U1148, Cardiovascular Bio-Engineering, X. Bichat Hospital, Université Paris Diderot, Université Paris 13, Sorbonne Paris Cité, France

Vilos Critian Laboratory of Nanomedicine and Biomaterials, Department of Anesthesiology, Brigham and Women's Hospital, Harvard Medical School, 75 Francis St., Boston, MA 02115, USA. Universidad Andres Bello, Facultad de Medicina, Center for Integrative Medicine and Innovative Science (CIMIS), Echaurren 183, Santiago, Chile

Vizirianakis Ioannis S. Department of Pharmacology, School of Pharmacy, Aristotle University of Thessaloniki, Thessaloniki GR-54124, Greece

Werstler David Laboratory of Nanomedicine and Biomaterials, Department of Anesthesiology, Brigham and Women's Hospital, Harvard Medical School, 75 Francis St., Boston, MA 02115, USA., University of Waterloo, Canada

Whyte Andrew Laboratory of Nanomedicine and Biomaterials, Department of Anesthesiology, Brigham and Women's Hospital, Harvard Medical School, 75 Francis St., Boston, MA 02115, USA., University of Waterloo, Canada

Wu Yun Laboratory of Nanomedicine and Biomaterials, Department of Anesthesiology, Brigham and Women's Hospital, Harvard Medical School, 75 Francis St., Boston, MA 02115, USA

Yameen Basit Laboratory of Nanomedicine and Biomaterials, Department of Anesthesiology, Brigham and Women's Hospital, Harvard Medical School, 75 Francis St., Boston, MA 02115, USA

INDEX